DIAGNOSIS CRITICAL

DIAGNOSIS CRITICAL

The Urgent Threats Confronting Catholic Health Care

Leonard J. Nelson, III

Our Sunday Visitor Publishing Division
Our Sunday Visitor, Inc.
Huntington, Indiana 46750

Nihil Obstat: Rev. Michael Heintz, Ph.D.
Censor Librorum

Imprimatur: ✠ John M. D'Arcy
Bishop of Fort Wayne-South Bend
April 14, 2009

The *Nihil Obstat* and *Imprimatur* are official declarations that a book or pamphlet is free of doctrinal or moral error. No implication is contained therein that those who have granted the *Nihil Obstat* or *Imprimatur* agree with the contents, opinions, or statements expressed.

The Scripture citations used in this work are taken from the *Second Catholic Edition of the Revised Standard Version of the Bible* (RSV), copyright © 1965, 1966, and 2006 by the Division of Christian Education of the National Council of the Churches of Christ in the United States of America. Used by permission. All rights reserved.
English translation of the *Catechism of the Catholic Church* for the United States of America copyright © 1994, United States Catholic Conference, Inc. — Libreria Editrice Vaticana.
English translation of the *Catechism of the Catholic Church: Modifications from the Editio Typica* copyright © 1997, United States Catholic Conference, Inc. — Libreria Editrice Vaticana.

Every reasonable effort has been made to determine copyright holders of excerpted materials and to secure permissions as needed. If any copyrighted materials have been inadvertently used in this work without proper credit being given in one form or another, please notify Our Sunday Visitor in writing so that future printings of this work may be corrected accordingly.

Copyright © 2009 by Our Sunday Visitor Publishing Division,
Our Sunday Visitor, Inc. Published 2009.

14 13 12 11 10 09   1 2 3 4 5 6 7 8 9

All rights reserved. With the exception of short excerpts for critical reviews, no part of this work may be reproduced or transmitted in any form or by any means whatsoever without permission in writing from the publisher. Contact:

Our Sunday Visitor Publishing Division
Our Sunday Visitor, Inc.
200 Noll Plaza
Huntington, IN 46750
1-800-348-2440
bookpermissions@osv.com

ISBN: 978-1-59276-070-1 (Inventory No. T121)
LCCN: 2009923182

Cover design by Tyler Ottinger / Cover photo: Shutterstock
Interior design by Sherri L. Hoffman

PRINTED IN THE UNITED STATES OF AMERICA

Contents

Dedication and Acknowledgments — 7

Introduction — 9

PART ONE. Moral Foundations — 21

CHAPTER ONE: The Catholic Natural-Law Tradition — 23
CHAPTER TWO: Challenges to the Catholic Natural-Law Tradition — 27
CHAPTER THREE: The Reassertion of Absolute Norms — 33
CHAPTER FOUR: Secular Bioethics versus Catholic Bioethics — 42
CHAPTER FIVE: Ethical and Religious Directives — 53

PART TWO. Catholic Identity — 79

CHAPTER SIX: Transformation of the Catholic Hospital from Religious Ministry to Business Enterprise — 84
CHAPTER SEVEN: Catholic Hospitals and Canon Law — 90

PART THREE. The Struggle to Maintain Catholic Identity as Reflected in Two Health Care Systems — 101

CHAPTER EIGHT: Providence Health System — 103
CHAPTER NINE: Ascension Health — 118

PART FOUR. Catholic Health Care and the Right of Conscientious Objection — 131

CHAPTER TEN: Protection of Conscientious Objection — 138
CHAPTER ELEVEN: Mandated Contraceptive Coverage — 151
CHAPTER TWELVE: Emergency Contraception Laws — 163

PART FIVE. End-of-Life Care — 175

CHAPTER THIRTEEN: Catholic Teaching on End-of-Life Care — 178

CHAPTER FOURTEEN: The Controversy over Withdrawing Artificial
    Nutrition and Hydration from Patients in a Persistent
    Vegetative State   182
CHAPTER FIFTEEN: A Case Study in End-of-Life Care: Terri Schiavo   196

PART SIX. Social Justice and Health Care Reform   201

CHAPTER SIXTEEN: The United States Health Care System   204
CHAPTER SEVENTEEN: Health Care Reform Proposals   213

Conclusion   223

Notes   231

Index   345

Dedication and Acknowledgments

I dedicate this book to my wife, Janice, in appreciation for her patience and support during the many hours I spent writing it.

Ann Carey, a Catholic journalist, encouraged me to write this book, provided information to me, and commented on a draft manuscript.

I also appreciate the efforts of the following in reading and commenting on various drafts of this book or portions thereof: Professor Brannon Denning, Cumberland School of Law, Samford University; Professor Thomas Berg, St. Thomas University School of Law; Professor Dennis Sansom, Samford University; Monica Nelson Fischer, health care attorney; and Kurt Fischer, a law student at Cumberland School of Law. Finally, thanks to Dean John Carroll and Associate Dean H.C. "Corky" Strickland of the Cumberland School of Law for the research grants to support my work on this book. The views expressed herein are my own, and any errors are my responsibility.

Chapters Ten, Eleven, and Twelve are adapted from "God and Woman in the Catholic Hospital," 31 *J. Legis.* 69 (2004). Chapters Thirteen, Fourteen, and Fifteen are adapted from "Catholic Bioethics and the Case of Terri Schiavo," 35 *Cumb. L. Rev.* 543 (2005). Chapters Sixteen and Seventeen are adapted from "A Tale of Three Systems: A Comparative Overview of Health Care Reform in England, Canada, and the United States," 37 *Cumb. L. Rev.* 513 (2006-2007).

I also wish to thank the following centers and institutes for permitting me to give lectures that served as forerunners for this book: the Biotechnology and Law Center at Samford University, the Health Care Ethics and Law Institute at Samford University, the Institute for Professional Ethics and Responsibility at Benedictine College, and the Notre Dame Center for Ethics and Culture.

Introduction

In his encyclical *Evangelium Vitae*, John Paul II highlighted the contemporary struggle between a "culture of life" and a "culture of death."[1] A primary bastion for the cultivation and preservation of a "culture of life" in our society has been the Catholic hospital. But, unfortunately, the distinctive mission of the Catholic hospital is in grave danger of extinction due to "a confluence of powerful environmental forces."[2] Cultural, religious, economic, and political forces seem to be working in tandem to erode the identity of Catholic hospitals. A coalition of powerful forces now view the Catholic presence in health care as an obstacle to making abortion a more readily available mainstream medical procedure. And, during his campaign for the presidency, Barack Obama promised to sign the Freedom of Choice Act (FOCA), proposed legislation that as presently written could remove virtually all limitations on access to abortion and set aside existing conscience-clause protection for individuals and institutions.[3]

During the past thirty years, there has been a transition to lay leadership in Catholic health care systems as the numbers of religious have drastically declined. At one time, Catholic hospitals were managed by members of the sponsoring orders. Now, they are managed by laypersons — many of whom are not Catholic. While there has been a concerted effort to preserve the mission of these Catholic hospitals and inculcate the values of the founding order in lay employees, it is too soon to tell whether these efforts will be successful.[4]

In addition, health care has become a highly competitive business. Hospitals now compete with each other on the basis of price and quality to obtain contracts with private health care plans. With respect to publicly financed healthcare, there is constant pressure on hospitals to contain costs while improving outcomes. Increased emphasis on pay-for-performance in both public and private insurance will undoubtedly enhance competition. It is essential for hospitals to have adequate access to capital in order to compete successfully in this environment. For nonprofit hospitals, this requires good bond ratings, which in turn require cost-effective delivery of health care. In light of these developments, serious questions are now being raised as to whether nonprofit hospitals have any continuing legitimate role, and whether they act any differently than for-profit hospitals. Simultaneously, there has emerged a threat to the tax-exempt status of Catholic hospitals, based on allegations that they don't provide an adequate amount of health care services to the poor, and, in fact, provide less indigent care than non-Catholic facilities.[5]

Women's religious orders founded and fostered the development of most Catholic hospitals in the United States, and, ironically, issues related to women's reproductive rights may provide the most difficult challenges to the ongoing struggles by the sponsors of these hospitals in terms of preserving their Catholic identity. Catholic hospitals in the United States are currently under vigorous attack by well-organized "pro-choice" groups[6] seeking to force them to provide access to a full range of "reproductive health services."[7] Articles in popular magazines have contended that the Catholic character of particular hospitals prevents them from adequately serving the reproductive needs of their communities.[8]

In response to intense lobbying by "pro-choice" groups, several states have adopted laws that will require Catholic hospitals to provide emergency contraception for rape victims.[9] Simultaneously, there has also been a very successful campaign by these "pro-choice" groups to promote state legislation mandating that employers include contraceptive coverage in health insurance policies while limiting the ability of religious organizations to avoid the mandate.[10] Some Catholic leaders believe the "true goal [of the contraceptive coverage mandate] is to set the stage for mandated coverage of all so-called reproductive services, including abortion."[11] In a report issued in 2002, the American Civil Liberties Union's Reproductive Freedom Project called for legislation that would require Catholic hospitals to provide access to a full range of reproductive services.[12] In some states, legislation has already been proposed to force Catholic hospitals to provide either abortion referrals or abortions.[13]

Abortion is now widely available in specialized clinics and some non-Catholic hospitals, but this has not been sufficient for "pro-choice" activists. They seek to make abortion services available even in Catholic hospitals.[14] As Professor Lynn Wardle has noted, there has been a shift in tactics by liberal "pro-choice" activists: originally they "argued that they merely desired to give women the private choice to select abortion," but now "they try to compel hospitals, clinics, provider groups, and health care insurers to provide facilities for, personnel for, and funding for abortion."[15] There is an ongoing effort by several "pro-choice" groups to force all hospitals to provide abortions.[16] This acceleration of attacks on hospitals may be seen in a 1997 decision by the Supreme Court of Alaska that forced a private nonprofit hospital in Alaska to provide abortions.[17] Indeed, it has long been a goal of abortion rights supporters to "mainstream" abortion — i.e., to make it into a routine medical procedure by the strategy of relocating the performance of abortions from specialty clinics to general acute care hospitals.[18] As one feminist author has observed:

> North American abortion clinic violence has left North American feminists in search of effective strategies — both theoretical and practical — to keep adequate number of abortion clinics open for business. The strategy most of them have chosen is the mainstreaming of abortion provision into other health services for women. Burying women's abortion services in mainstream medical clinics goes hand in hand with redefining abortion from being an ethical issue to a health issue.[19]

In a 1998 panel discussion on Catholic Identity sponsored by the Catholic Health Association, Fr. Brian Hehir, then a Professor at Harvard Divinity School, noted: "A fundamental disagreement between Catholic providers and their opponents is whether reproductive choices should be public or private issues. . . ."[20] Mary Healey-Sedutto, Director of Health and Hospitals, Archdiocese of New York, another participant in this panel discussion, was somewhat more specific in her comments. In discussing bills pending at the time in the New York legislature that would have required Catholic hospitals to provide a full range of reproductive health services in violation of Catholic ethical norms, she stated:

> I am in shock at the rapidity with which these issues have developed. . . . In the past months, five bills have moved through the assembly into the senate that will fundamentally challenge our ability to remain in healthcare. . . . Our opponents have a frightening and insidious strategy. . . . They have learned how to use our own strengths against us. . . . They speak of their mission, of their core values, their ministry. They attend our meetings and participate in the discussion. They praise us with great flourish, but then move on to the one "deficit:" that we are preventing society from having access to what they see as societal rights.[21]

Under federal and state conscience-clause legislation, individuals and institutions have been protected from having to perform medical procedures such as abortion.[22] But these protections are currently under attack. Groups such as the ACLU contend that conscience-clause legislation has given Catholic institutions too much protection and this has resulted in unwarranted restrictions in the availability of reproductive health services.[23] The argument of these groups is that because Catholic hospitals operate in the public sector and receive public funds, they should not be permitted to impose restrictions on the availability of reproductive health services.[24]

Catholic hospitals are governed by the *Ethical and Religious Directives for Catholic Health Care Services*[25] (*ERD*s), a set of norms adopted by the National Conference of Catholic Bishops and most recently updated in 2001. Those reproductive services deemed morally wrong by the *ERD*s, and thus not to be provided in Catholic hospitals, include contraception,[26] direct sterilization,[27] and direct abortion.[28] Catholic health care leaders acknowledge that the passage of legislation linking the receipt of federal funds to the provision of reproductive services prohibited by the *ERD*s will effectively destroy Catholic health care.[29]

Politicians, and especially Democrats, have become increasingly receptive to demands for legislation to require all hospitals to provide reproductive health services to their patients and insurance coverage for such services to their employees. While the Catholic Church has typically disagreed with Democrats over issues such as abortion, they have agreed on many other social justice issues.[30] Traditionally, Catholic voters were an important part of the New Deal coalition, and leading Democrats had a close relationship with Church leaders, but now prominent Democrat politicians are willing to defy the teachings of the Catholic Church by promoting legislation that would compel Catholic institutions to provide reproductive health services in violation of Catholic moral teaching.[31]

The complicity of Catholic politicians in the continued expansion and protection of the abortion right undermines arguments by Catholic institutions and individuals for conscience protection. It is more difficult for Catholic leaders to argue for conscience-clause protection of Catholic health care institutions and individuals when leading politicians who publicly identify themselves as Catholics are working to expand and protect the right to abortion. The stance of these politicians is in direct conflict with the Church's teaching that the protection of the life of the unborn child from abortion is a basic human right.[32] In contrast, "pro-choice" Catholic politicians seem to view access to abortion as a fundamental right.[33]

Thus, instead of working diligently to limit the constitutional right recognized in *Roe v. Wade*, "pro-choice" Catholic legislators argue that since Catholics live in a pluralistic society, we cannot impose our views about abortion on others.[34] They present the Church's teaching on abortion as a peculiarity of Catholic doctrine rather than as a basic human right derived from the precepts of natural law through the use of reason.[35] And they also refer to prudential limitations that counsel against the imposition of a ban on abortion that would be practically unenforceable.[36] But if one views abortion as immoral, these prudential concerns should not prevent attempts to limit access to abortion by such means as parental involvement laws and Medicaid funding, restrictions that have been shown to be effective in reducing abortion.[37]

In the past two presidential election cycles, the Catholic bishops in the United States have struggled with developing a coherent response to "pro-choice" Catholic politicians. On the one hand, Archbishop Raymond L. Burke, formerly of St. Louis, Missouri (and, since 2008, Prefect of the Supreme Tribunal of Apostolic Signatura in the Vatican),[38] has argued that Catholic politicians who publicly support abortion rights should be denied Communion. In 2003, while serving as Bishop of LaCrosse, Wisconsin, he notified Catholic politicians who supported abortion rights that they should not present themselves for Communion.[39] One of the affected politicians, David Obey (D-WI), responded in an essay published in *America*, stating that he viewed Bishop Burke's action as an improper attempt to coerce him into violating his conscience by supporting legislation that would undermine the constitutional right of access to abortion.[40]

Burke subsequently became Archbishop of St. Louis, and, in 2004, he announced he would not give Communion to John Kerry, a "pro-choice" Catholic and the Democratic candidate for President in 2004.[41] He also issued a pastoral letter indicating that it was a "grave sin" to vote for a "pro-choice" candidate unless all the candidates in the race supported abortion rights.[42] But other bishops, such as Cardinal Theodore McCarrick, the former Archbishop of Washington, DC, have indicated they are not willing to exclude pro- "choice" Catholic politicians from Communion.[43] Donald Wuerl, the current Archbishop of Washington, DC, has also indicated his unwillingness to deny Communion to "pro-choice" Catholic politicians.[44] Although he has condemned support for abortion rights by Catholic politicians, Archbishop Wuerl has stated that the denial of Communion is the responsibility of the local bishop of a national political figure's home diocese.[45] He has also argued that the decision to receive Communion is primarily that of the individual Catholic, based on their own conscience.[46]

In 2004, the United States Conference of Catholic Bishops adopted *Catholics in Political Life*,[47] a statement that left the question of denial of Communion to "pro-choice" Catholic politicians up to the prudential judgment of individual bishops. In response to this document, Archbishop Burke published an essay opining that the United States Bishops had acted improperly in this regard.[48] He concluded that "consistent canonical discipline" required ministers of Holy Communion to deny Communion to Catholic politicians who have obstinately and publicly persisted in their support of abortion rights and have been warned not to present themselves for Communion.[49]

The activities of "pro-choice" Catholic Democrat politicians also emerged as an issue in the 2008 presidential campaign. Controversy resulted from the mischaracterization of Catholic teaching on abortion by two prominent Catholic politicians. First, Speaker of the House Nancy Pelosi (D-CA), in an appearance on *Meet the Press*, cited St. Augustine and argued that Church teaching was unclear on the morality of direct abortion in the first trimester of pregnancy.[50] Her comments provoked a response from the United States Conference of Catholic Bishops, stating that since the first century, the Church has taught that procured abortions at any stage of development are "gravely immoral."[51]

Two weeks later on *Meet the Press,* the Democratic Party candidate for Vice President, Senator Joe Biden (D-DE), also a Catholic, cited St. Thomas Aquinas in support of his assertion that the Church's views on abortion have been a matter of longstanding debate, and that the question of when human life begins is a "personal and private matter."[52] This also provoked a response from the bishops: "Today embryology textbooks confirm that a new human life begins at conception. . . . The Catholic Church does not teach this as a matter of faith; it acknowledges it as an objective fact."[53] The reaction of two bishops to Biden's comments illustrates the disagreement among bishops on the issue of withholding Communion from "pro-choice" politicians: the Bishop of Scranton, Pennsylvania (Biden's hometown), announced that Biden could not receive Communion, but the bishop of Wilmington, Delaware (where Biden lives and worships), announced that he could.[54]

The bishops have also struggled with providing coherent guidance to voters about the abortion issue. While some bishops have pushed for clearly instructing the faithful that they cannot vote for a "pro-choice" candidate where there is an acceptable pro-life alternative, others have sought to preserve the option to vote for a "pro-choice" candidate based on his or her positions on other issues. In preparation for the 2008 election, the bishops revised the brochure prepared every four years to provide guidance to Catholic voters.[55]

At least partly because the 2004 version had been criticized for treating a candidate's position on abortion as merely one issue of many,[56] the 2008 version is less equivocal on the abortion issue. It states that "intrinsically evil" actions such as abortion could not be equated with other issues.[57] It also states that Catholics who vote for "pro-choice" candidates because of their position on abortion "would be guilty of formal cooperation in evil."[58] Further:

> The direct and intentional destruction of innocent human life from the moment of conception until natural death is always wrong and is not just one issue among many.[59]

But, nonetheless, it leaves the door slightly ajar for voters to vote for "pro-choice" candidates "for other morally grave reasons."[60] And the document further states, "At the same time, a voter should not use a candidate's opposition to intrinsic evil to justify indifference or inattentiveness to other important moral issues."[61]

Notwithstanding the apparent consensus in support of the 2008 voters' guide, the disagreement among bishops over the importance of the abortion issue became evident during the 2008 election campaign. Most bishops merely distributed the voter guide without further comment; a few indicated that abortion is just one issue among many that a voter should consider; and several others argued that abortion was the issue of overriding importance in the election.[62] In the "abortion is just one issue" camp was Gabino Zavala, an auxiliary bishop in the Archdiocese of Los Angeles, who stated:

> What I believe, and what the church teaches, is that one abortion is too many. That's why I believe abortion is so important. But in light of this, there are many other issues we need to bring up, other issues we should consider, other issues that touch the reality of our lives.[63]

On the other hand, Archbishop Burke opined that the Democratic Party in the United States was at risk of becoming "a party of death."[64] Bishop Martino of Scranton, Pennsylvania, issued a letter to parishioners warning that voting for a "pro-choice" candidate was tantamount to endorsing homicide.[65] Cardinal George of Chicago issued a letter to parishioners stating: "One cannot favor the legal status quo on abortion and also be working for the common good."[66] And in an article in *First Things*, Bishop Charles Chaput of Denver stated:

> *The right to life is foundational.* Every other right depends on it. Efforts to reduce abortions, or to create alternatives to abortion, or to foster an environment where more women will choose to keep their unborn child, can have great merit — *but not if they serve to cover over or distract from the brutality and fundamental injustice of abortion itself.* We should remember that one of the crucial things that set early Christians apart from the pagan culture around them was their rejection of abortion and infanticide. Yet for thirty-five years I've watched prominent "pro-choice" Catholics justify themselves with the kind of moral and verbal gymnastics that should qualify as an Olympic event. All they've really done is capitulate to *Roe v. Wade*.[67]

An additional feature of the 2008 campaign was the endorsement of Barack Obama by some prominent pro-life Catholic academics. Douglas Kmiec, a former Dean of Catholic University School of Law, publicly endorsed Obama notwithstanding his disagreement with him on the issue of abortion, indicating that he believed Obama was not "closed to opposing points of view and, as best as it is humanly possible, he will respect and accommodate them."[68] And Nicholas Cafardi, a former Dean of Duquesne University School of Law, announced that he was endorsing Obama in part because "we have lost the abortion battle permanently."[69] Cafardi pointed to Obama's endorsement of measures to reduce abortion as a justification for his support.[70] He also argued that the expansion of social welfare programs in an Obama presidency could result in a decrease in the numbers of abortions.[71] In an article criticizing these endorsements, George Weigel noted:

> The bishops already find themselves defending the Catholic integrity of Catholic hospitals under pressures from state governments; those pressures, as well as pressures on doctors and other Catholic health-care professionals, will increase in an Obama administration, especially if FOCA succeeds in knocking down state conscience-clause protections for Catholic health-care providers and institutions. And should an Obama administration reintroduce large-scale federal funding of abortion, the bishops will have to confront a grave moral question they have managed to avoid for decades, thanks to the Hyde amendment: does the payment of federal taxes that go to support abortion constitute

Introduction

a form of moral complicity in an "intrinsic evil"? And if so, what should the conscientious Catholic citizen do?[72]

In response, Kmiec and Cafardi, joined by Cathleen Kaveny, a theology professor at Notre Dame, argued:

> Promoting a culture of life is necessarily interconnected with a family wage, universal health care and, yes, better parenting and education of our youth. This greater appreciation for the totality of Catholic teaching is at the very heart of the Obama campaign; it is scarcely a McCain footnote.[73]

Despite the efforts by some bishops to focus the attention of Catholics on the singular importance of the abortion issue, exit polls indicated that a majority of Catholics casting ballots in the 2008 presidential election voted for Barack Obama, an ardent supporter of abortion rights.[74] Accordingly, Peter Steinfels characterized the bishops as among "the big losers" in the election.[75] Unfortunately, that characterization may prove to be prophetic. The 2008 election could usher in a new era in Catholic life in the United States where abortion will be fully funded by the government or private health insurers and Catholic health care institutions will be required to provide abortions.

The threat posed by the Obama administration's pro-abortion agenda was a topic at the annual fall assembly of the United States Conference of Catholic Bishops, held in November 2008, shortly after the election. At the meeting, Auxiliary Bishop Thomas Paprocki warned the bishops that the passage of FOCA, legislation that President Obama had promised to sign, "would reduce religious freedom" and have "a significant and adverse effect."[76] He continued, "The next step would be for federal law to require abortion by all hospitals, including Catholic hospitals, which we cannot do."[77] And further: "We'd need to consider taking the drastic step of closing our Catholic hospitals completely."[78] Cardinal George agreed that the loss of federal funds would put Catholic hospitals out of business.[79] The bishops indicated that they would view the enactment of FOCA as an "attack on the Church."[80] And they authorized Cardinal George to draft a statement.[81]

The final statement issued by Cardinal George forcefully presented the bishops' position, but stopped somewhat short of characterizing the possible enactment of FOCA as an attack on the Church, instead stating: "Aggressively pro-abortion policies, legislation, and executive orders will permanently alienate tens of millions of Americans, and would be seen by many as an attack on the free exercise of their religion."[82] The statement noted that FOCA would invalidate state laws imposing restraints on abortion, coerce Americans into supporting abortion "with their tax dollars," and further:

> FOCA would have an equally destructive effect on the freedom of conscience of doctors, nurses and health care workers whose personal convictions do not permit them to cooperate in the private killing of unborn children. It would threaten Catholic health care institutions and Catholic Charities. It would be an evil law that would further divide our country, and the Church should be intent on opposing evil.

Some commentators characterize the bishops' statement as an overreaction because FOCA is unlikely to pass in 2008.[83] But others think that it may pass, take seriously the bishops' threat to close Catholic hospitals, and are concerned about its potential adverse impact on health care reform.[84]

Moreover, the adoption of comprehensive health care reform could itself pose a threat to Catholic health care. The Democratic Party is committed to expanding access to abortion. The commitment to unlimited abortion access "regardless of ability to pay" was a plank in both the 2004 and 2008 Democratic Party platforms.[85] The Democratic Party is also committed to comprehensive reform to provide universal access to health care.[86]

With the election of Barack Obama, it is probable that federal legislation will be proposed to achieve universal access to health care for all Americans. That legislation could mandate private insurance coverage for abortions and require all hospitals to provide a full range of reproductive services as a condition of receiving federal monies. While the adoption of a health care system providing universal access has been supported by the Catholic Health Association as a matter of social justice,[87] this call for social justice as implemented by a Democratic administration could include universal access to contraception, sterilization, and abortion to be provided at all hospitals.[88]

This book focuses on the ongoing struggle to preserve a distinctively Catholic health care system in the United States. Part One discusses the moral foundations of Catholic health care. I review the Catholic natural-law tradition and challenges to that tradition. Controversies among Catholic theologians over the proper role of Catholic hospitals and the influence of the secular bioethics movement on Catholic health care are examined. Various versions of the *ERDs* are reviewed, with particular attention to their treatment of abortion, contraception, sterilization, and end-of-life treatment. The concept of material cooperation is also reviewed.

Part Two discusses the transformation of Catholic hospitals from religious ministries to large-scale business enterprises. The religious origins of Catholic hospitals in the United States are reviewed. I discuss the difficulties that Catholic hospitals have in remaining true to their religious mission in an increasingly competitive marketplace and in a culture that is increasingly permeated by the sexual revolution and the "culture of death." Catholic identity and the related concepts of canonical status and sponsorship are discussed. Part Three reviews the struggle of two health care systems to maintain their Catholic identities.

Part Four discusses the role of conscience in health care, particularly the problem of the accommodation of conscientious objection for Catholic health care providers. I review the impact of United States Supreme Court precedents that have undermined constitutional protection for Catholic hospitals that may in the near future be required to provide services that are prohibited under the *ERD*s. Conscience-clause legislation is discussed. The controversy over mandated contraceptive coverage is reviewed. A Washington state attorney general's opinion and recent cases from California and New York dealing with the constitutionality of a contraceptive coverage, mandate as applied to employee health plans sponsored by Catholic institutions, are analyzed. Recent legislation requiring Catholic hospitals to provide emergency contraception is discussed. Studies on the current practices in Catholic hospitals with respect to emergency contraception are reviewed. A recent American College of Obstetricians and Gynecologists (ACOG) opinion that would require doctors to refer for abortion is analyzed. And the possible impact of the enactment of FOCA is discussed.

Part Five discusses end-of-life care issues with a particular focus on the controversy over withdrawing assisted nutrition and hydration [ANH] from patients in a persistent vegetative state [PVS] and the case of Terri Schiavo. Part Six focuses on social justice and health care reform with particular attention to the role of Catholic health care organizations in advocating reforms, and the threats posed by the adoption of universal health care. Finally, I conclude that Catholics may have to focus their future efforts on the creation of alternatives to acute care hospitals such as free clinics, specialized centers for reproductive medicine, and hospices for end-of-life care that could reinvigorate the religious health care ministry.

Part One

Moral Foundations

Cultural and religious changes have had a significant impact on Catholic health care as traditional Catholic teachings on human sexuality and reproduction have become increasingly countercultural. And, since the Second Vatican Council, there has been substantial controversy among Catholic theologians over the morality of contraception, sterilization, and even abortion, under certain circumstances. Through the 1950s, many priests relied on manuals on medical moral issues written by such authors as Gerald Kelly, Charles J. McFadden, and Thomas J. O'Donnell, all scholars working in the Catholic natural-law tradition.[1]

In the 1960s, however, there arose a fundamental split between Catholic moral theologians relying on traditional natural-law methodology, and revisionist moral theologians, some of whom have been referred to as proportionalists or consequentialists, advocating an accommodation between Church teaching and the prevailing culture through the development of a more contextual, practical approach and the eschewal of reliance on transcendent, pre-existing absolute moral norms. This split was initially occasioned by the issuance of *Humanae Vitae*[2] and its rejection by many Catholic moral theologians, but the divide between traditionalists and revisionists deepened as disputes moved on to other issues such as sterilization and abortion. Catholic health care was also influenced by the secular bioethics movement, which had its origins during this period and resulted in a decreased emphasis on absolute moral norms in favor of more casuistic and pragmatic approaches to ethical issues.

David Kelly, a critic of the traditional approach, which he describes as "physicalism," has delineated three stages in the development of the methodology of Catholic medical ethics: traditional (1100-1960), transitional (1960-1970), and contemporary (1970-present).[3] During the traditional stage, the primary focus was on "the purpose of the act biologically or physically."[4] Thus under this approach, artificial contraception is considered an intrinsic evil because the purpose of human sexuality is procreation.

In the transitional phase, greater emphasis was placed on "the personal or human dimensions of the acts in their circumstances."[5] While the conclusions of these moralists were typically the same as the traditionalists, their reasoning differed. For example, artificial contraception was still considered to be immoral — but not because of the physical nature of the act; rather, because it frustrated the purpose of marriage, — i.e., "unrestricted self-giving."[6]

In the contemporary stage, the focus is on "the human, social, spiritual, psychological consequences of the act."[7] David Kelly further notes:

> Revisionist moral theologians are apt to find that when they examine the personal dimensions of human nature and human behavior, the conclusions are not the same as those arrived at by the traditional or transitional moralists.

These theologians have rejected the notion that there are intrinsically evil acts without reference to context or consequences. They tend to evaluate the morality of an act by looking to its effect on the human person, an approach described as "personalism."[8] Accordingly, they would permit artificial contraception in order to enhance the marital relationship.[9]

Ultimately, however, two encyclicals issued by John Paul II repudiated the approach taken by revisionist theologians who questioned the existence of moral absolutes,[10] and reaffirmed traditional proscriptions on direct abortion and euthanasia as intrinsically evil acts.[11] The traditional approach continues to be the basis for the moral norms set forth in the various versions of the *ERDs*.

Chapter One

The Catholic Natural-Law Tradition

The Church has traditionally used a natural-law methodology in addressing medico-moral issues. Until the 1960s, this traditional natural-law approach was seldom questioned within the ranks of the Church. Since then, however, there has been ongoing dispute within the Church over whether this tradition, particularly its insistence on moral absolutes, continues to be relevant in the modern world. Revisionist theologians have urged that the teaching of the Church and the practice of Church institutions should accommodate to an increasingly post-Christian socio-legal environment that has rejected the sanctity-of-life ethic and embraced contraception, abortion, and physician-assisted suicide. These arguments have, in turn, been refuted by moral theologians loyal to the Magisterium.[1] In this chapter, I will describe the Catholic natural-law tradition as it has been used to develop a moral foundation for clinical ethics.

The Received Tradition: The Existence of Moral Absolutes

In the Catholic natural-law tradition, certain actions are deemed intrinsically immoral, notwithstanding potentially beneficial consequences.[2] William May, drawing on the writings of St. Thomas Aquinas, summarizes the traditional approach by noting that there are three levels of natural-law precepts: 1) self-evident first principles (e.g., good is to be pursued and evil avoided); 2) a second set of more specific precepts that can be readily derived from first principles through the use of natural reason; and 3) more "remote conclusions," i.e., specific moral norms, known only to the "wise, or those perfected in the virtue of prudence."[3]

Traditional Catholic moral theologians such as Professor May argue that the Magisterium of the Church has infallibly taught certain core moral precepts, such as those summarized in the Decalogue, "precisely *as these precepts have been traditionally understood within the Church.*"[4] This would include the traditional proscription on direct abortion.[5] In addition, there are specific

PART ONE: *Moral Foundations*

moral norms, e.g., the proscription on artificial contraception, that have been authoritatively proposed by the Magisterium but may not have been infallibly proclaimed.[6] Traditionalists such as May argue that even as to these precepts, however, dissent among Catholic theologians is not permissible.[7]

Benedict Ashley and Kevin O'Rourke note that Catholic natural-law reasoning is oriented to the ultimate goal of "happiness, which is found only in friendship with God and our neighbor."[8] Thus natural-law reasoning involves making a determination as to whether our actions are a proper means of fulfilling this ultimate goal.[9] Ashley and O'Rourke make an important distinction between *finis operis*, the moral object of the act, and *finis operantis*, the motive of the actor.[10] They conclude that no matter how good the motive of the actor may be, it cannot make the moral object good if that object is intrinsically immoral: "That is why we may not 'do evil for good to come of it' and why 'the end does not justify the means.'"[11]

Ashley and O'Rourke give an example of a physician who gives a suffering patient a lethal injection in order to end the suffering. In such a case, the moral object (*finis operis*) is killing the patient and the motive (*finis operantis*) is the desire to end suffering. They conclude that the intent to end the suffering cannot justify the act because killing an innocent human being is an intrinsically evil act, regardless of the motive.[12] They summarize the methodology of natural reasoning as including the following three steps:

A. Act toward the right ultimate goal, that is, friendship with God and neighbor.

B. Choose an effective means to achieve that goal. Thus, acts that are intrinsically evil must be rejected. Help in selecting good actions and in avoiding bad actions is offered in various moral codes of the church; e.g., Ten Commandments and *Ethical and Religious Directives*.

C. If the act chosen is an appropriate means to an ultimate end, then one must have an honest intention, and all other circumstances must contribute to the good moral effect.[13]

The principle of double effect has also had a significant role in the traditional Catholic natural-law approach. The principle of double effect treats indirect abortions or sterilizations — i.e., abortions or sterilizations that result as unintentional by-products of medical treatments for serious pathological conditions — as morally licit. Under the principle of double effect, the administration of morphine to treat the pain of a terminally ill cancer patient would be permissible even if it had the unintended effect of shortening that patient's life by depressing respiration. Gerald Kelly noted that under the principle of double effect, an action is deemed morally licit if the following requirements are met:

> 1) The action, considered by itself and independently of its effect, must not be morally evil . . . 2) The evil effect must not be the means of producing the good effect. The principle underlying this condition is that a good end cannot justify the use of an evil means . . . 3) The evil effect is sincerely not intended, but merely tolerated. . . 4) There must be a proportionate reason for performing the action, in spite of its evil consequences. In practice, this means that there must be a sort of balance between the total good and the total evil produced by an action. Or, to put it another way, it means that, according to a sound prudential estimate, the good to be obtained is of sufficient value to compensate for the evil that must be tolerated.[14]

David Kelly has noted that "the principle of double effect was the primary operational principle" of the traditionalist approach in Catholic medical ethics and is still widely used in both Catholic and secular bioethics.[15] It provides the basis for the distinction between direct and indirect abortions, direct and indirect sterilizations, and direct and indirect euthanasia. Those acts considered direct are always wrong, while those determined to be indirect may be morally licit.[16]

The Manuals

Albert Jonsen notes that the approach taken by Catholic moral theologians through the middle of the twentieth century was typified by "an exposition of fundamental moral principles derived from natural law and divine revelations, followed by a casuistic analysis of specific topics."[17] It was also characterized by deference to the Magisterium.[18] This approach may be seen in manuals such as *Medical Ethics* by Charles J. McFadden, O.S.A. — a text originally designed for teaching Catholic nurses, later modified for use in teaching ethics to pre-medical students, nurses, medical students, and physicians.[19] In the introduction to McFadden's work, Fulton J. Sheen emphasized the importance of doctors and nurses having "a moral sense of oughtness."[20]

McFadden clearly explicated his belief in "absolute" moral norms that are "immutable" and "universal," i.e., binding at all times and in all places on all people.[21] He defined natural law in the traditional Thomistic sense as humanity's participation in the eternal law through the use of reason.[22] He also emphasized the importance of "true conscience," a conscience that is properly formed and directs actions in accordance with the precepts of the natural law.[23] Noting the difficulty in ascertaining the precepts of the natural law, McFadden referred to "[t]he Moral Law" that "is to be found in tradition, in Sacred Scripture, and in the teaching of Christ's infallible Church."[24] He concluded, "It is this law known both by reason and Divine Revelation which should be cherished by doctor and nurse alike as the source and basis of their moral ideals."[25]

As to contraception, McFadden noted that by the 1940s, the use of contraception was already widespread even among Catholics.[26] Nonetheless, he stated that "[i]n contraception, man completely perverts the order of nature and acts contrary to the will of the Creator."[27] As to oral contraceptives, he stated:

> These drugs, taken orally or in any other manner, are aimed at preventing the conjugal act from achieving its natural end and as such, their use constitutes a perversion of nature.

He concluded with the following instruction to Catholic nurses and doctors: "No instruction on the methods of using contraceptives of any type may be given to any person, regardless of religion, by a doctor or nurse."[28]

In accordance with traditional teaching, McFadden condemned all direct sterilizations, i.e., surgical sterilizations of a man or woman for the purpose of preventing future pregnancies, as "mutilation[s]" not permitted by the moral law.[29] On the other hand, in accordance with the principle of double effect, he recognizes that "therapeutic sterilizations," i.e., procedures resulting in sterility where "the primary objective is the removal of a diseased organ and the preservation of the health and life of the patient" rather than where the "[d]esire to effect sterilization" is the motive, may be morally licit.[30]

As to abortion, in conformity with Catholic tradition, McFadden condemned all "direct abortions," defined as procedures "employed to procure the expulsion of fetus."[31] This condemnation would include "therapeutic abortion," defined as abortions that are "directly induced as a means of safeguarding the health and life of the mother."[32] On the other hand, he recognizes that under the principle of double effect, "indirect abortion[s]," defined as "any instance in which a treatment or operative procedure is performed for some other purpose but incidentally and secondarily does cause the expulsion of the fetus," are morally licit.[33]

CHAPTER TWO

Challenges to the Catholic Natural-Law Tradition

There are a number of "revisionist theologians"[1] within Catholicism (some of whom have been described as proportionalists or consequentialists) that have rejected a fundamental principle of the Catholic natural-law tradition in medical ethics: i.e., they deny that the violation of a specific norm, such as the prohibition on direct abortions, direct sterilizations, or artificial contraception, may be considered an intrinsically immoral act, regardless of its consequences and context.[2] Many of these theologians would nonetheless acknowledge that there are some absolute principles; i.e., the obligation to always "act in conformity with love of God and neighbor."[3] They would also generally acknowledge that norms using "morally evaluative language" may be absolute, e.g., a prohibition on murder rather than a prohibition on direct killing.[4] But they would not acknowledge that all direct abortions or direct sterilizations are immoral per se.

Fr. Thomas O'Donnell, S.J., a one-time Georgetown University professor and medical-moral consultant to the U.S. Catholic Conference who was primarily responsible for the preparation of the 1971 version of the *ERDs*, discussed *infra*, once told me in a conversation that he regarded the distinction between *finis operis* (the moral object) and *finis operantis* (the motive of the actor) as fundamental to the differences in approach between traditional Catholic moral theologians and revisionist theologians. That is, in his view, revisionist theologians had rejected the notion that acts such as the killing of an innocent human being or abortion were intrinsically evil acts, and were essentially arguing instead that the good motive of the actor could transform these acts into morally good acts.

Professor May has summarized the major principles underlying the arguments of revisionist theologians as follows: "(1) the requirements of the 'preference principle' or 'principle of proportionate good'; (2) the existence of a human act as a totality; and (3) the historicity of human existence."[5] May notes that as to the "principle of proportionate good," revisionist theologians argue that in articulating norms it is necessary to take into account the effect of the norms on "human goods or values."[6] Under this approach, acts such as direct abortion, direct sterilization, and contraception could be considered moral if "done for the sake of a proportionally greater good."[7] The totality argument is closely related to the proportionality argument, and proposes that the morality of an act can only be appraised by taking account of the totality of its effect.[8] This also requires an appraisal of the intention of the actor.[9] Thus under this view, contraceptive sterilization — when undertaken because of concern that a future pregnancy might endanger a mother's life — would be viewed as appropriate for the purpose of stabilizing the marriage.[10] Finally, the historicity argument is based on the observation that specific moral norms develop in particular historical contexts and are subject to revision, based on continuing human experience.[11]

Professor Christopher Kaczor has noted that the controversy between Catholic traditionalists and the proportionalists parallels to some extent the divide between deontologists and teleologists. In appraising the morality of particular acts, deontologists, focusing on pre-existing transcendent norms, accept the notion that certain acts are intrinsically evil notwithstanding their seemingly beneficial consequences. Teleologists, on the other hand, focus on whether a proportionate good is brought about by the act in question.[12] Traditionalist theologians view the Catholic natural-law approach as predominantly deontological, while proportionalists argue that it is for the most part teleological.[13] Indeed, proportionalists argue that with the exception of norms such as the prohibition of artificial contraception and direct killing, most norms in the Catholic tradition have been "teleologically parsed."[14] The primary focus of the activity of the proportionalists has been in rejecting the traditionalists' characterization of contraception and sterilization as intrinsically evil acts that are always and everywhere wrong under any circumstances.[15]

Benedict Ashley and Kevin O'Rourke have, however, characterized the Catholic natural-law tradition as being teleological in the sense that it is "based on the choice of means suitable to achieve the true goals of human life," rather than deontological, i.e., "merely based on obedience to law."[16] Indeed, in *Veritatis Splendor*, John Paul II noted:

> The moral life has an essential *'teleological' character*, since it consists in the deliberate ordering of human acts to God, the supreme good and ultimate end (*telos*) of man . . . [b]ut this ordering to one's ultimate end is not something subjective, dependent solely upon one's intention.[17]

And *Veritatis Splendor* condemns the teleologism used in consequentialism or proportionalism insofar as:

> The former claims to draw the criteria of the rightness of a given way of acting solely from a calculation of foreseeable consequences deriving from a given choice . . . [and] [t]he latter . . . focuses rather on the proportion acknowledged between the good and bad effects of that choice, with a view to the "greater good" or "lesser evil" actually possible in a particular situation.[18]

Revisionist theologians also contend that it is permissible for Catholic theologians to publicly dissent from non-infallible teachings proposing specific moral norms, such as the proscription of artificial contraception.[19] Following the Second Vatican Council, this controversy over the nature of moral reasoning within the Catholic tradition became public, as seen in the reaction to *Humanae Vitae*,[20] the papal encyclical rejecting artificial contraception. William May argues that the "roots of the rejection of moral absolutes" by revisionist theologians may be found in the Majority Report on the issue of contraception issued by the Papal Commission for the Study of Population, the Family, and Natality.[21]

The Majority Report recommended a change in Church teaching: i.e., that contraception no longer be considered intrinsically evil and that the Church permit the use of artificial birth control methods where there are serious reasons to avoid pregnancy.[22] There was a also a second report authored by members of the commission arguing that artificial birth control methods should not be permitted.[23] In *Humanae Vitae*, Pope Paul VI rejected the use of artificial birth control methods including direct sterilization, but did permit recourse to intercourse during infertile periods where there are serious reasons to avoid pregnancy.[24]

Although revisionist theologians are a disparate group, virtually all of them reject the Catholic Church's ban on artificial birth control methods, and it is difficult to understand the movement apart from the controversy over this issue.[25]

Eventually, those who dissented from *Humanae Vitae* realized that the traditional natural-law approach did not provide a satisfactory basis for their dissent and began to develop alternative approaches.[26] Building on the principle of double effect, they developed a new approach to medical bioethical issues that deemphasized the application of absolute moral norms.[27]

While some revisionist theologians focused on reforming the Catholic natural law tradition by using a teleological approach, others, such as Charles

Curran, seem to have completely rejected the Catholic natural law tradition, at least as applied to medical morals.[28] For example, in a 1970 book, Curran outlines the "Points of Dissatisfaction" with the Catholic natural-law tradition.[29] His basic position is that the adherence to the Catholic natural-law tradition in the provision of health care services is untenable because it is based on the existence of pre-existing, absolute medico-moral norms.[30] Curran has opined that the Catholic natural-law tradition has been a major flashpoint of disagreement between Protestant and Catholic theologians and called for a "critical appraisal of natural-law theory," noting that the questioning of the Church's position on contraception has led to a questioning of the entire system of natural law on which it was based.[31]

Curran has noted that Catholic natural-law theory has received wide support "from many men of goodwill" in the area of social justice, but in the area of medical morals, it has not been well received.[32] According to Curran, the primary defect in regard to the Catholic natural-law tradition's approach to issues such as abortion, contraception, sterilization, and artificial insemination has its unfortunate focus on "the physical structure of the act itself."[33] He has therefore argued that it is preferable to view an act in its "total human context" rather than just focusing on its physical attributes.[34]

Curran has also criticized traditional natural-law theory as embracing an archaic "classicist world view" that focuses on the immutable, instead of a "historical world view" that focuses on change and evolution.[35] According to Curran, these two world views in turn have created two different theological methodologies: the classicist focuses on preexisting abstract principles, while the historicist focuses on the context of the act.[36] Although he has acknowledged that Vatican II did not officially adopt either view, he sees the primary thrust of Vatican II to be tilted toward the historicist view, noting its emphasis on the importance of entering into dialogue with the modern world.[37]

Regarding the teachings of the Magisterium of the Church, he has opined that, unfortunately, many Catholics still accept them "in a somewhat fundamentalist manner."[38] Instead, he has argued that they should be viewed "in light of the historical, cultural, and scientific circumstances of the time in which they were composed."[39]

Curran treats contraception and sterilization as related questions: once one accepts the notion that reproduction may be prevented, other than the permanence of the procedure, there is little basis for distinguishing between "interfering with the act of sexual intercourse (contraception) or interfering with the reproductive faculty (anovulant pills, sterilizing operations)."[40] On this basis, he has argued that the rejection of the natural-law basis for the prohibition on the use of contraception by married couples, as advocated by the Majority Report of the Papal Commission, also necessitates a rejection of any limitation on direct sterilization.[41] Curran has also questioned the traditional absolute prohibition on direct abortions.[42] He has argued that the traditional teaching should be modified to permit an abortion where it is necessary to save the life of the mother.[43] Curran has even suggested that direct abortion could be considered a moral option to be provided by Catholic hospitals because of concerns about the impact of the pregnancy on the mental health of the mother.[44]

Curran criticizes the use of the principle of double effect in traditional Catholic natural-law teaching, noting that it has been typically used to distinguish between situations where the evil effect is merely permitted for proportionate reasons (deemed morally licit) rather than intended (deemed morally illicit).[45] Curran is critical of the traditional use of the principle of double effect in its focus on the "sole immediate effect" of the procedure in question without reference to other values.[46] Thus, although it would permit termination of an ectopic pregnancy by removal of the fallopian tube where the purpose of the procedure is to prevent the rupture of the tube, it would not permit removal of the fetus alone.[47] Curran, however, would extend this principle so as to permit removal of the fetus without removal of the tube in order to preserve the woman's fertility.[48]

Clearly, the influence of the revisionists has been significant: in 1977, the Catholic Theological Society of America published a study stating that artificial contraception, sterilization, and masturbation could not be considered intrinsically immoral acts.[49] Indeed, the issuance of *Humanae Vitae* marked the beginning of an era of public dissent where large numbers of people remained in the Church despite their rejection of its teaching on matters related to human sexuality.[50] There were also well-known Catholic theologians who argued that Catholic hospitals operating in a pluralistic society should provide procedures such as contraceptive sterilizations that are considered morally permissible by large segments of the population.[51] These same theologians have argued that an obligation to provide sterilizations and contraception flows from the receipt of public funds.[52]

By the 1970s, an era of open dissent from Church teachings from within the Church had become very public. In 1973, the "pro-choice" group Catholics for a Free Choice was founded "as an offshoot of the National Organization for Women" for the purpose of advocating abortion rights.[53] In 1986, Charles Curran was told that he could no longer teach moral theology at Catholic University because of his heterodox views.[54] The same year, two nuns were "warned by the Vatican that they will be thrown out of their order unless they recant[ed] their view that there is diversity of thought on abortion."[55] Public opinion polls during the mid-1980s indicated that a majority of Catholics favored the use of artificial birth control (68%) and the legality of abortion in cases of rape or incest (55%).[56]

The issuance of *Humane Vitae* and the ensuing dissent was a "watershed" event in Catholicism in the United States that led to widespread rejection of Church teachings concerning human sexuality.[57] In terms of its practical effect, the widespread prevalence of dissent among both religious and lay Catholics may make it more difficult for Catholic health care institutions to persuade policymakers that they should be exempt from laws of general application requiring the provision of sterilizations and abortions. And, of course, the situation of Catholic health care institutions has become even more precarious since it has become commonplace for high-profile Catholic politicians to be openly and avowedly "pro-choice."[58]

Chapter Three

The Reassertion of Absolute Norms

In the 1970s and 1980s, there was a vigorous debate "between *proportionalists* — moral theologians who wanted to forge a new direction in Catholic morality by emphasizing the prominence of proportionate reason in the Catholic tradition — and *traditionalists* — those who insisted that attributing such centrality to proportionate reason would undermine the absolute norms that prohibit 'intrinsically evil acts.'"[1] Beginning in the 1970s, some Catholic theologians — a variegated group commonly referred to as proportionalists — embraced a principle whereby the morality of acts was to be judged by their proportionate good.[2] From this viewpoint, acts such as direct sterilization to preserve the health of the mother against the threat of future pregnancies and the use of artificial contraception could be justified as enhancing or preserving family stability.[3]

The *Catechism of the Catholic Church*[4] and two papal encyclicals issued in the 1990s reaffirmed traditional Catholic teaching on the existence of absolute moral norms. In *Veritatis Splendor* (1993),[5] John Paul II condemned the approach taken by the proportionalists. And in *Evangelium Vitae* (1995),[6] John Paul II pointed out the dangers posed by a pervasive "culture of death." These developments have, in turn, had an influence on the 1994 and 2001 versions of the *ERDs*, discussed *infra*.

a. The *Catechism of the Catholic Church*

The *Catechism* embraces the traditional Catholic natural-law approach:

> There are concrete acts that it is always wrong to choose, because their choice entails a disorder of the will, i.e., a moral evil. One may not do evil so that good may result from it.[7]

The *Catechism* also reasserts traditional Church teaching on abortion, sterilization, and contraception. Paragraph 2270 states, "Human life must be respected and protected absolutely from the moment of conception."[8] Paragraph 2271 further states:

Since the first century the Church has affirmed the moral evil of every procured abortion. This teaching has not changed and remains unchangeable. Direct abortion, that is to say, abortion willed either as an end or a means, is gravely contrary to the moral law.[9]

Under Paragraph 2272 of the *Catechism,* the penalty for formal cooperation in the procurement of an abortion is automatic excommunication.[10] This is one of the few infractions that results in automatic excommunication under the Code of Canon Law. Paragraph 2366 condemns both artificial contraception and contraceptive sterilization by providing that "it is necessary that each and every marriage act remain ordered *per se* to the procreation of life."[11] It further notes: "This particular doctrine, expounded on numerous occasions by the Magisterium, is based on the inseparable connection, established by God, which man on his own initiative may not break, between the unitive significance and the procreative significance which are both inherent to the marriage act."[12]

The *Catechism* also reasserts traditional teaching on euthanasia. Direct euthanasia is condemned as "morally unacceptable" notwithstanding "motives and means."[13] Thus, an act or omission undertaken for the purpose of ending the life of a handicapped, sick, or dying person is considered murder, even if it is motivated by a desire to end suffering.[14] In accordance with traditional teaching, the *Catechism* further recognizes the permissibility of refusing aggressive medical treatment that is disproportionately burdensome.[15] Similarly, the *Catechism* recognizes that it is morally acceptable to administer a non-lethal dose of pain-control medication to a dying person, even if its unintended result is to shorten that person's life.[16] Indeed, "palliative care" is encouraged as "a special form of disinterested charity."[17]

b. *Veritatis Splendor*

Veritatis Splendor was issued by John Paul II in August of 1993 for the purpose of responding to the arguments of the proportionalists, and "with the intention of clearly setting forth certain aspects of doctrine which are of crucial importance in facing what is certainly a genuine crisis."[18] The encyclical was occasioned by the need to restate "certain fundamental truths of Catholic doctrine which in the present circumstances, risk being distorted or denied."[19] Specifically, it was occasioned by the phenomenon of public dissent within the Church that rejected the "Church's moral teachings" and the authoritative role of the Magisterium.[20] It has been among the most controversial encyclicals issued by John Paul II.[21]

Chapter One of the encyclical begins with a meditation on the dialogue of Christ with the rich young man, who asks, "What good must I do to inherit eternal life?" and Jesus' response, which is to "keep the commandments."[22] In this chapter, *Veritatis Splendor* affirms the authority of the Magisterium to establish absolute norms governing moral conduct.[23]

In Chapter Two of *Veritatis Splendor* — perhaps its most controversial section — John Paul II notes that, since Vatican II, "there have developed certain interpretations of Christian morality which are not consistent with 'sound teaching.'"[24] In this chapter, John Paul II notes that, in contemporary ethical discourse, there has been a strong tendency to separate freedom from truth and to place excessive emphasis on individual autonomy.[25] He also notes these trends in Catholic moral theology.[26]

After referring to the extravagant emphasis on individual autonomy in contemporary ethical discourse, the encyclical condemns the work of moral theologians who reject the existence of absolute moral norms:[27]

> No one can fail to see that such an interpretation of the autonomy of human reason involves positions incompatible with Catholic teaching.[28]

Veritatis Splendor restates the traditional definition of the natural law as being the participation by human beings in the eternal law by the use of reason.[29] It rejects arguments that the traditional approach focuses too much on physicalism, i.e., the biological nature of acts such as contraception and direct sterilization, rather than on the historical and social context of such acts.[30] In rebuttal, it states:

> A doctrine which dissociates the moral act from the bodily dimensions of its exercise is contrary to the teaching of Scripture and Tradition.[31]

And it reaffirms the existence of moral absolutes, "*negative precepts* of the natural law," governing human conduct that are valid always and everywhere.[32] Noting that some moral theologians have emphasized the cultural context in order to question the immutability of specific moral norms, it responds, "There is something in man that transcends those cultures."[33] It condemns an approach that legitimizes departures from moral norms as so-called "pastoral solutions."[34] While acknowledging the important role of conscience, it emphasizes the role of the teachings of the Church in forming the consciences of Christians.[35]

Perhaps most significantly, in Chapter Two, *Veritatis Splendor* emphatically rejects the arguments of moral theologians who would judge the morality of acts "on the basis of a technical calculation between the 'premoral' or 'physical' goods and evils which actually result from the action."[36] In this encyclical, John Paul II acknowledges that moral life is teleological in the sense that all moral life is ordered toward God as its end,[37] but specifically condemns two teleologisms: proportionalism and consequentialism. He defines proportionalism as an approach that "by weighing the various values and goods being sought, focuses rather on the proportion acknowledged between the good and bad effects of that choice, with a view to the 'greater good' or 'lesser evil' actually possible in a particular situation."[38] He also rejects the consequentialist position because it "claims to draw the criteria of the rightness of a given way of acting solely from a calculation of foreseeable consequences deriving from a given choice."[39]

Instead, *Veritatis Splendor* reemphasizes the continuing validity of the traditional natural-law teaching that "the morality of the human act depends primarily and fundamentally on the 'object' rationally chosen by the deliberate will."[40] It reiterates that acts such as contraception and direct abortion are intrinsically evil, regardless of circumstances.[41] Finally, as to the phenomenon of public dissent from the Magisterium by moral theologians, it states:

> Moral theologians are to set forth the Church's teaching and to give, in the exercise of their ministry, the example of loyal assent, both internal and external, to the Magisterium's teaching in the areas of both dogma and morality.[42]

In response to *Veritatis Splendor*, Professor Richard McCormick, S.J., a professor at the University of Notre Dame and a prominent proportionalist, claimed that the encyclical had misrepresented his views and the views of other proportionalists. He stated:

> The encyclical repeatedly states of proportionalism that it attempts to justify morally wrong actions by a good intention. . . . I wish the Pope's advisors had been more careful here. No proportionalist that I know would recognize her/himself here. . . . I think it misses the point of what proportionalists are saying. When contemporary theologians say that certain dismalness in our actions can be justified by a proportionate reason, they are not saying that morally wrong actions . . . can be justified by the end. They are saying that an action cannot be qualified simply by looking at the material happening, or at its object in a very narrow and restricted sense. This is precisely what the tradition has done in the categories exempted from teleological assessment (e.g., contraception and sterilization). It does this in no other area.[43]

In response to this claim by McCormick, Professor Janet Smith noted that the key point in this exchange is that proportionalists justify the morality of certain acts (i.e., contraception and sterilization) that the Magisterium has taught are to be considered intrinsically evil, and this is precisely the accusation made against proportionalists in *Veritatis Splendor*.[44] Professor Smith further noted:

> The source of disagreement is that the tradition thinks some actions are intrinsically evil by their object and the proportionalists think that no actions are intrinsically evil by their object; they are only premoral evil (object here means the action itself apart from the circumstances and intention of the agent).[45]

Although he was harshly critical of much of Chapter Two in the encyclical, Professor McCormick acknowledged that it quite properly condemned "contemporary relativism and individualism," and the tendency in contemporary ethics to detach freedom from truth.[46] McCormick also conceded that there has also been an excessive emphasis on individual autonomy in contemporary medicine that has followed in the wake of the overthrow of medical paternalism. This, in turn, had led to an extravagant notion that the only thing that counts is what the patient wants in a given situation and the absence of "any sense of an objective moral order."[47] Of course, McCormick did not concede that the proportionalists have in any way contributed to this phenomenon, but surely their public dissent from the teachings of the Magisterium declaring certain absolute moral norms (primarily those dealing with sexual issues such as contraception and sterilization) does have a tendency to undermine this sense of an objective moral order.

c. *Evangelium Vitae*

Evangelium Vitae was written by John Paul II to defend the right to life "from the moment of conception to until the moment of natural death."[48] It also seeks to combat the prevalence of a "culture of death" that is "excessively concerned with efficiency" and accordingly devalues the lives of those who impose burdens on others.[49] John Conley has noted that John Paul II employs three strands of analysis in the encyclical: scriptural narrative, neo-scholastic, and cultural critique.[50]

The scriptural narrative builds on the story of Cain and Abel to reassert the sanctity of life.[51] The neoscholastic strain of analysis reasserts the traditional absolute norms embraced by the manualists on direct abortion and euthanasia.[52] But perhaps the most compelling portion of the encyclical is its cultural critique of contemporary Western society. The encyclical focuses on a conflict between a "culture of death" and a "culture of life" and situates it in the context of a systemic disregard for human life based on a utilitarian ethic.[53] The encyclical even refers to the unleashing of a "conspiracy against life" that has undermined the family as well as "relations between peoples and States."[54] There is also a critique of contemporary democracy, with its extravagant emphasis on individual autonomy, its failure to protect the weak, and its ethical relativism.[55]

Evangelium Vitae reasserts the traditional teaching on the immorality of contraception and condemns a "contraceptive mentality" that strengthens the temptation to resort to abortion when an unwanted life is conceived.[56] While acknowledging that abortion and contraception are distinctly different — the former undermining the procreative nature of the sexual act and the latter destroying human life — it refers to them "as fruits of the same tree" that are "rooted in a hedonistic mentality."[57] It expresses alarm at the fact that "attacks on life are spreading" and these attacks "receive widespread and powerful support from a broad consensus on the part of society" as well as "widespread legal approval and the involvement of certain sectors of health care personnel."[58]

Evangelium Vitae notes that "various techniques of artificial reproduction" are morally unacceptable, insofar as they separate the procreative from the unitive; moreover, these techniques typically result in the creation of "spare embryos" that are ultimately destroyed.[59] Similarly, "prenatal diagnosis" is deemed morally unacceptable when it serves as a prelude to "eugenic abortion."[60] And the encyclical notes that now, even *infanticide* is proposed as a possible measure in some cases, thereby returning us to a form of barbarism thought to be consigned to the past.[61]

Evangelium Vitae also notes with concern the spread of euthanasia, both "disguised and surreptitious, or practised openly and even legally," due to a cultural context that sees no value in prolonging suffering and a "Promethean attitude" that gives rise to a desire to control the timing of the end of life.[62] Euthanasia is also "sometimes justified by the utilitarian motive of avoiding costs which bring no return and which weigh heavily on society."[63] The encyclical further notes proposals "to eliminate malformed babies, the severely handicapped, the disabled, the elderly, especially when they are not self-sufficient, and the terminally ill."[64]

Evangelium Vitae traces the current attacks on human life to a concept of freedom that places an excessive emphasis on individual autonomy and emancipation "from all forms of tradition and authority."[65] It refers to an ongoing struggle between a "culture of life" and a "culture of death."[66] Furthermore, referring to the "unspeakable crime" of abortion, it condemns all direct abortions.[67] It further emphasizes that human life is to be protected from the time of fertilization of the ovum.[68] As to abortion, in *Evangelium Vitae*, John Paul II concludes:

> Therefore by the authority which Christ conferred upon Peter and his Successors, in communion with the Bishops . . . *I declare that direct abortion, that is abortion willed as an end or as means, always constitutes a grave moral disorder*, since it is the deliberate killing of an innocent human being.[69]

Evangelium Vitae recognizes that euthanasia must be distinguished from the refusal of "aggressive medical treatment" that imposes disproportionate burdens on the patient — thus retaining the traditional distinction between ordinary (proportionate) and extraordinary (disproportionate) treatment.[70] It also recognizes the continuing propriety of the application of the principle of double effect, which permits the administration of nonlethal doses of narcotic pain medication when the intent is to ease suffering, even though its administration may hasten death.[71] In *Evangelium Vitae*, John Paul II concludes by condemning euthanasia in the same terms he used in condemning abortion:

> Taking into account these distinctions, in harmony with the Magisterium of my Predecessors and in communion with the Bishops of the Catholic Church, I confirm that euthanasia is a grave violation of the law of God, since it is the deliberate and morally unacceptable killing of a human person. This doctrine is based upon the natural law and upon the written word of God, is transmitted by the Church's Tradition and taught by the ordinary and universal Magisterium.[72]

Similarly, suicide is adjudged equivalent to murder, and assisted suicide is condemned as "an injustice which can never be excused, even if it is requested."[73]

The language that John Paul II used in condemning euthanasia and abortion has raised the question of whether these statements meet the criteria set out in Vatican II for the invocation of the universal and ordinary infallibility. If that is the case, then continuing dissent from these norms by moral theologians claiming to be Catholic is problematic. William May notes that, as a prelude to his condemnation of abortion, John Paul II reviews the consistent teaching of the church on this matter with references to Scripture, Tradition, papal encyclicals, and canon law.[74] He thus concludes:

PART ONE: *Moral Foundations*

Clearly, here, John Paul II affirms that the teaching on the grave immorality of direct abortion has been infallibly proposed by the ordinary and universal magisterium.[75]

He reaches the same conclusion with respect to the condemnation of euthanasia.[76]

Francis Sullivan has said, "There are some good reasons for thinking that in this encyclical John Paul II intended to invoke, not the infallibility which Vatican I attributed to papal definitions, but the infallibility which Vatican II attributed to the teaching of the "ordinary and universal magisterium.""[77] Sullivan also noted, however, that at the time the encyclical was issued, Cardinal Ratzinger stated that John Paul II had considered making infallible declarations on abortion and euthanasia in *Evangelium Vitae*, but had decided against it because these teachings were already clearly "evident" in Christian faith and tradition.[78]

While Sullivan acknowledges that papal infallibility has never previously been invoked with respect to moral teaching, he opined that this does not preclude it from being invoked in this encyclical.[79] Nonetheless, Fr. Sullivan concludes that infallibility had not yet been "clearly established" at the time of his analysis because the exercise of the ordinary Magisterium requires a consensus among theologians that the doctrine was being infallibly taught, and this had not yet occurred.[80] He acknowledges that John Paul II "wanted all Catholics to hold definitively" these beliefs.[81] Yet he also opines that, even if infallibility attaches to the statements on abortion and euthanasia, it would not attach to the remainder of *Evangelium Vitae*, including its condemnation of contraception.[82]

The teachings of *Evangelium Vitae* are clearly intended to be applied by individuals as well as health care institutions. As to individuals, the encyclical states:

> Abortion and euthanasia are thus crimes which no human law can claim to legitimize. There is no obligation in conscience to obey such laws; instead there is a grave and clear obligation to oppose them by conscientious objection.[83]

And further:

> Absolute respect for every innocent human life also requires the exercise of conscientious objection in relation to procured abortion and euthanasia.[84]

As to health care institutions, *Evangelium Vitae* states:

> In particular, the role of hospitals, clinics and convalescent homes needs to be reconsidered. These should not merely be institutions where care is provided for the sick or the dying. Above all they should be places where suffering, pain and death are acknowledged and understood in their human and specifically Christian meaning. This must be especially evident and effective in institutes staffed by Religious or in any way connected with the Church.[85]

Chapter Four

Secular Bioethics versus Catholic Bioethics

Although the term *bioethics* was not coined until 1971,[1] the discipline of secular bioethics has, to a large extent, already supplanted religiously-based approaches to medical moral issues. The field includes both a theoretical wing — in which scholars have developed various theoretical approaches to ethical dilemmas — and an applied wing, which involves consultants (bioethicists) providing advice to hospitals on the formulation of policies and the application of ethical norms in specific cases.[2] Some secular bioethical theorists claim that their approaches are based on a cross-cultural, universal common morality that will facilitate the reaching of a consensus among persons of various backgrounds, both secular and religious, as to the solution of ethical dilemmas arising in medicine.[3] And bioethicists have been compared to a "secular priesthood" in their claim to provide authoritative guidance in applying the "holy texts of bioethics."[4]

The claims of both theoretical and applied bioethics have been subject to substantial criticism in recent years. Nonetheless, it has already had a significant impact on Catholic health care. Physicians and nurses affiliated with Catholic hospitals are exposed to secular bioethics as part of their education and training and through attendance at conferences. In some instances, Catholic health care institutions have hired staff bioethicists with training in this relatively new discipline. In this chapter, I provide a brief history of secular bioethics, question its moral coherence, examine the role of bioethicists, and call for a renewed emphasis on the development of a distinctive Catholic bioethics.

A Brief History of Secular Bioethics

Beginning in the 1960s, the secular discipline of bioethics began to emerge and supplant religious approaches to medico-moral issues. Albert Jonsen, a pioneer in the bioethics movement, a former Jesuit priest and theology professor at the University of San Francisco, traces the beginning of bioethics to the development of a shunt by Belding Scribner at the University of Washington that permitted persons with kidney failure to receive long-term dialysis.[5] In the case of the development of dialysis, the Seattle Artificial Kidney Center had more patients than it could possibly treat, and a committee was formed to determine, out of those determined to be medically suitable, "who shall live and who shall die."[6] The committee made its determination through the use of so-called "social worth criteria."[7] The activities of the Seattle committee occasioned significant controversy and discussion among prominent ethicists and theologians.[8]

Eventually, the new secular discipline of bioethics was organized and promoted through several conferences in the 1960s and the emergence of centers such as the Kennedy Institute at Georgetown, the Hastings Center, and the Society of Health and Human Values.[9] Dr. Edmund Pellegrino has noted that the field of "bioethics was 'baptized' in the early 1970s virtually simultaneously at the Kennedy Institute at Georgetown University and at the University of Wisconsin."[10] At the Kennedy Institute at Georgetown, "It was viewed primarily as a branch of philosophy . . . [and] its major orientation was to normative ethics."[11] At Wisconsin, bioethics was conceived of as a more broadly scientific and interdisciplinary pursuit.[12]

In the wake of *Humanae Vitae*, a number of Catholic moral theologians, including Jonsen, decided that they could no longer defend the Church's traditional positions on abortion and contraception.[13] According to Jonsen, the debate within the Catholic Church on the morality of contraception "inadvertently promoted the growth of bioethics by increasing the ranks of the new bioethicists."[14] Moreover, "It drove others away from their original home in Catholic moral theology into the new field of bioethics."[15] And questions as to the morality of abortion, sterilization, and contraception eventually disappeared altogether from the agenda of the new bioethicists.[16]

Later, the *Belmont Report*, a government-commissioned study focusing on developing ethical norms for research on human subjects, identified three governing principles of secular bioethics: "respect for persons, beneficence, and justice."[17] Ultimately, these "principles found their way into the general literature of the field, and, in the process, grew from the principles underlying the conduct of research into the basic principles of bioethics."[18] Accordingly, ethical decisions in particular situations were to be arrived at by balancing these competing ethical principles; no one principle trumps the others.[19]

In 1976, in the Quinlan case, the Supreme Court of New Jersey authorized the withdrawal of a respirator from a patient in a persistent vegetative state, indicating that this could be done without fear of liability where the

PART ONE: *Moral Foundations*

withdrawal has been approved by a hospital ethics committee.[20] The court's decision in *Quinlan* resulted in an increased interest in the establishment of hospital ethics committees. In 1992, the Joint Commission on Accreditation of Health Care Organizations (JCAHO) required hospitals to establish "some mechanism for addressing ethical concerns."[21]

By 2001, ethics committees were in place in over in 90 percent of hospitals.[22] These committees are typically used to develop policies concerning DNRs, withdrawal of treatment, treatment of anencephalic infants, and organ donation.[23] They also educate staff, provide counsel to physicians, and review and make recommendations in particular cases.[24] In a few hospitals, they are empowered to render binding decisions in specific cases.[25] In the 1990s, however, "hospitals moved away from unwieldy ethics committees, favoring instead the more user-friendly professional consultant."[26] Larger hospitals may also have in their employ bioethics consultants.[27] The secular bioethics movement has resulted in the creation of an association, the American Society of Bioethics and Humanities,[28] that has defined the core competencies required of bioethicists.[29]

The Marginalization of Religion by Secular Bioethics

Secular bioethics has traditionally "marginalized" religion and religious reflection on ethical issues.[30] Professor David Smolin has argued that secular bioethics, unlike a system of ethics based on religion, does not provide "answers."[31] He notes that in our Western philosophical tradition — indeed, in our culture as a whole — the secular discipline of ethics has been denuded of any metaphysical or theological content.[32] Similarly, he contends, "A bioethics built on this sort of secular ethics is virtually a hopeless enterprise,"[33] and that the field of secular bioethics as it has developed in the United States has been largely dominated by an academic discourse that evinces skepticism toward moral absolutes and views norms as essentially subjective preferences.[34] Professor Smolin argues that this prevailing attitude of ethical relativism is coupled with a pervasive emphasis on individual autonomy as the trump value that provides the rationale for most academic discourse in the field of secular bioethics.[35]

Notwithstanding this skepticism and ethical relativism, secular bioethical theorists do make claims of moral truth — and occasionally, these claims are accompanied with a very explicit rejection of Christian values.

For example, Peter Singer, now a professor at Princeton University and a leading bioethical theorist, has called for the rejection of the sanctity-of-life ethic and of its replacement with a quality-of-life ethic. In a 1983 article, he acknowledged that the sanctity-of-life ethic was being undermined by the prevalence of late-term abortions, the practice of denying nutrition to defective neonates, and the refusal to provide corrective surgery to children with Down syndrome — but then asked: "Is the erosion of the sanctity of life really so alarming?"[36]

Singer contends, "We can no longer base our ethics on the idea that human beings are a special form of creation, made in the image of God, singled out from all other animals, and alone possessing an immortal soul."[37] Indeed, Singer, an advocate of increased recognition of the rights of animals, argues that speciesism, i.e. — the preferential treatment of members of the species *Homo sapiens* — is immoral. In this regard, he would prefer to preserve the life of a dog or pig over the life of a severely defective human infant.[38]

In a subsequent book, Singer acknowledges that his approach is essentially utilitarian, but unlike classical utilitarianism with its focus on increasing pleasure and reducing pain, he focuses on "what, on balance, furthers the interests of those affected."[39] In some ways, reading Singer is refreshing — his arguments have such clarity — but it is also chilling because of its complete rejection of the sanctity-of-life ethic, which he characterizes as a distinctive contribution of Christianity that is no longer relevant.[40] Indeed, Singer gives us a complete moral blueprint for bioethics in a post-Christian world.

For example, he opines that, with respect to abortion, "At least within the bounds of non-religious ethics, there is a clear cut answer and those who take a different view are simply mistaken."[41] Singer identifies the central "conservative" argument against abortion: i.e., it is immoral because it is the killing of innocent human beings.[42] He then rejects the traditional "liberal" arguments that attempt to find some morally significant dividing line between the fetus and a child for the purpose of claiming that a fetus is not a human being.[43] He notes that "there is no obvious sharp line that divides the fertilised egg from the adult."[44] He acknowledges that neither viability nor birth provide any meaningful dividing line for the purposes of determining the morality of abortion.[45] He also rejects liberal arguments that concede the humanity of the fetus, but argue that abortion is morally permissible because of the difficulties of enforcing abortion laws, or because abortion is a "victimless" crime and thus in the realm of private morality.[46] And he even questions the feminist argument that insists on a woman's right to abortion, regardless of the consequences, because of the role of the mother as an autonomous moral decision maker.[47]

Singer, however, also rejects the traditional conservative argument that bases the immorality of abortion on the categorization of the fetus as a human person. While he acknowledges that a human fetus is a human being in the sense of being a member of the species *Homo sapiens*, he denies that this has any moral significance.[48] And he argues the fetus is not a "person" because it is not rational, or "self"conscious.[49] He then concludes that we should not accord the fetus any "greater value than the life of a non-human animal at a similar level of rationality."[50]

Perhaps not surprisingly, Singer also endorses active euthanasia in certain circumstances.[51] He posits that being "a member of the species *Homo sapiens* is not relevant to the wrongness of killing. . . . rather, it is characteristics like rationality, autonomy and self-consciousness that make a difference."[52] He argues that it is morally permissible to end the life of some, regardless of their inability to consent. For example, since infants are "neither rational nor self conscious,"[53] whether disabled or not, they do not have "as strong a claim to life as being capable of seeing themselves as distinct entities, existing over time."[54] While he doesn't advocate the direct killing of normal infants — primarily because of the impact on the parents — he does conclude that there is nothing immoral about intentionally killing disabled infants.[55] Likewise, non-voluntary active euthanasia is morally permissible in the cases of older persons who no longer have the capacity to consent because they are in a permanent coma or persistent vegetative state.[56]

For rational, "self" conscious, competent adult patients who have requested to die, Singer supports the morality of active euthanasia and endorses the example of the Netherlands as providing an appropriate legal regime that will prevent it from spreading beyond its proper purview.[57] Under the guidelines adopted in the Netherlands, euthanasia is acceptable where a patient "with an irreversible condition causing [unbearable] protracted physical or mental suffering" makes a "well-informed, free and durable" explicit request for euthanasia.[58] There must also be no "reasonable alternative" available for the alleviation of the patient's suffering, and another independent doctor must confirm the decision.[59] Justice Rehnquist, however, in his opinion for the court in *Washington v. Glucksberg*,[60] is somewhat less sanguine about the success of the Netherlands guidelines:

> The Dutch government's own study revealed that in 1990, there were 2,300 cases of voluntary euthanasia (defined as "the deliberate termination of another's life at his request"), 400 cases of assisted suicide, and more than 1,000 cases of euthanasia without an explicit request.

In addition to these latter 1,000 cases, the study found an additional 4,941 cases where physicians administered lethal morphine overdoses without the patients' explicit consent.... This study suggests that, despite the existence of various reporting procedures, euthanasia in the Netherlands has not been limited to competent, terminally ill adults who are enduring physical suffering, and that regulation of the practice may not have prevented abuses in cases involving vulnerable persons, including severely disabled neonates and elderly persons suffering from dementia.[61] [citations omitted]

In his 1983 article, Singer rejects the slippery-slope argument against active euthanasia, arguing that societies that have practiced euthanasia "have been able to hold the line around those categories of beings that could be killed, so that the lives of other members of these societies were at least as well protected as the lives of citizens of the United States."[62] While he mentions ancient Greece and the Eskimos as exemplars of such societies,[63] his 1983 article neglects to mention Nazi Germany, where the killing spread from the disabled and retarded in state institutions to the mass extermination of Jews, Gypsies, and others in Auschwitz and other camps.

In his later book, Singer confronts the slippery-slope notion more fully, particularly the example of the Nazi euthanasia program — but then claims that the Nazi program was distinct from modern euthanasia programs in that it was not motivated by a "concern for the suffering" and was often involuntary.[64] In addition, he notes that the Nazis took into account racial factors and "the ability to work" in the selection of patients to be killed.[65] But the differences may not be as great as he supposes. A seminal study by Robert Lifton makes it clear that the practice of active euthanasia, as it developed in Germany in the 1920s and '30s, was motivated at least in part by the desire to use killing as a means of "healing" and was embraced by leading members of the medical profession in Germany prior to the Nazi regime's co-option of the movement for its own purposes.[66] As to its progression under the Nazis, he states:

> Of the five identifiable steps by which the Nazis carried out the principle of "life unworthy of life," coercive sterilization was the first. There followed the killing of "impaired" children in hospitals; and then the killing of "impaired" adults, mostly collected from mental hospitals, in centers especially equipped with carbon monoxide gas. This project was extended (in the same killing centers) to "impaired" inmates of concentration and extermination camps and, finally, to mass killings, mostly of Jews, in the extermination camps themselves.[67]

PART ONE: *Moral Foundations*

The Unsuccessful Attempts to Develop a Universally Acceptable Normative Framework for Bioethics

Secular bioethics is an enterprise with an ambitious agenda: developing a set of normative principles for the resolution of moral issues related to "the application of biotechnology in human life."[68] It has placed a great deal of emphasis on the development of a consensus on these issues.[69] Its attempts to develop a universally accepted normative framework for bioethical decision making have, however, been frustrated by the lack of a common morality in contemporary society.[70]

Professor Tristram Englehardt has noted that the failure to develop this common morality is the "fundamental catastrophe of contemporary secular culture,"[71] a failure that "frames the context of contemporary bioethics."[72] As a result, he argues, our world is populated by "moral strangers," unable to reach consensus through rational argumentation or appeals to some external moral authority.[73]

Fr. Kevin Wildes, S.J., has provided a useful survey of methodologies of the secular bioethics movement that organizes them into three categories — foundationalism, principlism, and casuistry — and sees these different methodologies as being reflective of "the moral pluralism in secular societies."[74] Foundationalism encompasses various theories that claim to provide a universal, normative framework not based on religion for the resolution of bioethical issues.[75] Within this category, Wildes includes such diverse approaches as utilitarianism, virtue theory, natural-law theory, and contractarian theory.[76] He argues, however, that due to the moral pluralism of contemporary society, these approaches cannot provide a sufficient basis for a consensus on bioethical issues:

> One strength of the foundational method — its universality — is also its weakness. The universal needs to address bioethical issues. But with the content comes particularization.[77]

And of course, with particularization comes disagreement over such issues as abortion and physician-assisted suicide.

In discussing the next category, principlism, Wildes observes that due to the difficulty of reconciling the variant meta-ethical underpinnings of the foundationalist methodologies, other bioethicists have attempted to sidestep the problem by developing an approach to resolving bioethical issues that focuses on the application of mid-level principles — i.e., respect for autonomy, nonmaleficence, beneficence, and justice — rather than foundational principles.[78] Wildes, however, argues that this approach also falls short in providing a basis for a bioethical consensus because it also depends on the existence of a common morality that is elusive.[79]

Finally, Wildes analyzes casuistry, an approach that seeks to develop a consensus on the resolution of paradigm cases. In this category, Wildes focuses on the work of Albert Jonsen and Stephen Toulmin who have proposed a methodology that borrows the casuistic approach used by the Catholic Church in the High Middle Ages but is shed of its traditional context within a particular religious community.[80] Wildes, however, argues that while the casuistry of the Middle Ages was coherent within a "communal context that possesses moral and juridical authority," it cannot be expected to provide "like service in a morally pluralistic world."[81]

The Practice of Bioethics in the Clinical Setting

There is continuing controversy over whether bioethics consultation should be considered a legitimate profession,[82] in that applied bioethics may be an "elitist enterprise."[83] One commentator has, in fact, referred to bioethicists as "philosopher kings."[84] Applied bioethics, as developed in academic medical centers, is a "problem-solving methodology for the vexing day-to-day troubles of modern medicine."[85] Bioethicists are involved in both formulating institutional policies and resolving ethical dilemmas in particular cases, where there may be some disagreement among the patient, family members, and health care providers.

In the case context, the role of the bioethicist is to assist family members in understanding the factual context, and then to facilitate the health care providers, the patient (if competent), and family members in reaching an amicable solution. It is assumed that this consensus is achievable in most cases, as long as those concerned act rationally. But from the perspective of the bioethicist, there is a problem with religion: it potentially interjects elements of irrationality and stubbornness into a situation that "should" be mediated and handled rationally. Not surprisingly, there are anecdotal accounts of bioethicists denigrating the religious beliefs of a patient's family.[86]

Many bioethicists use a casuistic approach that uses paradigm cases as precedents for the resolution of particular cases. This approach is perhaps best captured in the popular book *Clinical Ethics*, written by Albert Jonsen with Mark Siegler and William J. Winslade.[87] This book is designed for use by clinicians at the bedside in making ethical decisions in particular cases.[88] It provides a framework for analysis and series of questions for use in ethical

PART ONE: *Moral Foundations*

analysis. Originally designed for specialists in internal medicine, it avoids discussing ethical issues in obstetrics and reproductive medicine, noting: "The problems there involve an enigmatic third party, the fetus, and thus, they require a more complex approach than this book provides."[89]

Jonsen, Siegler, and Winslade posit that ethical analysis should focus on four topics: medical indications, patient preferences, quality of life, and contextual features.[90] They recognize that the religious beliefs of the patient should be considered as part of "patient preferences."[91] They also recognize, under contextual features, that "religious belief and teaching may be relevant to medical care."[92] And further that "Catholicism and Judaism both have extensive teachings about medical care that may dictate or prohibit certain interventions."[93] Nonetheless, although they recognize that religious counseling plays a significant role in the health care system, they characterize the relationship between religion and scientifically based Western medicine as problematic and distant.[94] And their case examples suggest that they view the religious beliefs of the patient or the patient's family primarily as an idiosyncrasy or potential problem to be dealt with by the rational, science-oriented physician.[95]

Catholic Bioethics

Edmund Pellegrino has noted that the sources and methodology of Catholic bioethics differ from secular bioethics: Catholic bioethics is premodern, based on Scripture and the natural law as revealed in the work of moral theologians and the teachings of the Magisterium,[96] including papal encyclicals.[97] Pellegrino contrasts it with a modernist, secular bioethics that finds its origins in the Enlightenment, rejects religion and metaphysics, and focuses primarily on autonomous human reason.[98] And he also distinguishes it from a postmodernist approach that rejects modernist rationalism and any attempts at constructing a coherent, overarching moral philosophy.[99]

While secular bioethics is concerned more with procedural issues,[100] Catholic bioethics has traditionally been concerned with the norms of good moral decision making rather than with the identity of who makes the decision.[101] A 1991 statement by the Catholic Bishops of Pennsylvania asserts that religiously grounded bioethics provides unique insights on issues that secular bioethics cannot provide:

> Bioethics based on philosophy and legal principles provides some guidance through the maze of problems in health care. Yet it is also clear

that philosophy and law alone do not adequately address all of the real concerns and pertinent issues. Religious bioethics makes an invaluable contribution to contemporary moral debates by offering insights into human nature, the purpose of life, the meaning of suffering and education to true virtue. These considerations assist doctors and patients alike to make wise choices both in everyday practice and in the most difficult cases. Religiously grounded bioethics leads people to place their attention on the right thing to do and frees the autonomy of choice from a vision which can easily become narrow and even dreadfully wrong. We can humanize the face of technology by giving it a moral evaluation in reference to the dignity of the human person, who is called to realize the God-given vocation to life and love.[102] (Footnotes omitted.)

Unfortunately, however, secular bioethics has had a significant influence on Catholic hospitals, particularly on hospital ethics committees and the bioethicists Catholic hospitals employ.[103] While the bioethics movement may have been helpful in developing an increased sensitivity to ethical issues in the clinical setting, its influence also poses a significant danger to the preservation of distinctively Catholic health care. Generally, academic discourse on bioethics has been carried on in "a religion-free zone."[104] And it is a tenet of some liberal Catholic bioethicists that the Church should drop its traditional teachings on absolute moral norms governing abortion, sterilization, and contraception in order to be relevant to contemporary society and acceptable to educated elites.[105] Indeed, as observed by one commentator who is a reform Jew, "many Roman Catholic theologians . . . [have been] bent on reducing [the] substantive moral content of their religion to what they took to be the general requirements of moral rationality."[106]

One of the effects of Vatican II in the United States was the acceleration of a trend among Catholics to assimilate and accommodate to predominant cultural influences. Some Catholic moral theologians saw Vatican II as a call to cast off the traditional Catholic natural-law approach and to suppress the distinctive nomos in Catholic hospitals. In the realm of Catholic institutions, Vatican II was seen as a green light for the secularization of Catholic higher education and health care. These trends were exacerbated by the increasing availability of federal funding for these institutions (for hospitals, this included Hill-Burton funding for capital improvements, as well as Medicare and Medicaid reimbursement for patient care) and the belief that secularization was necessary in order to secure that funding. In the past four decades, however, the danger of this approach for the future of Catholic health care

PART ONE: *Moral Foundations*

has become increasingly obvious. As Tristram Engelhardt has noted, we live in a post-Christian age where "[a]n old and once more vigorous pagan moral vision is resurfacing, bringing with it its own accounts of birth, reproduction, suffering and death, which are at loggerheads with traditional Christianity."[107] In such an age, a distinctive Catholic health care will only survive if it continues to emphasize its commitment to its rich, content-thick particularity of Catholic moral teaching.

Thus, while it is certainly appropriate for Catholic health care leaders to participate in public discourse with secular bioethicists on ethical issues, even this must be done with some caution.[108] It is vital that, in this discourse, a clear distinction be preserved between practices prevalent in non-Catholic institutions and those practices that are morally permissible in Catholic institutions. There is an understandable tendency among Catholic health care leaders to present Catholic hospitals as being mainstream institutions that are in sync with the tenets of the secular bioethics movement. There are, however, practices such as abortion, sterilization, physician-assisted suicide, and euthanasia currently available, or potentially available, in non-Catholic hospitals that should never be permitted in Catholic hospitals. And it is unlikely that adherents of the secular bioethics movement, with their aspirations to universality, heavy emphasis on individual autonomy, ethical relativism, and religious skepticism, will generally be supportive of the right of Catholic hospitals to continue to adhere to the moral norms governing Catholic hospitals as set forth in the *Ethical and Religious Directives for Catholic Health Care Services*.[109]

Chapter Five

Ethical and Religious Directives

The influence of the traditional Catholic natural-law approach to bioethical issues may be seen in the *Ethical and Religious Directives for Catholic Health Care Services* (*ERD*s), a set of norms adopted by the United States Conference of Catholic Bishops and most recently revised in 2001.[1] "The directives describe procedures that are judged morally wrong by the National Conference of Catholic Bishops and the United States Catholic Conference."[2] Those procedures judged morally wrong include artificial contraception,[3] direct sterilization,[4] direct abortion,[5] and direct euthanasia.[6]

These prohibitions are based on absolute norms. Thus, artificial contraception and direct surgical sterilizations performed for contraceptive purposes are deemed immoral, notwithstanding substantial reasons for limiting fertility. Direct abortions are adjudged immoral, notwithstanding the potential effect of the pregnancy on the life or health of the mother. And direct euthanasia — i.e., acts or omissions intended to end a human life — is deemed immoral, notwithstanding a benign motive to prevent further suffering. This traditional natural-law approach may be seen in all versions of the *ERD*s.

Not surprisingly, however, in light of the widespread acceptance of contraception, abortion, and sterilization within our culture, compliance with the *ERD*s by Catholic hospitals has been, at times, problematic. One observer has noted:

> The provision of abortion and other reproductive-altering services prohibited by the religious directives would violate its moral commitments and thus would not be offered by Catholic hospitals.[7]

Nonetheless, while Catholic hospitals have generally refrained from providing direct abortions, compliance with the *ERD*s has been uneven when it comes to contraception and sterilization. Typically, obstetrician-gynecologists practicing in Catholic hospitals and physician office buildings owned by Catholic hospitals provide prescriptions for contraceptives to their patients. An anonymous survey of Catholic hospitals in the 1970s revealed that 20

PART ONE: *Moral Foundations*

percent of the hospitals were providing "medically indicated sterilizations," and even more were providing contraceptive services in their hospitals.[8] And abortion referrals have been provided in community health care facilities that have been merged with Catholic hospitals.[9]

Compliance with the *ERDs*' prohibition of direct sterilizations has been particularly problematic. In some instances, bishops have clearly stated that direct sterilizations cannot be performed within Catholic hospitals located in their dioceses and even requested physicians practicing in adjacent buildings to observe the *ERDs*.[10] But other Catholic hospitals have been accused of attempting to circumvent the *ERDs* by cooperating with non-Catholic health care providers to offer sterilization services.[11] Moreover, because of "an excessive focus on the bottom line," some Catholic hospitals provide direct sterilizations in their facilities in conjunction with repeat Caesarean sections.[12] And some have apparently misinterpreted the *ERDs* to permit the performance of direct sterilizations where future pregnancies could endanger a woman's health.[13]

Recently, a whistleblower report alleged that six Catholic hospital systems operating in Texas were routinely allowing direct sterilizations, and perhaps even some direct abortions, to be performed in their facilities.[14] On November 21, 2008, Bishop Alvaro Corrada, S.J., of Tyler, Texas, issued a statement acknowledging that "many direct sterilizations had been done" at two Catholic hospitals in his diocese in violation of the *ERDs* and apologized for his failure of oversight.[15] He attributed the situation to a "serious misinterpretation of the *ERDs*."[16] In a subsequent statement issued on December 1, 2008, Bishop Corrada clarified the distinction between indirect sterilizations, which are permitted by the *ERDs*, and direct sterilizations, which are forbidden by the *ERDs*.[17] But apparently, at least one hospital in his diocese continues to insist that sterilizations are permissible under the *ERDs* when deemed "medically necessary," i.e., in order to alleviate health problems that could be exacerbated by future pregnancies.[18]

The past forty years have seen an ongoing controversy over the meaning of the ban on direct sterilizations; several attempts have been made to clarify and reaffirm the Church's teaching on this point through revision of the *ERDs* and statements issued by the Congregation for the Doctrine of the Faith (CDF).[19] In a 1975 document responding to questions posed by United States bishops concerning whether exceptions could be made to the ban, the CDF replied that sterilizations for contraceptive purposes were forbidden, even if done for the purpose of avoiding medical problems that could result from future pregnancies.[20]

The same point was reiterated in a 1993 response issued by the CDF.[21] Even critics of the traditional teaching, such as David Kelly, have acknowledged that under the principle of double effect, only indirect sterilizations are permitted — e.g., removal of a cancerous or otherwise diseased uterus — while direct sterilizations — e.g., performance of a tubal ligation to avoid health problems from future pregnancies — are forbidden.[22] Nonetheless, many involved in Catholic health care, including some bioethicists, still hold to a mistaken belief that tubal ligations at the time of repeat Caesarean sections are permissible under Directive 53 of the *ERDs*.[23] Directive 53 states that sterilizations are permitted only for treatment of a "serious pathology" when "a simpler treatment is not available."[24] Clearly, "the possibility of a future pregnancy is not a serious pathology."[25]

Complicating the situation is the fact that *ERDs* are not effective in a particular diocese until they are promulgated by the local bishop,[26] and the bishop is responsible for monitoring compliance with the *ERDs* in his diocese.[27] In the United States, conformity with the *ERDs* may provide a litmus test for determining the degree to which a hospital is serious about preserving its Catholic mission.[28] Indeed, the thrust of the *ERDs* is to require Catholic hospitals to preserve their distinctively Catholic mission.[29] If the *ERDs* are not observed by a particular Catholic health care facility, then the local bishop could withdraw recognition of the hospital's identity as a Catholic institution.[30] This, in turn, could result in closure of a facility controlled either by the diocese or the members of a religious order through their reserved powers.[31] If the facility is actually owned by a civil corporation and controlled by a lay board of trustees, then it could continue operations, shorn of the recognition of its Catholic character by the local bishop.[32]

1921 Code of Ethics

A code of medical ethics for Catholic hospitals in the United States was initially a project of the Catholic Hospital Association, the forerunner of today's Catholic Health Association of the United States (CHA).[33] The Catholic Hospital Association was founded on April 8, 1915, at a meeting that took place at Marquette University.[34] Although the first president was a Jesuit priest, it was seen primarily as a "sisters' organization," and sisters from the various women's religious orders that sponsored Catholic hospitals played a significant role in the organization from its inception.[35]

In the 1920s, "standardization" was a significant movement in Catholic health care.[36] "Standardization" refers to the compliance with the standards adopted by the American College of Surgeons (ACS). Fr. Moulnier, the first president of the Catholic Hospital Association, believed that it was essential that Catholic hospitals meet ACS standards.[37] A code of ethics was first adopted by the association in 1921, at the height of the standardization movement, in order to defuse a controversy over the role of the ACS in accrediting Catholic hospitals.[38] This code was based on a paper, presented by Fr. Michael Bourke at the 1919 Catholic Hospital Association convention, that focused primarily on "moral issues related to surgery."[39] Fr. Bourke then compiled a set of ethical norms for health care facilities in the Archdiocese of Detroit.[40] The norms prohibited destruction of fetal life and sterilization.[41]

Some Catholic physicians believed that accreditation by ACS portended greater secular control over Catholic hospitals and threatened their religious mission.[42] In response to these concerns, Moulnier wanted to adopt Fr. Bourke's code in order to calm "fears that Catholic moral principles could be jeopardized by the secular accrediting agency."[43] Moulnier believed it was important that Catholic hospitals meet the standards set forth by secular accrediting agencies such as ACS.[44] Eventually, the 1921 code was "accepted verbatim by many dioceses, and slightly modified by others."[45]

The 1949 *ERDs*

The 1921 code was replaced by a revised code titled the *Code of Ethical and Religious Directives for Catholic Hospitals*, published in 1949 by the Catholic Hospital Association.[46] Through the 1940s, Gerald Kelly, S.J., regularly addressed medico-moral issues in a column published in *Hospital Progress*, a Catholic Hospital Association publication, and it was primarily through his efforts that the code was revised.[47] Fr. Kelly, a professor of theology, used a traditional natural-law approach to analyze ethical issues. He headed a committee that developed the 1949 *ERDs*.[48] The revised code was primarily motivated by the obsolescence of various provisions of the 1921 code due to medical advances that had improved the safety of some surgical procedures.[49] In addition, since Catholic hospitals were collaborating more frequently with public agencies, it was deemed necessary "to articulate clear positions on issues such as birth control and contraceptive methods."[50] "The new code was also broader than its predecessor, addressing issues such as x-ray treatments, artificial insemination, and birth control information."[51]

The 1949 *ERDs* were paired with the 1954 *Code of Medical Ethics for Catholic Hospitals*.[52] The 1949 *ERDs* served as the basis for the development of the 1954 code, a document prepared at the request of several bishops, which became the official code in many United States dioceses.[53] The 1954 code did not have canonical force until approved by a local bishop for his diocese;[54] it was merely a more succinct form of the 1949 *ERD*s that could be hung on the operating room wall.[55] A revised edition of the 1949 *ERD*s was published by the Catholic Hospital Association in 1956, containing "new material on professional secrecy, ghost surgery, psychotherapy, and spiritual care for non-Catholics."[56]

The focus on moral absolutes was made clear in the introduction to the 1949 *ERD*s, where it was specifically stated: "The principles underlying or expressed in this code are not subject to change."[57] In *Medico-Moral Problems*, a book published by the Catholic Hospital Association in 1958, Fr. Kelly examined the 1949 *ERD*s and defended their approach.[58] Indeed, Kelly specifically refuted the notion that the ends could justify the means.[59] In doing so, he appealed to both the natural law and divine law:[60]

> It must be admitted that those who are not soundly trained in the science of morality are much inclined to judge things as if a good end did justify an evil means. Thus there are sincere defenders of such things as therapeutic abortion, masturbation to obtain semen for analysis, donor insemination, and so forth. Our objection to these and similar things is that, though the ultimate purposes are certainly good (e.g., to save a mother's life, to promote fertility), the means used to attain these purposes are morally evil and never permitted.[61]

Although the 1949 *ERD*s were premised on the notion that there are moral absolutes, some procedures such as indirect abortions and indirect sterilizations were permitted under the principle of double effect when the end (abortion or sterilization) is neither desired nor intended.[62] It was also acknowledged that the underlying moral principles might "grow and change as theological investigation and the progress of medical science open up new problems or throw new light on old ones."[63] Moreover, it was acknowledged that the 1949 *ERD*s were not comprehensive in their coverage. Thus, the Introduction states: "The Directives prohibit only those procedures, which, according to present knowledge of facts, seem certainly wrong."[64] Otherwise, with respect to procedures that were the subject of legitimate theological debate, physicians were left free to follow "the principles of sound medicine."[65] When the morality of a particular procedure was "doubtful," and the *ERD*s did not cover the situation or their application was unclear, physicians were required to seek consultation from consultants selected by the hospital unless there was an emergency requiring immediate action.[66]

PART ONE: *Moral Foundations*

In a section titled "Procedures That Involve Serious Risk to, or Destruction of Life," the 1949 *ERD*s first articulated "Principles," and then turned to "Particular Applications."[67] Three general principles were set out:

1. The direct killing of any innocent person, even at his own request, is always morally wrong. . . .
2. *Risk* to life and even the indirect taking of life are morally justifiable for proportionate reasons. . . .
3. Every unborn child must be considered as a human person, from the moment of conception.[68]

Particular applications were then set out, including specific provisions dealing with abortions, Caesarean sections, ectopic pregnancies, euthanasia, hysterectomies, post-mortem examinations, premature delivery, pregnancy tests, and radiation therapy.[69]

Direct abortions were prohibited, even when necessary to save the life of the mother.[70] No exceptions to this norm were recognized, and it was further stated: "Every procedure whose sole immediate effect is the termination before viability is a *direct* abortion."[71] "*Cranial* operations for the destruction of fetal life" were also forbidden.[72] With respect to ectopic pregnancies, the 1949 *ERD*s provided: "Any direct attack on the life of the fetus is morally wrong."[73] Kelly noted that these provisions were primarily directed to the prohibition of "therapeutic abortion[s]" — i.e., "a direct abortion which is deliberately induced for the purpose of saving the life of the mother."[74] He noted that the explicit prohibition on "therapeutic abortion" had remained unchanged since 1884, when the Holy See was first asked for a statement on the question of its morality.[75]

The application of the principle of double effect as it pertains to indirect abortions may also be seen in the 1949 *ERD*s. In the case of ectopic pregnancies, it disallowed any "direct attack on the life of fetus," but allowed removal of "[t]he affected part of an ovary or fallopian tube even where that resulted in an indirect termination of the pregnancy where the operation cannot be postponed without notably increasing the danger to the mother."[76] According to David Kelly, prior to 1933, Catholic medical ethics only permitted surgery to be performed where the fallopian tube had already ruptured, and this resulted in additional danger to the life of the mother.[77] But in 1933, T. Lincoln Bouscaren, S.J, argued in a doctoral dissertation that a salpingectomy (removal of the fallopian tube with the fetus inside) was an indirect abortion under the principle of double effect.[78] He described the act as being the removal of the diseased tube rather than the removal of the fetus.[79] He also rejected the morality of salpingostomy, i.e., the slitting open of the fallopian tube and the removal of the fetus.[80]

Treatments for "serious pathological conditions" in the mother were permitted when they "[could] not be safely postponed" until viability even if they may "indirectly" result in abortion.[81] Similarly, pre-viability treatments "primarily designed" for treatment of hemorrhages were permitted, even if they resulted in an "indirect" abortion.[82] A hysterectomy for treatment of a medical condition was permitted, even in the presence of a pregnancy and pre-viability, in cases where "the operation cannot be safely postponed till the fetus is viable."[83] The induction of labor post-viability that would result in premature delivery was permitted, but only for "a very serious reason."[84] Procedures "primarily designed to empty the uterus" were permissible only where "the physician is reasonably sure that the fetus is already dead or already detached."[85]

"Euthanasia in all its forms" was explicitly "forbidden."[86] Moreover, "the failure to supply the ordinary means of preserving life" was treated as euthanasia.[87] Although not actually stated, this provision carried with it an implicit recognition that the declination or failure to provide extraordinary treatment was morally permissible when it would impose a disproportionate burden on the patient. The traditional application of the principle of double effect was also evident insofar as it was not considered euthanasia "to give a dying person sedatives merely for the alleviation of pain, even to the extent of depriving the patient of the use of sense and reason, when this extreme measure is judged necessary."[88] These sedatives were not to be given to a patient who has not "properly prepared for death," and, for a Catholic patient, this meant that the patient must have received the "Last Sacraments."[89] Moreover, sedatives were also not to be given to "patients who are able and willing to endure their sufferings for spiritual motives."[90]

A second section governed "Procedures Involving Reproductive Organs and Function."[91] The principles set forth at the beginning of the section provided that masturbation was prohibited "even for a laudable purpose" and that "[c]ontinence, either periodic or continuous" was the only morally acceptable form of birth control. In addition, direct sterilization was always forbidden.[92] Indirect sterilization was permitted only under strictly circumscribed conditions.[93] Gerald Kelly opined that under the 1949 *ERDs*, sterilizations could only be justified on the basis of sound medical indications.[94] Accordingly, based on the principle of double effect, indirect sterilizations were permissible for the treatment of a serious pathological condition where no "simpler remedy" was "reasonably available" and the resultant sterility was "an unintended and unavoidable effect."[95]

This second section also dealt with artificial insemination, castration, contraception, hysterectomy in the absence of pregnancy, and sterility tests.[96] Castration was permitted for treatment of "a serious pathological condition"; "oophorectomy or irradition of the ovaries" was permitted for treatment of breast cancer; and orchidectomy was permitted for the treatment of prostate cancer, with a further caveat that "[I]n all cases the procedure least harmful to the reproductive organs should be used."[97]

The 1949 *ERD* excluded the use of artificial contraception as well as surgical sterilization for the purposes of preventing conception, no matter how grave the reasons.[98] There was a specific prohibition on advising or encouraging the use of contraceptives in the hospital setting.[99] The 1949 *ERD*s, however, further stated that "[c]ontinence is not contraception" and physicians were encouraged "to explain the practice of periodic continence to those who have need of such knowledge."[100]

Likewise, "hysterectomy, in the absence of pregnancy" was permitted as a treatment for uterine prolapse or as "a necessary means of removing some other serious pathology."[101] It was not, however, permitted as a routine matter after a series of Caesarean sections or for contraceptive purposes.[102] Even after childbearing was no longer possible in the woman, a hysterectomy was still considered mutilation and thus could only be performed for "sound medical reasons."[103]

The 1971 *ERDs*

The 1949 *ERD*s were not "an authorized version"; and some commentators contended that, in practice, they resulted in "geographical mortality," particularly with respect to the performance of contraceptive sterilizations in Catholic hospitals.[104] Theologians at this time disagreed over the morality of sterilizations performed for clinical reasons to avoid pathologies that could result from future pregnancies.[105] In some dioceses, sterilizations were deemed morally permissible if a future pregnancy could result in serious health problems in a woman; other dioceses, however, treated all sterilizations performed to avoid health problems resulting from future pregnancies as direct sterilizations and forbade them as such.[106] In the 1960s, due to the influence of revisionist theologians, the bishops in some dioceses began to interpret the Directives to permit direct sterilizations and distribution of contraceptives in Catholic hospitals.[107] Therefore, "[b]ecause of the problem of 'geographical mortality'," the CHA asked the NCCB to compose one set of directives for the whole country.[108]

In 1971, the National (U.S.) Conference of Catholic Bishops approved a revised version of the *ERDs*.[109] This revision was primarily motivated by the need to address issues such as the availability of sterilization, contraception, and artificial insemination in Catholic hospitals in the aftermath of challenges to traditional teaching in these areas.[110] The revised directives were formulated and adopted during a time of vocal dissent from *Humanae Vitae*, the papal encyclical restating traditional Church teaching on artificial birth control issued in 1968.[111] At this time, there was increasing discontent among Catholic moral theologians with, and dissent from, the traditional natural-law approach to medico-moral issues as found in the 1949 *ERDs*.

Criticism of the 1971 *ERDs* by Dissenting Theologians

Many Catholic theologians were sharply critical of the 1971 *ERDs*.[112] Upon publication of the 1971 *ERDs*, noted bioethicist Richard A. McCormick, S.J., attacked them as being too rigid because they prohibited Catholic hospitals from providing direct sterilization, contraceptives, and artificial insemination.[113] McCormick was particularly critical of the directives dealing with abortion and artificial insemination, noting that very few theologians would subscribe to absolute bans on direct abortion or masturbation to obtain seminal specimens.[114] McCormick and others also criticized the 1971 *ERDs* for their failure to take account of the pluralistic nature of contemporary society and the changing nature of Catholic hospitals.[115] Instead, they advocated relaxation of the traditional prohibition on material cooperation with evil so that Catholic hospitals could provide those reproductive health services that had been traditionally prohibited by Catholic teaching.[116] In this regard, McCormick argued:

> Finally, Catholic health facilities themselves have undergone subtle but discernible changes in their self-image. Increasingly, they have become community hospitals, often with heavy non-Catholic staff and clienteles. They were frequently financed through public funds or by appeal to the whole community, and still often enough the only health facility reasonably available to a community. In this climate the concept of a "Catholic hospital" becomes problematic.[117]

McCormick criticized the ecclesiology "implicit in the code's preamble" in its position that the local bishop has the authority to decide "difficult moral questions by fiat."[118] He suggested that many bishops are simply not up to this task.[119] He also faulted the way in which the 1971 *ERDs* dealt with material cooperation, particularly those provisions of the 1971 *ERDs* that held the hospital responsible for permitting the performance of immoral procedures within its facility. Instead, he suggested that the primary ethical actors were the physicians and patients and that, in some circumstances, a hospital should tolerate the use of its facility for prohibited procedures. In support of this, he referred to "well-known principles of cooperation" that involve balancing the harm against the good that would come from enforcement of the prohibition.[120] McCormick argued it was morally permissible for a hospital to permit immoral procedures when it served "the total good of its patients."[121] By way of example, he suggested that a prohibition on post-partum sterilization would be unjustified if it would result in the closure of an obstetrics-gynecology department.[122] He thus concluded that "the revised code does not adequately deal with the phenomenon of cooperation."[123]

McCormick also criticized the manner in which the 1971 *ERDs* dealt with the "phenomenon of dissent" following the public controversy over *Humanae Vitae*. In this regard, he acknowledged the potential problem of scandal, but asserted that Catholic hospitals could allow the performance of immoral procedures and still prevent scandal by making careful distinctions between policies and practices.[124] He argued that the 1971 *ERDs* would go "too far" if they take the position that any departure from the *ERDs* was to be considered a source of possible scandal.[125]

Finally, McCormick disagreed with the assertion in the preamble, quoted *infra*, that the 1971 *ERDs* were based on unchangeable "moral absolutes."[126] He acknowledged the existence of moral absolutes at a very "general and indefinite" level — i.e., "human life must be respected" or "all patients must be treated justly."[127] But he asserted that there could be no moral absolutes in particular cases without reference to context and circumstances. In particular, he referred to the prohibition on artificial contraception. He noted that other theologians shared his views on this matter and criticized the drafters of the preamble for inappropriately adopting "a single theological position" as the "teaching of the Church."[128]

Another critic of the 1971 *ERDs* was Warren T. Reich, then a Senior Research Scholar in Medical Ethics at Georgetown's Kennedy Center for Bioethics.[129] Reich's rejection of the existence of moral absolutes was at the heart of his critique. His advocacy of changes in Church teaching on medical moral issues was coupled with his desire to accommodate the practices of Catholic institutions to trends in American culture. Reich believed that the 1971 *ERDs* could provoke "an acute confrontation of forces in the American Church and American Society."[130] He asserted that the approach taken by the 1971 *ERD*s might result in institutional policies that would stifle further development and innovation in the field of medical ethics.[131] Reich faulted the 1971 *ERD*s for focusing too much on issues of sex and reproduction, while neglecting justice issues and failing to come to grip with "recent biomedical breakthroughs."[132] He accused the bishops of having "closed an eye to the more recent scholarly natural-law reflection on the principle of double effect and the principle of totality."[133]

Reich noted the widespread prevalence of dissenting views among Catholic theologians on the morality of artificial contraception, sterilization, and artificial insemination. He advocated a "right to conscientious dissent in moral matters" based on "changed attitudes towards [sic] the authority of the moral magisterium," and the preeminent role of individual conscience in making moral decisions.[134] He even suggested that it was immoral for Catholic hospitals to refuse to provide access to procedures prohibited under the 1971 *ERD*s in light of their receipt of public funds.[135] He referred to a peculiarly "'Catholic' morality" in contradistinction with the general and prevailing morals of the community.[136] Reich argued that imposing "Catholic moral teachings" on non-Catholics violated the teachings on religious freedom and freedom of conscience found in the teachings of Vatican II.[137] He concluded that in the 1971 *ERD*s, "moral teaching was subordinated to the pressures of administrative policy-making."[138]

Reich identified the most significant fault of the 1971 *ERD*s as their insistence that they were binding on physicians, patients, board members, and administrators.[139] He argued that the 1971 *ERD*s promoted "geographical morality" insofar as its provisions were less open-textured and flexible than the guidelines approved by the Canadian bishops in 1970. Indeed, he noted with approval the Canadian bishops' statement that their guidelines were not to be taken as commands, and that the judgment of the individual conscience was the ultimate authority.[140] Reich observed that "geographical morality" could result from divergent opinions among U.S. bishops.[141] He argued that the 1971 *ERD*s represented a throwback to "the days of Galileo" because they recognized the ultimate role of the local bishop in evaluating the morality of scientific advances and he questioned the competence of the bishops to make these determinations.[142]

Reich surmised that the motivation behind the bishops' decision to adopt "a very restrictive moral teaching" was a desire to maintain the distinctive identity of Catholic hospitals.[143] He questioned the wisdom of making ethical norms into institutional policy on the basis that such generic policies could not properly be applied across the board without reference to "the

PART ONE: *Moral Foundations*

complexity of the modern hospital, the right to a free exercise of conscience, and the fact of changing norms."[144] His conclusion:

> One result of the promulgation of the national code will be a harmful and unnecessary intensification of the alienation of American hierarchy from both the medical world and the theological world.[145]

Adoption of the 1971 *ERDs* by the Bishops

Despite the negative reaction of many well-known theologians, the National Conference of Catholic Bishops (NCCB) overwhelmingly voted to approve the 1971 version of the *ERDs*.[146] Their subsequent widespread adoption by local bishops was further encouraged by the 1973 *Roe v. Wade* decision and the fact that, as noted by John Cardinal Krol, Archbishop of Philadelphia and president of the NCCB, Catholic hospitals might not be able to take advantage of recently adopted conscience-clause legislation unless rules were in place that prohibited them from performing abortions.[147] Widespread adoption of the *ERDs* was also encouraged by the issuance of an injunction by a U.S. District Court in Montana, in October of 1972, that enjoined a Catholic hospital from prohibiting a physician from performing a tubal ligation on a patient.[148]

In sharp contrast with McCormick's and Reich's flexible approaches to ethical issues, the preamble to the 1971 *ERDs* reiterated the acceptance of the existence of moral absolutes:

> These *Directives* prohibit those procedures which, according to present knowledge, are recognized as clearly wrong. The basic moral absolutes which underlie these Directives are not subject to change, although particular applications might be modified as scientific investigation and theological development open up new problems or cast new light on old ones.[149]

In a 1972 article in the *Linacre Quarterly*, Thomas J. O'Donnell, S.J., a consultant involved in drafting the 1971 *ERDs*, responded to the criticism of the *ERDs*:

> The controversy is basically about the teaching of the Catholic Church on abortion and contraception.[150]

He defended *Humanae Vitae's* condemnation of contraception as the authentic teaching of the Church, and rejected the notion that Catholics who disagreed with this teaching were free to follow their own consciences.[151] As to those who argued that it was permissible to allow contraceptive sterilization and abortion in Catholic hospitals under the principles of material cooperation, Fr. O'Donnell responded that their arguments amounted to "moral casuistry."[152]

O'Donnell defended the role of the local bishops in providing authoritative guidance on medico-moral issues.[153] He rejected the charge of "geographical morality," a charge that had been leveled against 1949 *ERDs* as well as the 1971 *ERDs*.[154] The "geographical morality" criticism of the 1971 *ERDs* focused primarily on the possibility of differing interpretations and applications of the principles of material cooperation by local bishops, but the preamble to the 1971 *ERDs* confirmed the role of the local bishop in making prudential judgments:

> Any facility identified as Catholic assumes with this identification the responsibility to reflect in its policies and practices the moral teachings of the Church, under the guidance of the local bishop.[155]

While Fr. O'Donnell acknowledged that local bishops had the responsibility of making prudential judgments on these issues, he argued that this approach was consistent with the Catholic natural-law tradition.[156] In this regard, he noted that it was appropriate to provide for prudential judgment to be exercised by the local bishop where the question is whether a particular institution may call itself Catholic rather than on the morality of particular procedures.[157] He also noted the irony of those criticizing the 1971 *ERDs* on the basis of "geographic morality" being the same people who advocated that moral absolutes be ignored in favor of a "situation ethic."[158]

Fr. O'Donnell went on to explain that the controversy over the 1971 *ERDs* was not due to diverging opinions on what the Church taught on abortion and contraception, but a disagreement over whether those teachings should be followed by Catholic institutions.[159] He presciently concluded:

> The road ahead for the Catholic hospital — partly supported by public funds in a pluralistic, and to a great extent, contraceptive and abortion-oriented society — is fraught with dangers to its corporate endurance, and even its continued existence.[160]

The preamble further provided that it was the responsibility of the Boards of Trustees of Catholic health care facilities "to prohibit those procedures which are morally and spiritually harmful."[161] Thus, the 1971 *ERDs* rejected the argument that, because of their receipt of federal funds, Catholic hospitals should provide access to procedures such as direct sterilization that were accepted by large segments of the community.[162] Accordingly, they were subject to ongoing criticism by theologians advocating a more flexible approach by Catholic hospitals in such matters.[163]

In his 1976 text, O'Donnell argued that pluralism did not necessarily require adherence to a common morality, but rather could mean a "coexistence of varying theological attitudes (including that of a Catholic hospital)."[164] He added that many dissenting theologians advocated the provision of sterilizations in Catholic hospitals but not abortions — although the logic of their argument would support provision of both procedures.[165] He also noted that receipt of public funds did not carry with it either a moral or legal obligation to provide sterilizations and abortions, as evidenced by conscience-clause legislation.[166]

Treatment of Abortion under the 1971 *ERDs*

As to abortion, the 1971 *ERDs* reaffirmed the traditional prohibition on all direct abortions. Directive 12 specifically prohibited "the directly intended destruction of a viable fetus."[167] Material cooperation in the provision of abortion was also forbidden.[168] This prohibition extended also to "the interval between conception and implantation of the embryo." Directive 24 specifically provided: "curettage of the endometrium after rape to prevent implantation of a possible embryo is morally equivalent to abortion."[169] Directive 11 emphasized, "[a]ny deliberate medical procedure, the *purpose* of which is to deprive a fetus or an embryo of its life, is immoral."[170]

Fr. O'Donnell defended these prohibitions against charges that Catholic hospitals and obstetricians routinely preferred the life of the child over the life of the mother by reiterating that, in principle, direct killing of either mother or child was prohibited by Catholic teaching.[171]

The 1971 *ERDs* also reaffirmed traditional applications of the principle of double effect in the abortion context. Under Directive 13, it was permissible to provide treatment that indirectly resulted in an abortion where the intent was "the cure of a proportionately serious pathological condition of the mother" and the treatment could not be "safely postponed until the fetus is viable."[172] With respect to an extrauterine pregnancy, the 1971 *ERDs* permitted, with certain limitations, removal of "the dangerously affected part of the mother . . . even though fetal death may be foreseen."[173] Directive 16 seemed to require removal of the affected part of the mother rather than permit removal of the fetus only, an approach criticized by Charles Curran because it would fail to preserve the fertility of the woman.[174] Thus, the 1971 *ERDs* accepted the arguments of Bouscaren that it was morally licit to perform a salpingectomy for treatment of an ectopic pregnancy, but not a salpingostomy.[175] In addition, a Caesarean section for removal of a viable fetus was permitted "even with risk to the child, when necessary for the safety of the mother."[176]

Treatment of Contraception and Sterilization under the 1971 *ERDs*

Traditional prohibitions on contraception and direct sterilization were also reaffirmed by the 1971 *ERDs*. Directive 18 prohibited contraceptive sterilization, "whether permanent or temporary."[177] Also prohibited was "every action which, either in anticipation of the conjugal act, or in its accomplishment, or in the development of its natural consequences, proposes, whether as an ends or as a means, to render procreation impossible."[178] This would appear to have been intended to prohibit Catholic health care institutions from providing access to artificial contraception in any form.

O'Donnell, in his 1976 text, argued that it was not morally permissible for Catholic hospitals to tolerate the performance of contraceptive sterilizations or a birth control clinic in a hospital-owned professional office building because of the risk of scandal.[179] Nonetheless, there was some continuing controversy concerning the permissibility of sterilization for contraceptive purposes even under the 1971 *ERDs*.[180] Directive 18 prohibited "[s]terilization, whether permanent or temporary, for men or for women . . . as a means of contraception."[181] Procedures that resulted in sterility were permitted where the intention was not contraceptive.[182] Directive 19 prohibited actions taken for the purpose of rendering "procreation impossible."[183] But Directive 20 provided that procedures that indirectly resulted in sterility were permitted where the intention was not contraceptive and the procedure was necessary for treatment of a "serious pathological condition."184 Directive 20 provided that procedures that indirectly resulted in sterility were permitted where the intention was not contraceptive and the procedure was necessary for treatment of a "serious pathological condition."[184]

Some moral theologians argued that Directive 20 was to be read in conjunction with Directive 6, which stated: "Ordinarily the proportionate good that justifies a medical or surgical procedure should be the total good of the patient."[185] They contended that the allowance of sterilization in Directive 20 for the treatment of "serious pathological conditions" under certain conditions should be read in light of the principle of totality set forth in Directive 6, and, therefore, sterilization was permissible for the good of the patient based on clinical indications.[186] Thus, under this interpretation, sterilization would be justified where the patient was suffering from cardiac or renal disease that could make future pregnancies dangerous.[187]

On the other hand, in his 1976 text, O'Donnell contended, "The principle of totality cannot be used to justify direct sterilization, and this is precisely the reason for the word 'ordinary' in Directive Six."[188] Furthermore, he argued that various provisions of the 1971 *ERD*s were intended to prohibit all direct sterilizations — i.e., sterilizations for the purpose of preventing pregnancy — regardless of the therapeutic justification for the procedure.[189] Ultimately, the controversy "was referred to the Vatican by the NCCB, and the Congregation for the Doctrine of the Faith (CDF) offered the theological opinion that sterilizations of this type were contraceptive, and, therefore, prohibited in Catholic health care facilities."[190]

Treatment of End-of-Life Issues in 1971 *ERD*s

Consistent with the Catholic natural-law tradition, the 1971 *ERD*s explicitly forbade "euthanasia ('mercy killing') in all its forms."[191] It also reiterated the traditional distinction between extraordinary and ordinary treatment by stating that the "failure to supply the ordinary means of preserving life is equivalent to euthanasia," but that "neither the physician nor the patient is obliged to use extraordinary means."[192] And the 1971 *ERD*s reiterated the traditional application of the principle of double effect by noting that it was permissible "to give a dying person sedatives and analgesics" for pain relief, even if their effect was to hasten death.[193]

The 1971 *ERD*s included, for the first time, provisions relating to organ transplantation in response to significant developments in that field.[194] In 1968, the National Conference of Commissioners on Uniform State Laws had issued the Uniform Anatomical Gift Act in 1968 to facilitate organ donations.[195] In that same year, the Ad Hoc Harvard Committee issued a report setting forth a revised definition of death that included brain death, a concept subsequently embraced by the President's Commission for the Study of Ethical Problems in Medicine and Biomedical and Behavioral Research.[196] In 1980, the National Conference of Commissioners for Uniform State Laws promulgated the Uniform Determination of Death Act and defined death to include "irreversible cessation of the functions of the entire brain, including the brain stem."[197]

The 1971 *ERD*s permitted the harvesting of organs from living donors "when the anticipated benefit to the recipient is proportionate to the harm done to the donor, provided that the loss of such organ(s) does not deprive the donor of life itself nor of the functional integrity of his body."[198] Under this provision, it was permissible to harvest a kidney from a living donor for transplant as long as the proportionality test was met.[199] As for harvesting organs from cadavers, it was not permitted "until death has taken place" and death was determined "in accordance with responsible and commonly accepted scientific criteria."[200] There was also a requirement that the determination of death was ordinarily to be made by a physician who was not part of the transplant team.[201]

The 1994 *ERDs*

A revised and expanded text of the *ERDs* was "developed by the Committee on Doctrine of the National Conference of Catholic Bishops and approved as the national code by the full body of bishops at their November 1994 General Meeting."[202] The approval of the 1994 *ERDs* was accompanied by a recommendation that the diocesan bishops adopt them.[203] The 1994 *ERDs* were adopted after "a consultative process that spanned seven years and included input from hundreds of persons involved in the Church's health ministry."[204] Beginning in July of 1988, five agencies were consulted by subcommittee of the Committee on Doctrine of the NCCB with regard to revisions of the *ERDs*: CHA, the Pope John XXIII Center (now the National Catholic Bioethics Center), the Center for Health Care Ethics at St. Louis University, the Medical-Moral Board of the Archdiocese of San Francisco, and the Kennedy Institute of Ethics at Georgetown University.[205] The final version was submitted to the NCCB in fall 1994, after several drafts and a review by the Congregation for the Doctrine of the Faith.[206]

The preamble to the 1994 *ERDs* noted the "extraordinary change" that had taken place in health care in the United States and in the Church.[207] Among the changes noted were "technological advances," "significant changes in religious orders and congregations," and "the increased involvement of lay men and women."[208] The preamble stated: "Now, with American health care facing even more dramatic changes, we reaffirm the Church's commitment to health care ministry, and the distinctive Catholic identity of the Church's institutional health care services."[209] The 1994 *ERDs* focused primarily on "institutionally based Catholic health care services" but it was noted that they could "also . . . be helpful to Catholic professionals engaged in health care services in other settings."[210]

Moreover, the preamble to 1994 *ERDs* stated: "They address the sponsors, trustees, administrators, chaplains, physicians, health care personnel, and patients or residents of these institutions and services."[211] The drafters of the 1994 *ERD*s and the bishops were well aware that by this time many of those "serving as trustees, administrators, or health care professionals in Catholic facilities are not Catholic."[212] Accordingly, they clearly intended that both Catholics and non-Catholics with management roles in Catholic health care facilities should act in accordance with the *ERD*s.[213] Indeed, deBlois and O'Rourke argue that this was appropriate because if non-Catholics could not in good conscience follow the *ERD*s, then they were "free to disaffiliate from the Catholic institution."[214]

The 1994 *ERD*s were divided into six parts: "The Social Responsibility of Catholic Health Care Services"; "The Pastoral and Spiritual Responsibility of Catholic Health Care"; "The Professional-Patient Relationship"; "Issues in Care for the Beginning of Life"; "Issues in Care for the Dying"; and "Forming New Partnerships with Health Care Organizations and Providers."[215] There is a general introduction, focusing on the theological underpinnings of Catholic health care,[216] and an appendix, titled "Principles Governing Cooperation."[217]

Obviously, the necessity of taking specific steps to preserve the religious identity of Catholic health care institutions was among the most important goals of the 1994 *ERD*s. The introduction recognized that laypersons and many non-Catholics are involved in Catholic health care.[218] It was noted that their participation was essential for the continuation of the Catholic health care mission.[219] Perhaps not coincidentally, the introduction also recognized the unique responsibility of the local bishop in preserving the religious identity of Catholic health care in his diocese: "These responsibilities will require that Catholic health care providers and the diocesan bishop engage in ongoing communication on ethical and pastoral matters that require his attention."[220] Certainly, at this time it was appropriate that the role of the bishop be emphasized in light of the continuing decline in the numbers of religious involved in the health care ministry. Indeed, greater involvement of the bishop in the supervision of the health care ministry may have been viewed as an essential means of preserving Catholic identity in such an environment.

There was also a recognition that adherence to the directives was necessary for the purpose of maintaining Catholic identity. In order to reinforce the importance of the 1994 *ERD*s in preserving religious identity, Directive 5 required that Catholic institutions adopt them as policy, require adherence to them by employees and the medical staff, and provide instruction on them for administrators and staff members.[221] Also included was a specific requirement: "Employees of a Catholic health care institution must respect and uphold the religious mission of the institution and adhere to these directives."[222] Moreover, in an apparent response to critics who have argued that Catholic health care institutions in a pluralist society have the obligation to provide procedures that violate Catholic moral teaching, the introduction to the section on social responsibility specifically stated: "Catholic health care does not offend the rights of individual conscience by refusing to provide or permit medical procedures that are judged morally wrong by the teaching authority of the Church."[223]

The 1994 *ERD*s also placed greater emphasis on social justice issues such as access to health care and the rights of employees as compared with prior versions. The section titled "The Social Responsibility of Catholic Health Care Services" contained a specific recognition of a right to adequate health care. Accordingly, Directive 3 provided that "Catholic health care should distinguish itself by service to and advocacy for those people whose social condition puts them at the margins of our society and makes them particularly vulnerable to discrimination. . . ."[224] And Directive 7 required Catholic health care institutions to treat their employees justly and recognize their collective bargaining rights.[225]

The 1994 *ERD*s also, for the first time, included a section specifically dealing with the pastoral and spiritual responsibilities of Catholic health care providers — probably to address concerns arising from the decline in the numbers of religious working in health care. The introduction to this section recognized that Catholic health care institutions must address the spiritual needs of patients and their families. In light of the shortened nature of hospital stays, however, it was recognized that most pastoral care would be provided at the parish level before and after the hospital stay.[226] There was a requirement that those involved in providing pastoral care, including laypersons, must have an understanding of the 1994 *ERD*s.[227] The appropriateness of appointing non-Catholics to the pastoral care staff of Catholic hospitals was recognized, but, in order to safeguard the religious identity of the institutions, the director of pastoral care was required to be a Catholic; any exception from that requirement had to be approved by the local bishop.[228]

The 1994 *ERD*s specifically addressed the care to be given to victims of sexual assault. The 1971 *ERD*s had treated the use of curettage of the endometrium after rape as the equivalent of abortion, and thereby prohibited it.[229] But Directive 36 of the 1994 *ERD*s recognized that the victim of a rape should be able to defend herself against conception and authorized treatment with medication to "prevent ovulation, sperm capacitation, or fertilization."[230] The Directive, however, prohibited "treatments that have as their purpose or direct effect the removal, destruction, or interference with the implantation of a fertilized ovum."[231] An accompanying footnote recommended "that a sexually assaulted woman be advised of the ethical restrictions that prevent Catholic hospitals from using abortifacient procedures."[232] Also included was a reference to guidelines issued by the Pennsylvania Catholic Conference for the treatment of victims of sexual assault.[233]

The section "Issues in Care for the Beginning of Life" dealt with abortion, contraception, artificial insemination, and sterilization in a manner similar to previous versions of the *ERD*s, and it also dealt with newer topics such as genetic counseling, prenatal diagnosis, and surrogate motherhood.[234] The treatment of abortion was unchanged from the 1971 *ERD*s — i.e., direct abortions were never permitted.[235] Abortion was defined to include "[e]very procedure whose sole immediate effect is the termination of pregnancy before viability . . . which . . . includes the interval between conception and implantation of the embryo."[236] Directive 47 permitted treatment interventions to treat a serious pathological condition in the mother, even where it would result in the death of a non-viable fetus.[237] Sr. Jean deBlois and Fr. Kevin O'Rourke emphasized that the appropriate application of this directive required adequate data about the nature of the medical conditions of both mother and fetus, as well as data on the effect of the proposed intervention on their medical condition.[238]

As in the 1971 *ERD*s, discussed *supra*, there was a specific admonition that Catholic hospitals were not to provide abortion services "even based upon the principle of material cooperation."[239] There was a further admonition concerning the "need to be concerned about the danger of scandal in any association with abortion providers."[240] In addition, and perhaps in recognition of the widespread prevalence of abortion in the wake of *Roe v. Wade*, Catholic health care providers were encouraged to provide: "compassionate physical, psychological, moral, and spiritual care to those persons who have suffered from the trauma of abortion."[241]

The 1994 *ERD*s permitted early induction of labor, post-viability, but only for "proportionate reasons."[242] This topic had not been addressed in the 1971 *ERD*s. As to extrauterine pregnancies, intervention was not permitted by the 1994 *ERD*s if it constituted a direct abortion.[243] By implication then, intervention would be permitted if intended for the purpose of treatment. This subject was treated with more brevity in Directive 48 of the 1994 *ERD*s as compared with the 1971 *ERD*s. Under the 1971 *ERD*s, removal of the affected part of the mother (e.g., cervix, ovary of fallopian tube) was permitted, but the separation of the fetus from its site was not permitted.[244] Charles Curran criticized this approach and argued that the removal of the affected part should not be required in order to preserve the fertility of the mother.[245]

Sr. Jean deBlois and Fr. Kevin O'Rourke argued that Directive 48 of the 1994 *ERD*s could be construed to permit removal of the fetus without removal of the affected part, i.e., a salpingostomy, for the purpose of curing the pathological condition.[246] On the other hand, David F. Kelly has conceded that a salpingostomy would not be permitted under Directive 48.[247] But he also noted John Tuohey's argument that since a salpingostomy involves the detachment of the outer layer of cells that become the placenta (trophoblast), rather than the inner layer of cells that become the fetus (the cytobast),[248] it could be morally permissible under the principle of double effect to remove the fetus from the tube.[249]

Directive 52 of the 1994 *ERD*s prohibited Catholic health care institutions from promoting or condoning contraceptive practices, and encouraged them to provide instruction on natural family planning.[250] This provision was more succinct than the treatment of the matter in the 1971 *ERD*s.[251] The reference to the promotion of Natural Family Planning in the context of the prohibition on promoting or condoning contraception may be due to the recognition that by this time, contraceptives were being routinely prescribed and dispensed in professional office buildings owned by Catholic hospitals. A Catholic hospital could then counteract the impression that it was condoning contraception and dilute the risk of scandal [252] by providing instruction on Natural Family Planning. Moreover, deBlois and O'Rourke argued that there was some greater flexibility under Directive 52 than under prior versions of the *ERD*s. For example, they suggested that physicians at an inner-city clinic sponsored by a Catholic hospital could prescribe birth-control pills for unmarried teenagers involved in drug abuse or for those who had a history of pregnancies ending in abortions.[253]

The treatment of sterilization in the 1994 *ERD*s was similar to prior versions of the *ERD*s. Directive 53 prohibited "[d]irect sterilization . . . whether permanent or temporary" in Catholic health care institutions.[254] Consistent with prior versions of the *ERD*s, procedures that induced sterility were, however, permitted where "their direct effect is the cure or alleviation of a present pathology and a simpler treatment is not available."[255] These provisions appear to have followed Fr. O'Donnell's interpretation of the 1971 *ERD*s, discussed *supra*, in that they implicitly prohibited all direct sterilizations, regardless of a possible justification based on the impact of future pregnancies on the woman's health.

PART ONE: *Moral Foundations*

Part Five of the 1994 *ERD*s was titled "Issues in Care for the Dying."[256] The directives in this part restated traditional Catholic teaching on end-of-life issues. The introduction to this section states "[a]bove all . . . a Catholic health care institution will be a community of respect, love, and support to patients or residents and their families as they face the reality of death."[257] The introduction emphasized the importance of effective pain management for those nearing death.[258] While it recognized that there was a duty to preserve life, it also recognized that this duty was not absolute and that it was morally permissible to "reject life-prolonging procedures that are insufficiently beneficial or excessively burdensome."[259] It also stated that "[s]uicide and euthanasia are never morally acceptable options."[260] It called for the avoidance of two extremes: the "insistence on useless or burdensome technology . . . and, on the other hand, the withdrawal of technology with the intent of causing death."[261]

In addition, the introduction included a separate paragraph dealing with medically assisted nutrition and hydration (ANH). It stated: "Some state Catholic conferences, individual bishops, and the NCCB Committee on Pro-Life Activities have addressed the moral issues concerning medically assisted hydration and nutrition."[262] It further states that ANH procedures "are not morally obligatory either when they bring no comfort to a person who is imminently dying or when they cannot be assimilated by a person's body."[263] There was also specific mention of the morality of withdrawing ANH from a patient in a persistent vegetative state ("PVS"), pointing "out the necessary distinctions between questions already resolved by the magisterium and those requiring further reflection."[264] This language suggests that the 1994 *ERD*s refrained from taking a definitive position on this issue because at the time there was no consensus among moral theologians and no authoritative determination by the Magisterium on the morality of withdrawing ANH from a PVS patient whose life could be sustained with this treatment.[265]

The directives (prescriptive norms) in Part Five reinforced the teachings set forth in the introduction. They restated the traditional distinction between ordinary and extraordinary treatment noting that "[a] person has a moral obligation to use ordinary or proportionate means" to preserve life; "means . . . that *in the judgment of the patient* offer a reasonable hope of benefit and do not entail an excessive burden or impose excessive expense on the family or the community."[266] On the other hand, it was permissible for a person to "forgo extraordinary or disproportionate means," i.e, "those that *in the patient's judgment* do not offer a reasonable hope of benefit or entail an excessive burden, or impose excessive expense on the family or the community."[267] The focus here on the individual judgment would seem to emphasize the role of individual conscience rather than on an objective standard in making this determination.

There is, however, a further qualification: an "informed judgment" by a "competent patient" as to the refusal of life-sustaining treatment was to be honored, but only if it was not "contrary to Catholic moral teaching."[268] Moreover, Catholic health care institutions were forbidden from condoning or participating "in euthanasia or assisted suicide in any way."[269]

The traditional application of the principle of double effect was reiterated:

> Medicines capable of alleviating or suppressing pain may be given to a dying person, even if this therapy may indirectly shorten the person's life, so long as the intent is not to hasten death.[270]

It was also recognized that while patients were to "be kept as free from pain as possible," they also had a "right to prepare for . . . death" and "should not be deprived of consciousness without a compelling reason."[271]

The 1994 *ERDs* included a section dealing specifically with the formation of new partnerships among Catholic and non-Catholic health care institutions.[272] The adoption of this section appears to have been motivated, at least in part, by concerns about the risk of scandal arising from such partnerships. The introduction to the new section states: "[N]ew partnerships can pose serious challenges to the viability of the identity of Catholic health care institutions and services, and their ability to implement these directives in a consistent way, especially when partnerships are formed with those who do not share Catholic moral principles."[273] It also mentioned the "risk of scandal."[274] Accordingly, Directive 687 required prior consultation with the local bishop before entering into partnerships that could have "serious consequences for the identity or reputation of Catholic health care services, or entail the high risk of scandal."[275] Directive 698 required that partnerships that could affect the identity or religious mission of Catholic health care institutions "must respect Church teaching and discipline."[276] It further provided: "Diocesan bishops and other church authorities should be involved as such partnerships are developed, and the diocesan bishop should give the appropriate authorization before they are completed."[277] If the partnership was involved in activities that would violate Church norms, then the Catholic institution was to limit its participation "in accord with the moral principles governing cooperation."[278] It was further emphasized, however, that the possibility of scandal may, however, in some circumstances, preclude cooperation that would otherwise be morally appropriate.[279]

Part One: *Moral Foundations*

Accompanying this new section on partnerships was an appendix titled "The Principles Governing Cooperation."[280] Although principles differentiating between formal and material cooperation have traditionally focused on individuals, this appendix focused on the activities of Catholic institutions. The principles set forth sought to distinguish the actions of the entity directly involved in the wrongdoing from the actions of the cooperating institution, i.e., the Catholic health care institution. The first distinction made was between formal and material cooperation. If the cooperating institution intended "the object of the wrongdoer[s]," then the cooperation was formal and thereby forbidden.[281] Formal cooperation did not have to be explicit, and was to be implied if "no other explanation can distinguish the cooperator's object from the wrongdoer's object."[282] If, on the other hand, the cooperating institution did not either explicitly or implicitly intend the object of the wrongdoer's activity, then the cooperation could be characterized as material and deemed morally licit.[283]

Second, a further distinction was made between mediate and immediate material cooperation. Immediate material cooperation was defined to encompass situations when the cooperator had the same object as the wrongdoer.[284] In the absence of duress, immediate material cooperation was treated as identical to formal cooperation.[285] Immediate material cooperation was deemed morally illicit in the absence of duress, but if duress was present, then it could be treated as morally licit.[286] If it was possible to distinguish the wrongdoer's intention from the cooperator's intention, then cooperation was characterized as mediate and could be deemed morally licit.[287] The principles further set out two other considerations in appraising the morality of material cooperation: (1) the requirement that "the object of material cooperation should be as distant as possible from the wrongdoer's act;" and a further requirement that (2) "any act of material cooperation requires a proportionately grave reason."[288] Finally, it was considered "essential that the possibility of scandal should be eliminated."[289]

The 2001 *ERDs*

In the spring of 2001, the Congregation for the Doctrine of the Faith (CDF) asked the National Conference of Catholic Bishops to revise Part Six of the 1994 *ERDs*.[290] The request was motivated by specific concerns regarding the misapplication of the principle of cooperation in three arrangements entered into by Catholic health care institutions in the United States.[291] The CDF "sought a clarification of the distinction between material and formal cooperation so as to exclude any possibility of proportionalist interpretations of the principle."[292] At its June 2001 meeting, the Catholic bishops in the United States approved revisions of the 1994 *ERDs*.[293] The revisions were not extensive, but, nonetheless, may have a significant impact on collaborative arrangements between Catholic and non-Catholic institutions.[294] Indeed, the revisions were occasioned by the Vatican's concerns about the "culpable cooperation" of Catholic health care institutions in the immoral conduct of non-Catholic institutions.[295]

After the adoption of the 1994 *ERDs* a number of Catholic hospitals had been accused of attempting to circumvent implementation of the *ERDs* by cooperating with non-Catholic health care providers to provide reproductive services that were prohibited under the *ERDs*. In 2001, the *ERDs* were modified to make it more difficult for Catholic hospitals to utilize cooperative arrangements to continue to provide reproductive services such as sterilizations that they would not be permitted to provide directly under the *ERDs*. This revision was primarily motivated by the Brackenridge Hospital case, discussed *infra*.

Most of the provisions of the 2001 *ERDs* are unchanged from the 1994 *ERDs*. The directives concerning abortion,[296] contraception,[297] and sterilization[298] are the same. As in the 1994 *ERDs*, Directive 49 of the 2001 *ERDs* provides: "For a proportionate reason, labor may be induced after the fetus is viable." By 2003, at least two Catholic hospital systems were performing early induction of labor under limited circumstances where the baby had a condition that would significantly shorten its life, such as anencephaly or agenesis.[299] Nonetheless, it seems clear that these policies are not morally licit under Directives 48 and 49 of the 2001 *ERDs*.[300]

The most significant change in the 2001 *ERDs* is the elimination of the appendix in the 1994 *ERDs* dealing with cooperation. The 2001 edition notes that the appendix is omitted because "the principles of cooperation that were presented there did not sufficiently forestall certain possible misinterpretations and in practice gave rise to problems in concrete applications of the principles."[301] In addition, a new directive, Directive 70, provides: "Catholic health care organizations are not permitted to engage in immediate material cooperation in actions that are intrinsically immoral, such as abortion, euthanasia, assisted suicide, and direct sterilization."[302]

In addition, an important statement added in a footnote to Directive 70 notes: "While there are many acts of varying moral gravity that can be identified as intrinsically evil, in the context of contemporary health care the most pressing concerns are currently abortion, euthanasia, assisted suicide, and direct sterilization."[303] The footnote then continues with a specific reference to a 1975 statement of the Sacred Congregation for the Doctrine of the faith, *Quaecumque Sterilizatio*, absolutely forbidding the provision of direct sterilizations in Catholic hospitals.[304] Finally, the footnote states that Directive 70 supersedes a previous commentary issued by the bishops.[305]

Part Two

Catholic Identity

The concept of Catholic identity is related to both the canonical status of Catholic hospitals and their sponsorship by Catholic religious orders.[1] There is no specific reference in the 1983 *Code of Canon Law* to health care institutions.[2] And there are no guidelines in the *Code of Canon Law* for determining the Catholic identity of health care institutions.[3] In fact, Catholic identity is not a term of art under canon law.[4] On the other hand, "[t]he name or title 'Catholic' cannot be used without the consent of the competent church authority."[5] The local bishop determines whether a particular hospital is considered Catholic, and this determination of Catholic identity carries with it an element of "accountability to ecclesiastical authorities."[6]

This accountability includes an expectation of adherence to the *ERDs*. All United States bishops have adopted the *ERDs*, thereby making them applicable to Catholic hospitals in their dioceses. Under canon law, the religious orders that sponsor hospitals do so "as representatives of the Church itself under the authoritative directives of the canon law," and "[t]hus they are not free to pick and choose among moral imperatives."[7] Moreover, "canon law positively prohibits officers and directors of church-affiliated hospitals from disguising their identity or allowing that identity to be eroded through contractual or personnel management decisions."[8] It is the local bishop who determines whether a particular institution within his diocese has lost its Catholic identity.[9] Ultimately, however, "aside from use of the name 'Catholic'," Catholic identity is more "a matter of public perception, rather than church law."[10]

Previously, bishops could rely "on religious congregations to operate and oversee" their health care institutions in accordance with Catholic ethical and moral standards.[11] When religious orders directly owned and operated their health care ministries, the bishop could exercise control through his "personal authority over particular congregation members."[12] But with the changing relationship between the religious congregations and their health care enterprises, and the increasing role of the laity, this type of direct and personal control is no longer feasible.[13] Instead, the preservation of Catholic identity in health care institutions must rely more on normative standards — i.e., the adherence of the institution to the norms set forth in the *ERD*s as interpreted and applied by the local bishop.[14]

Francis Morrisey has described three traditional approaches to ascertaining Catholic identity: a legal/institutional approach, a doctrinal approach, and a values-based approach.[15] The first, the legal/institutional approach, focuses primarily on the status under canon law of the institution conducting the activity and its relationship with the local bishop.[16] The second, the "doctrinal approach," focuses on the organization's purpose and public perceptions as to its Catholicity.[17] The third, the values-based approach, focuses on criteria such as the organization's commitment to providing health care to the poor, its adherence to Catholic values, and its attention to the spiritual dimensions of health care.[18] Morrisey acknowledges that under any of these approaches, Catholic identity requires the maintenance of a link to the local bishop.[19]

Morrisey proposes that in place of these traditional approaches, the following criteria be utilized to determine Catholic identity: mission, sponsorship, holistic care, and ethics.[20] It is questionable, however, whether some of these criteria are all that helpful in ascertaining Catholic identity. Mission can be stated at such a general level, i.e., providing care in a manner that is consistent with gospel values,[21] that it may not constrain organizations in practice. Some would contend that sponsorship, i.e., "operating . . . in the name of and under the authority of a given juridic person,"[22] is on the wane and may eventually disappear. Holistic care, i.e. "sensitivity to whole person,"[23] is also too vague to serve as any sort of meaningful restraint. Of these criteria, only ethics, and more particularly in the United States, compliance with the *ERD*s as interpreted and applied by the local bishop, provides any significant guarantee of continuing Catholic identity.

Ultimately, the preservation of Catholic identity requires continuing "commitment to the moral teachings and ethical norms of the church."[24] And this may be problematic since "[t]hese are at times, counter cultural stances, witnessing to respect for the integrity of human life in the face of abortion, sterilization, assisted suicide, euthanasia, and certain areas of research and experimentation."[25] Morrisey acknowledges that while all Catholic institutions "subscribe to the directives in theory, not all follow them in practice."[26] In this regard, he notes: "The question has frequently arisen recently in the restructuring of Catholic health care organizations: Who will be responsible for monitoring the application of directives? It is not enough to say that they will be followed: a person or process must make sure they are applied."[27]

Maintaining Catholic identity is complicated by the fact that contemporary Catholic health care operates in both the spiritual and secular worlds. The managers of Catholic hospitals have to balance spiritual and ethical commitments with the necessity of competing effectively in the marketplace. Generally, Catholic health care in the United States has been a business success story: according to a 2006 statistical survey by the American Hospital Association, there were 614 Catholic hospitals in the United States and 61 Catholic health care systems with approximately 5.5 million admissions annually.[28] During 2006, Catholic hospitals accounted for approximately 15.6 percent of all community hospital admissions in the United States, and "for more than one-fifth, or 20 percent, of admissions in 21 states and the District of Columbia."[29]

It is possible for Catholic hospitals to be both successful businesses and maintain their Catholic identity. Indeed, one study indicates that along with their business successes Catholic hospitals have also been successful in preserving their core mission of providing "comprehensive health care to vulnerable and underserved populations."[30] In addition, Catholic identity may in fact provide a comparative advantage in the marketplace. In 2003, the Catholic Health Association recognized the potential value of Catholic identity when it announced plans for a new initiative that would focus on branding Catholic health care in order to enhance its ability to compete in the market place.[31] It was thought that branding would increase public awareness of the provision of "state-of-the-art care" as well as "spiritual health care services" by Catholic hospitals.[32]

Notwithstanding the business successes of Catholic health care, however, the withering away of the sponsoring orders has resulted in uncertainty over the prospects for survival of the distinctively Catholic hospital.[33] This uncertainty has been exacerbated by other environmental factors — a pervasive "culture of death" overtly hostile to Catholic moral teaching, financial dependence on government programs, and the need to compete for contracts with private health plans. This identity crisis is further compounded by the ambiguous nature of Catholic hospitals: they are both community institutions and religious ministries. And as community hospitals, they are expected to supply whatever health care services the community demands, regardless of the *ERD*s.

Catholic hospitals were founded by religious orders as both religious ministries and community hospitals that provided treatment to patients from all backgrounds. As noted, *infra*, even in the nineteenth century, some Catholic hospitals received financial support from local governments and Congress. And of course, they later received federal support in the form of Hill-Burton funds in the 1940s and 1950s and Medicare and Medicaid payments beginning in the mid-1960s. Today they must compete with both for-profit and nonprofit systems for contracts with private health plans. Their financial dependence on continued governmental funding and contracts with private health plans has resulted in pressures being brought to bear on Catholic hospitals to provide reproductive services that violate the *ERD*s.

Due to these environmental factors, consistent compliance with the *ERD*s proscription on direct sterilizations has been particularly problematic for Catholic hospitals in the United States. While generally the managers of Catholic hospitals do not believe that the proscription against performing direct abortions affects them in the market place, some do believe that the proscription on performing direct sterilizations is a detriment to their ability to compete. In this regard, they are typically concerned about retaining business from the young families with health insurance who populate the upscale suburbs.

Not infrequently, a woman may request a postpartum sterilization because she doesn't want any more children and doesn't want to worry about using birth control. Some Catholic hospital managers believe the unavailability of sterilization under these circumstances is a handicap in marketing their childbirth and delivery services to affluent young couples with health insurance and in competing for contracts with health insurance plans.[34] Indeed, if postpartum sterilization is not available in Catholic hospitals, some couples may choose to avoid such hospitals for childbirth as well. Thus, Catholic hospitals have an economic incentive to facilitate access to sterilization services.

Catholic hospitals have dealt with sterilization in a number of ways. It is of course clear that Catholic hospitals must not permit direct sterilizations within the hospital itself under the *ERD*s. One approach to avoiding the impact of this ban on direct sterilization is to separate physically and fiscally the provision of sterilization services from the hospital. In some instances, this separation has been attempted by simply transporting the patient to a neighboring physician's office building or ambulatory surgery center that is not owned by the hospital for the performance of the sterilization procedure.

But some Catholic hospitals are actually performing direct sterilizations on their premises, in clear violation of the *ERD*s. For example, data collected by the Texas Department of Health Services and posted on the Web site Texas Price Point, a trade association representing Texas hospitals, indicates that several Catholic hospitals in Texas are performing direct sterilizations.[35]

In addition to the fact that the provision of direct sterilizations or "immediate material cooperation" in providing access to such services is a clear violation of the *ERD*s,[36] it strengthens the hands of those calling for the enactment of laws requiring Catholic hospitals to provide a full range of reproductive services.[37] Moreover, any involvement of Catholic hospitals in performing sterilizations has the potential to create scandal and causes both Catholics and non-Catholics to question whether the Catholic Church is sincere about enforcing its proscription of direct sterilization — or, for that matter, direct abortion. Entering into partnerships with entities that perform sterilizations or provide abortion referrals is the cause of scandal, even if these arrangements are structured in such a way as not to violate the *ERD*s. Even the appearance of complicity in facilitating access to direct sterilizations is not a prudent course of conduct in the current political environment.

This section begins with a brief recounting of the history of Catholic health care and an overview of the canonical status of Catholic hospitals and the sponsorship model. It will then review a particularly potent threat to Catholic identity: the sale of Catholic hospitals to for-profit corporations.

CHAPTER SIX

Transformation of the Catholic Hospital from Religious Ministry to Business Enterprise

The Early Years: Vision and Reason for the Catholic Hospital

Most Catholic hospitals in the United States were founded by religious orders,[1] and women's orders have been more active in the health care ministry than men's orders.[2] Catholic religious orders opened hospitals to care for the sick poor in Europe in the mid-nineteenth century, and these same religious orders were invited by bishops to open hospitals in the United States.[3] Following the cholera epidemic of 1849, there was a general recognition of the need for more hospitals in the United States.[4] Catholic bishops were particularly interested in opening Catholic hospitals during this period because of the widely prevalent anti-Catholicism and the tendency to proselytize in Protestant hospitals.[5] At this time, even in some public hospitals, Catholic priests were not permitted to minister to dying Catholic patients because of the objections of Protestant ministers.[6]

The founding of Catholic hospitals in urban areas of the United States during the 1850s stemmed largely from a desire to preserve the faith among the Catholic immigrant communities living in a hostile environment.[7] It was also motivated by discrimination against poor Irish Catholics in densely populated urban areas.[8] While religious prejudice was an important motivating factor in the founding of Catholic hospitals in the east, however, on the frontier it was less of a factor and interfaith cooperation was more common.[9]

During the Civil War, 617 sisters from 21 orders provided services to both sides.[10] It is generally accepted among historians that "the sisters' Civil War nursing dispelled religious prejudice . . . by demonstrating the practical viability of the vowed life . . . ."[11] Following the Civil War, from 1866 to 1917, women's religious orders opened 479 hospitals in the United States.[12] The provision of health care to the poor was viewed by these religious orders as "an extension of the ministry of the Church."[13] Initially, members of the religious order worked as managers and nurses in the hospital. These hospitals were a direct extension of the ministry of the religious orders.[14] Nonetheless, from the beginning these hospitals provided services to non-Catholics as well as Catholics.[15]

Catholic Hospitals as Semi-Public Community Institutions

In the late nineteenth century, some Catholic hospitals became "semi-public institutions partially underwritten with public funds."[16] For example, in 1897, Congress provided funds for Providence Hospital in Washington, DC, and this funding was challenged as a violation of the Establishment clause of the First Amendment.[17] In *Bradfield v. Roberts*, the U.S. Supreme Court rejected this challenge, relying on the fact that an Act of Congress had separately incorporated the hospital in 1864.[18] The court held that the hospital corporation was essentially secular in nature, even though its members were Roman Catholics and it was managed by a religious order.[19] *Bradfield* came to stand for the proposition that public funding of private religious hospitals does not violate the Establishment clause.[20]

During the period 1918-45, an additional 169 Catholic hospitals were opened by women's religious orders in the United States.[21] In many instances, local governments provided the initial physical plant for these hospitals and agreed to make fixed daily payments for indigent care.[22] The period 1946-65 proved to be an era of rapid expansion for the Catholic health care ministry.[23] The Hill-Burton Act, passed in 1946, provided federal funding for the construction and expansion of hospitals.[24] As a result of the impact of Hill-Burton, 123 new hospitals were opened by women's religious orders during the period 1946-65.[25] By 1965, there were a total of 808 general hospitals in the United States that were identified as Catholic.[26]

The Transition to Lay Management

Due to the precipitous decline in vocations following Vatican II,[27] most Catholic hospitals are now managed by laypersons rather than by members of their founding religious orders. In the late 1960s, as religious vocations declined, "lay men were appointed as administrators in religious institutes' hospitals."[28] Although relatively few hospitals closed as result of the decline in vocations, the number of sisters involved in health care ministry significantly declined.[29] A new relationship, one of sponsorship rather than direct control by the founding order, has evolved over the last few decades.[30]

This decline in religious vocations and change in the structure of Catholic health care organizations has changed the relationship between the Church and Catholic health care in the United States.[31] Prior to the Second Vatican Council, the relationship between the founding orders and Catholic hospitals was simple and straightforward: hospitals were managed and owned by religious congregations.[32] But "a paradigmatic shift occurred with Vatican II, when the onus of responsibility for church leadership moved from the clergy to the laity."[33]

In the 1940s, as a result of the abrogation of charitable immunity and the expansion of hospital liability in many jurisdictions, many religious orders separately incorporated their hospitals under state laws in order to protect themselves from malpractice lawsuits.[34] The creation of the Medicare and Medicaid programs in 1965 caused concern that Catholic hospitals could be disqualified from receiving federal funds if they were pervasively religious.[35] Accordingly, "hospitals were advised to expand their boards of directors to seek broader public participation, open their hiring policies for staff and administration, and blunt the religious imagery to dampen the appearance of religious influence."[36] This secularization impulse may also have been driven by a series of U.S. Supreme Court decisions that declared state aid to parochial schools to be a violation of the First Amendment, decisions that some scholars believe to have been motivated by anti-Catholicism of Supreme Court justices. [37]

Most Catholic hospitals are now organized as nonprofit, charitable corporations under state laws. Typically, "when a province of a religious institute sponsors several hospitals, it is likely that each hospital will be separately incorporated."[38] These are membership corporations with the members being designated representatives of the founding religious orders.[39] These members hold certain reserved powers,[40] but the management of these corporations is increasingly composed of laypersons.[41]

The corporations that own Catholic hospitals are typically qualified under IRC 501(c) (3)[42] as tax-exempt organizations; accordingly, they do not pay taxes on their profit, and donors may deduct donations from their federal income taxes. Prior to 1969, nonprofit hospitals were required to provide health care for the poor in order to qualify for exemption from federal income taxes, but in 1969, the Internal Revenue Service adopted the "community benefit" standard, "which did not require a hospital to treat indigent patients in order to qualify for exemption."[43] Instead, the charitable purpose that would serve as a basis for the exemption became the provision of "health care for the general benefit of the community."[44]

"No Margin, No Mission"

Catholic hospitals must generate profits in order to remain competitive in the marketplace — thus the frequently quoted refrain, "no margin, no mission."[45] They must generate a sufficient margin to be able to afford to adopt and deploy new technologies and offer new services in accordance with the demands of the health care marketplace. They must also provide the latest equipment and appropriate amenities to attract physicians to their staff in order to ensure a constant flow of patients into the hospital.

Managers of Catholic hospital systems have the difficult task of operating a financially viable enterprise nimble enough to adjust to ongoing changes in the health care marketplace, while adhering to Church directives concerning the moral aspects of the provision of health care. Catholic hospitals must cope with market pressures to become "more like" secular hospitals, while simultaneously managing their relationship with "the complex and hierarchical institutional environment of the Roman Catholic Church."[46]

The changing nature of the health care marketplace has had a significant impact on Catholic hospitals.[47] The shift to prospective payment in the Medicare program in 1980s placed additional pressures on hospitals to hold down costs. And, in the private sector, Catholic hospitals must compete for contracts with large health plans to provide services for the members of the plans.[48] Hospitals must be run in an economically efficient manner in order to remain competitive in their pricing structures when negotiating with health plans. Thus, Catholic health care facilities must be conducted as business entities, even if they are engaged in a religious ministry.[49] And the rise of consumer-directed health care places increased pressures on hospitals to focus on the preferences of their patient-consumers.[50]

Catholic hospitals, like most nonprofit organizations, also raise money for capital expenditures in the tax-exempt bond market. Favorable bond ratings depend upon a determination by investment banks of the financial viability of the organization. Accordingly, nonprofit health care systems must closely watch their bond ratings.[51] A lowering of a bond rating greatly increases the cost of raising capital funds and may have dire consequences for the nonprofit entity. Moreover, financial analysts could be concerned about a hospital that appeared to be too sectarian in its mission, if that quality makes the hospital unable to compete with other facilities in attracting contracts with health plans.

Mergers, Affiliations, and Sales

In the 1980s and '90s, economic pressures forced hospitals to participate in larger integrated systems in order to control costs and negotiate with health care plans. There have been several instances of mergers among Catholic-sponsored hospital systems in recent years in order to form larger, more efficient organizations capable of competing against for-profit systems.[52] In addition, Catholic health care systems have entered into contracts to manage community hospitals that they don't own, formed partnerships or joint ventures with non-Catholic hospitals,[53] acquired non-Catholic community hospitals, and sold hospitals to non-Catholic hospital systems.

Over the last two decades, "financial distress" has also brought about a number of mergers or affiliations between Catholic and non-Catholic health care facilities throughout the United States.[54] These affiliations can become particularly controversial where the Catholic facility becomes the sole provider as a result of a merger or acquisition. In some of these mergers, the non-Catholic facilities have been required to comply with the *ERD*s, and this has resulted in the discontinuation of reproductive health services that were not in conformity with Catholic moral teaching.[55]

Occasionally, in order to reduce opposition to a merger or affiliation, Catholic hospitals have entered into arrangements to allow continuation of services such as surgical sterilizations in separate facilities to be provided by unrelated organizations.[56] In other instances, proposed affiliations between Catholic and non-Catholic institutions have been blocked by Church authorities, despite attempts to avoid scandal by performing the prohibited services in separate facilities.[57] And some mergers have been called off because of controversy over the possible elimination of reproductive services.[58] On the other hand, when some Catholic hospitals have been sold to for-profit health care companies because of financial pressures, the buyer has agreed to continue to follow Catholic moral norms in the acquired facility.[59]

Notwithstanding the widespread outcry of concern by some groups about the adverse impact of affiliations between Catholic and non-Catholic facilities on the availability of reproductive services, one study indicates their actual impact may be minimal except with respect to a reduction in the availability of surgical abortions in those cases where the life of the mother is not in danger.[60] Nonetheless, in response to the demands of those concerned about the reduction in the availability of reproductive services due to acquisition of community hospitals by Catholic health care systems, the American Public Health Association adopted a policy recommending more government oversight of affiliations between Catholic and non-Catholic partners in order to ensure that reproductive health services are not discontinued.[61] And in 2003, California adopted legislation that prohibits the state attorney general — who has the authority under state law to block the sale of non-profit health care facilities — from consenting to the sale of a hospital where the seller makes the sale contingent on restrictions of the type of services the buyer will provide.[62]

Chapter Seven

Catholic Hospitals and Canon Law

Although there has been ongoing controversy over whether or not the incorporation of Catholic hospitals under civil law effectively ends direct control by the Church under canon law, the prevailing pattern in the United States is for hospitals to maintain their Catholic identity through the continuing influence of their sponsoring order. But more recently, due to the declining membership of religious orders, there is an increased emphasis on the role of the local bishop in supervising health care institutions and on the *ERDs* in establishing behavioral norms.[1] This chapter begins with a discussion of canonical status, continues with the McGrath-Maida controversy over the effect of civil incorporation, and concludes with a discussion of the evolving nature of the sponsorship model.

Canonical Status

Although canonical status (or its lack thereof) does not determine whether an organization is *de facto* pursuing a Catholic mission, the concept of Catholic identity is linked to canonical status. canon law recognizes three types of persons: physical persons, moral persons, and juridic persons.[2] Physical persons are individuals who have certain rights and duties in the Church by virtue of their baptism.[3] Moral persons — i.e., the Catholic Church and the Apostolic See — come into existence by virtue of divine law.[4] Juridic persons come into existence by virtue of the operation of canon law, either by decree by the competent authority or by virtue of a provision in the law itself.[5] There are two types of juridic persons under canon law: public and private.[6] They have been defined as follows:

> *Public juridic persons* operate in the name of the Church; their temporal goods are ecclesiastical goods; they represent the Church in the same sense that a diocese or religious congregation does.

Private juridic persons function in their own names; their goods are not considered ecclesiastical goods; and their works are considered more the *work of Catholics* than *Catholic works*.[7]

A 1993 publication by the Catholic Health Association described five organizational models of Catholic health care institutions that have been observed in the United States:

A. a health care facility established by public authorities that has been turned over to the Church or a public juridic institution of the Church to manage and operate;
B. a public authority that has established a health care facility containing a Catholic unit;
C. a hospital founded under Catholic auspices that is operated on a nondenominational basis;
D. a health care facility incorporated as a nonprofit civil corporation established by a religious institute and containing provisions in its articles of incorporation or bylaws providing certain reserved powers to the founding institute;
E. a health care institution recognized as a public juridic person under canon law.[8]

By far the most common of these arrangements in the United States is the fourth: a nonprofit civil corporation that maintains a relationship of sponsorship with its founding religious institute. Naturally, the shift to lay management in these organizations, along with the increasing number of affiliations between Catholic and non-Catholic hospitals, has inevitably raised questions on what it means to be a Catholic hospital. Moreover, with the continuing decline in vocations, it has been said that the Church's "'control' over the health care apostolate is . . . fast giving way to an 'influence' approach."[9]

In the United States, Catholic health care organizations have not traditionally operated as distinct juridic persons under canon law; many that are publicly regarded as Catholic have never been canonically recognized.[10] Originally, they were direct outreaches of particular religious orders or dioceses. Later, many were incorporated as separate civil corporations, sponsored by religious institutes, with certain powers reserved to members of the religious institute.[11] Typically, under civil law, "there are several corporations involved: the motherhouse corporation and each separate hospital corporation."[12] In contrast, under canon law, there is only one canonical public juridic person: the province. The separate hospital corporations are not considered separate

PART TWO: *Catholic Identity*

legal entities under canon law unless they have been specifically approved as public juridic persons.[13]

In addition to juridic persons, canon law also recognizes entities known as public associations of the faithful and private associations of the faithful.[14] Associations of the faithful may be formed to engage in apostolic works such as health care, but that is uncommon in the United States.[15] If they are engaged in work in a particular diocese, they are subject to the supervision of the bishop.[16] They cannot, however, use the name "Catholic" in their titles without the consent of the competent Church authority.[17]

There is some connection between the concept of Catholic identity and canonical status. According to Jordan Hite:

> If a group is recognized as a public juridic person or a public association of the faithful, by law it can act in the name of the church and, therefore, has Catholic identity. A private juridic person or a private association of the faithful needs to be recognized by the competent church authority to have Catholic identity even though it may not act in the name of the church. In addition, an organization that has no juridical status may have Catholic identity because its purpose and mission is to act in accord with Catholic principles and teaching.[18]

Recent years have seen a significant trend in Catholic health care toward combining and consolidating the health care operations of the various religious orders.[19] In some instances, this consolidation activity has resulted in the creation of new canonical structures.[20] It is now possible under canon law to constitute Catholic health care institutions as separate juridic persons, "the Church's counterpart to civil corporations."[21] According to Francis Morrisey, few private juridic persons have been established in health care,[22] but there have been several public juridic persons established in the health care field.[23]

The Holy See, a bishops' conference, or a local bishop may confer juridic status.[24] In the Vatican, the responsibility for the approval of petitions by religious institutes to create new juridic persons and their ongoing supervision has fallen to the Congregation for Institutes of Consecrated Life and Societies of Apostolic Life (CICLSAL).[25] Among the requirements imposed by CICLSAL for approval of a new public juridic person involved in health care is an "expressed commitment" in the proposed statutes "to the observance" of the *ERD*s.[26] When a public juridic person is created, the goods transferred to it remain within the Church, thus making it easier to obtain the necessary ecclesiastical approvals.[27] On the other hand, transfer of goods to a private juridic person would transfer them outside the Church; this makes their creation more problematic.[28] A public juridic person could operate in more than one diocese and could cover an entire health system.[29]

Ordinarily, the creation of a new public juridic person is preceded by a separate civil incorporation, and reserved powers would be included in both the documents pertaining to the new civil corporation as well as the statutes pertaining to the new public juridic person.[30] The powers are reserved to "the superiors and councils of religious institutes" involved in creating the new public juridic person.[31] Some religious congregations have requested the creation of new public juridic persons in order to safeguard the Catholic identity of their health care institutions and ecclesiastical goods against the time when members of the sponsoring group will no longer be available to manage their works or even provide formation for laypersons involved in their work.[32]

Nonetheless, at this time in the United States, most Catholic hospitals do not have separate canonical status. They are usually separately incorporated under civil law, but maintain a link with their founding order through a relationship referred to as sponsorship, discussed *infra*. The sponsoring religious order, however, as a public juridic person, is subject to canon law; it has a duty to operate the hospital, even though separately incorporated, "in conformity with the teachings of the Church."[33] Moreover, according to Maida and Cafardi, those persons responsible for overseeing the operations of the religious orders that sponsor Catholic hospitals are obligated to ensure that Catholic teachings are followed in these hospitals.[34] Under this approach, the lack of canonical status on the part of the separately incorporated hospitals is not significant with respect to Catholic identity. The purpose of the canon law is to maintain the distinctive Catholic identity of such entities, notwithstanding their separate civil incorporation.[35] Indeed, they are viewed as extensions of the religious orders that founded them.

The McGrath–Maida Controversy

In the 1960s and '70s, at the time that Catholic health care institutions were struggling with issues related to the transition to lay management and developing the concept of sponsorship, they were also attempting to resolve issues concerning the ecclesiastic control of property and the Church's control of civilly incorporated institutions.[36] Some religious orders came to believe that canon law had "lagged behind" theological and economic developments, and that traditional norms governing ecclesiastical control of property were outdated.[37] There was also increasing frustration over the tension between the requirements of civil law and canon law.[38]

Thus, a controversy emerged over the canonical status of Catholic hospitals in the United States and, in turn, had an impact on Catholic identity.[39] As noted by Christopher Kauffman, the opinions of McCormick and Reich, outspoken critics of the 1971 *ERD*s (see discussion in Chapter Five, *supra*), were premised on the notion that Catholic hospitals were essentially community hospitals and thus should not continue to emphasize their distinctiveness.[40] This view found support, *sub silentio*, in a book published in 1968 by canon lawyer J.J. McGrath, who opined that the effect of civil incorporation was to remove an institution from the Church's direct control.[41] The implications of the McGrath thesis was that for church-related hospitals, "[t]heir purposes, powers, rights, and obligations, including those relating to ownership of property, are to be determined solely by the applicable state and federal laws" rather than by canon law.[42]

In light of this purported effect of civil incorporation, McGrath then posed the question: "What makes the institution Catholic?"[43] His answer was that it was the continuing influence of the sponsoring order as exerted through: "(1) the charter and by-laws; (2) the board of trustees; (3) the administration; and (4) the staff of the corporation."[44] Accordingly, he advised that the religious sponsors should maintain their roles in these non-Catholic institutions through provisions in the corporate bylaws "for a definite number of the board of directors to be chosen from the sponsoring body."[45] He further noted, "The bylaws can require the board of trustees to choose the president and other officers of the institution from members of the sponsoring body."[46]

McGrath was also particularly concerned with maintaining a strict separation between the sponsoring religious congregation and the health care institutions incorporated under civil law.[47] For example, he suggested that members of the sponsoring order who worked in the institution should be employed under contracts with the institution and subject to "the same procedures used in employing or dismissing other employees."[48] And he advocated strict separation of "the administration of the institution . . . from the government of the religious community."[49] Not surprisingly, the McGrath thesis was embraced by those who favored a dilution of Catholic identity, as well as those concerned about maintaining governmental funding for Catholic hospitals.[50] But it is considered a "flawed" thesis in that it assumes that the decision to civilly incorporate a religious apostolate removes it from control of the Church and canon law, notwithstanding the lack of that intention at the time of the civil incorporation and the failure to obtain ecclesiastical permission for that purpose.[51] Daniel Conlin has observed:

> McGrath found in regard to Catholic hospitals, universities and colleges that it was not "the policy to erect them as canonical moral persons." Therefore, his conclusion was that those institutions did not belong to the Catholic Church. If an institution did not belong to the Church, then it would be reasonable to seek secular funding precisely by claiming it was not a religious institution.[52]

In a book published in 1975, A.J. Maida — now Cardinal Archbishop of Detroit — refuted the McGrath thesis, arguing that civil incorporation did not affect the Catholic nature of institutions, and that they were required to follow both civil and canon law, even after incorporation under civil law.[53] In other words, according to Maida, a hospital founded by a religious order remains Catholic and subject to canon law, notwithstanding its incorporation under civil law.[54] Nonetheless, despite this disagreement over the impact of civil incorporation, there was general agreement between the disputants that the sponsoring order should retain control through the reservation of certain powers at the time of civil incorporation.[55]

The McGrath–Maida controversy arose under the provisions of the 1917 *Code of Canon Law*.[56] With respect to the controversy, Professor Kennedy has observed that "both authors oversimplified the issue of canonical status under the 1917 code." He states further that the canonical status of Catholic institutions formed under the 1917 code "requires in each instance, detailed study of the facts surrounding the establishment and continued governance of the institution."[57] After the adoption of the revised 1983 *Code of Canon Law* promulgated by Pope John Paul II, this controversy was largely mooted because the revised code included "a more adaptable structure regulating temporal goods" that "gave considerable weight to local civil law and to a juridic person's proper law."[58] In addition, the Vatican rejected the McGrath thesis.[59]

The Evolution of the Sponsorship Model

The term "sponsorship" is used to describe the relationship between the founding religious institutes and their separate civil corporations that operate health care facilities.[60] Typically, sponsors are public juridic persons, i.e., religious institutes, who "carry out a ministry or apostolate in the name of the church."[61]

Beverly Dunn has delineated the evolution of the concept of sponsorship into three stages. The first stage of sponsorship began with the integration of laypersons into management positions in health care institutions and the separation of the governance of these institutions from that of the founding religious congregations.[62] The second stage involved the integration of laypersons into governing boards of institutions and emphasis on "mission education" for these persons.[63] The third phase involved the formation of collaborative ventures with other Catholic and non-Catholic sponsors to form integrated delivery systems.[64] As a result of these changes, "the focus of identity for Catholic health care institutions has shifted from their operation and governance by the founding religious congregations . . . to a broader ecclesial basis, highlighting their communion with the local bishop and the entire Church."[65]

As noted *supra*, most large Catholic health care systems do not have "distinct canonical status, but, rather, operate under the aegis of a sponsoring religious congregation or a society of apostolic life."[66] These sponsoring orders reserve certain powers at the time of the incorporation of the health care institution under civil law typically including the rights to: "1) establish the philosophy according to which the corporation operates, 2) amend the corporate charter and bylaws, 3) lease, sell, or encumber corporate real estate in excess of the approved sum, and 4) merge or dissolve the corporation."[67]

Under canon law, the sponsor (typically a religious order) has the responsibility of preserving the Catholic identity of its institutions and safeguarding the property used to further its mission.[68] Because of the decline in vocations, however, in the 1980s, the focus of the sponsoring orders shifted to "mission" as they attempted to clarify the fundamental values of Catholic health care and develop programs to inculcate those values in their lay employees.[69] "In many Catholic health care organizations, executive positions exist to promote and monitor the values of the sponsor."[70] Today, as the membership ranks of sponsoring orders continue to decline, increased attention is directed toward the formation of laypersons as sponsor representatives.[71]

In addition, since religious sponsors have delegated many of their powers to the governing boards of the health care institutions, the role of members of the corporate boards of trustees in ensuring faithfulness to the Catholic mission is receiving greater emphasis.[72] However, it's not clear at this time that these attempts will be sufficient to preserve the identity and mission of Catholic health care institutions, particularly in light of the legal assault by "pro-choice" groups and the increasing size and complexity of Catholic health care systems.[73]

The Sale of Catholic Hospitals to Non-Catholic Systems

On occasion, Catholic hospitals have been sold to non-Catholic systems because of financial pressures. For example, as discussed in Chapter Eight, *infra*, in 2002, Providence Hospital in Seattle — then the flagship institution of the Sisters of Providence — was conveyed to Swedish Hospital, a nonprofit, nonsectarian hospital, in a transaction described as joint venture. In 2007, the only Catholic hospital in Hawaii was sold to an alliance of local physicians and a Kansas-based hospital management company.[74]

By contrast, in 1998, the Vatican nixed a proposed merger in New Jersey between St. Peter's Hospital, a Catholic facility, and the Robert Wood Johnson Hospital. This denial, despite the approval of the local bishop, was reportedly due to concerns that the merger would eventually lead to the Catholic hospital profiting from direct sterilizations and abortions.[75]

In addition, there have been sales of academic health centers affiliated with Catholic universities to for-profit systems. Only four medical schools in the United States are affiliated with Catholic universities (Creighton, St. Louis, Loyola, and Georgetown), but the teaching hospitals at both Creighton University and St. Louis University have been sold to for-profit corporations.

In 1984, Creighton University's teaching hospital was sold to American Medical International (AMI), a for-profit chain, with the blessings of Archbishop Daniel Sheehan.[76] Then, in the early '90s, Creighton brought suit against AMI to regain some control over the hospital, resulting in Creighton reacquiring a 26% interest in it.[77] Subsequently, although the Chancellor of the Archdiocese of Omaha complimented Tenet Corporation (the for-profit corporate successor to AMI and then owner of the hospital) for its sensitivity to the hospital's Catholic mission and moral teaching,[78] the president of the Catholic Health Association criticized the hospital's management under Tenet for its "increased prices and reduced care for the indigent."[79]

Perhaps, the most high-profile sale occurred in 1994, when St. Louis University, a Jesuit institution, sold its teaching hospital to Tenet.[80] This transaction provoked considerable controversy because the president of St. Louis University, Lawrence Biondi, S.J., rejected a purchase offer for the hospital from other St. Louis-based Catholic health care systems in favor of a higher price from Tenet, against the wishes of St. Louis Archbishop Justin Rigali.[81] Biondi contended that the sale of the hospital was not subject to canon law; Rigali contended that it was.[82] According to Biondi, Vatican approval wasn't required for the sale because the hospital was owned by a civil corporation, governed by an independent board.[83] He also argued that, without the revenues from the sale, the St. Louis University School of Medicine would be forced to close within ten years.[84] And he noted that, in accordance with the agreement with Tenet, the hospital would continue to follow a Catholic mission and comply with the *ERDs*.[85]

However, Archbishop Rigali was concerned that the sale would compromise the hospital's Catholic mission and reduce the provision of care to the poor.[86] He opined:

> I continue to be preoccupied with the fact that — if the transaction is completed — this sale of the hospital will have a dramatic effect on the identity and mission of St. Louis University Hospital. It will cease to be a Catholic hospital. No matter what contractual commitments may have been made, it will be impossible for the hospital, after its sale, to preserve all of the values of Catholic health care. Notwithstanding its own upright and humanitarian character, any "for-profit" corporation is basically for profit.[87]

Three Cardinals (Hickey of Washington, DC, Law of Boston, and O'Connor of New York) joined Archbishop Rigali in condemning the sale to Tenet.[88] Cardinal O'Connor contended that the hospital was still Church property, despite its ownership by a civil corporation governed by a board predominantly composed of lay persons.[89] Sr. Jean DeBlois, Vice President for Mission Services of the Catholic Health Association, was also concerned about whether the hospital would be able to retain its Catholic mission after the sale.[90]

Eventually, the sale agreement between Tenet and St. Louis University was presented to the Holy See by the Superior General of the Jesuits, but formal approval by the Vatican was not sought.[91] Under the terms of the agreement with the university, Tenet was obligated to adhere to the *ERDs* and continue to provide charity care.[92] Concerns about the reduced level of charity care following the sale may have been unwarranted. In 2004, it was reported that the level of community benefit (including charity care) provided by St. Louis University Hospital was comparable to that provided by nonprofit hospitals in Missouri.[93]

Daniel Conlin has noted that the decision by St. Louis University not to involve canon law in the sale was "based on a wholesale acceptance of the significantly flawed McGrath thesis" and motivated by the fear that they would not obtain Vatican approval for the lucrative deal.[94] This dispute may have contributed to a proposal to require educational institutions sponsored by

Catholic religious to retain certain reserved powers in their corporate bylaws for the sponsoring order and include the statement, "This corporation shall at all times be operated in accordance with the Canon Law of the Roman Catholic Church."[95]

Despite all this, at times St. Louis University has continued to take the position that it is not a Catholic institution in any way subject to the control of the Catholic Church. In a 2007 decision, the Supreme Court of Missouri ruled that St. Louis University was not an institution that "was controlled by a religious creed" within the meaning of a Missouri Constitutional prohibition against public funding for religious entities.[96] This case arose from a challenge to public funding that St. Louis University was to receive from the city of St. Louis for the construction of a new basketball arena. The view of the University as to its Catholic nature was expressed in these excerpts from the brief it filed with the court:

> Saint Louis University is a corporation organized for higher educational purposes by the State of Missouri. As a result of changes in its corporate structure, the University is not now owned or controlled by the Society of Jesus. . . . The University's Board of Trustees is an independent, corporate lay-majority board. It consists of no fewer than 25 members and no more than 55 members. No fewer than six but no more than 12 of the members of the Board may be members of the Society of Jesus. . . . At the time of summary judgment, the University's Board of Trustees consisted of 42 trustees, of whom nine were Jesuit. The Board is comprised of people of all faiths and people with no particular religious affiliation. . . . Saint Louis University is not owned by the Catholic Church or by the Catholic Archdiocese of St. Louis. The University's Board of Trustees is not controlled by the Catholic Church, the Archdiocese, or any other church [citations to the record omitted].[97]

In support of its nonsectarian status, the university's brief in this case also refers specifically to the sale of St. Louis University Hospital, noting:

> The Church's lack of control over Saint Louis University and its board are shown by the sale of its hospital to Tenet Health Care in 1998. The sale was made directly against the strong and well publicized objection of the Catholic Archbishop of St. Louis. This specific fact confirms the more general and undisputed factual statement made by President Biondi in his Affidavit that the University Board is in fact independent. [citations to the record omitted][98]

PART THREE

The Struggle to Maintain Catholic Identity as Reflected in Two Health Care Systems

In this part, I focus on two Catholic health care systems and their sponsoring orders: Providence Health System and Ascension Health. Several common trends may be observed in these systems. In these systems, there has been a pronounced shift toward lay management since the 1960s. This development coincides with the decline in religious vocations. There has also been a concerted attempt to inculcate the values of the founding order in the lay employees. In both systems, networks of modest community hospitals founded and dominated by religious orders have become complex, large-scale nonprofit health care enterprises, with predominantly lay management, sponsored by religious orders.

These health care systems have accommodated to ongoing changes in the socio-legal environment and the health care marketplace. Nonetheless, they continue to emphasize the compassionate nature of their mission and its religious roots. They also continue to struggle with demands from external forces that they provide "reproductive health services" in violation of the *ERD*s. Continuing adherence to the *Directives* has been most problematic in the context of merger and acquisition transactions between Catholic and non-Catholic providers.

In some instances, these systems have entered into arrangements to provide services such as direct sterilizations and abortion referrals in conjunction with mergers or acquisitions of non-Catholic facilities. These arrangements, approved by local bishops, have become increasingly complex and nuanced. Unfortunately, there is an appearance that the *ERD*s — particularly their restrictions on reproductive services — are viewed by system managers as an impediment to the increased economies of scale to be achieved through mergers and acquisitions. The existence of such arrangements increases the risk of scandal and could embolden those who favor a mandate requiring all hospitals, including Catholic hospitals, to provide a full range of reproductive services.

CHAPTER EIGHT

Providence Health System

Providence Health and Services operates 26 acute care hospitals, "more than 35 non-acute care facilities," and a health plan in Alaska, California, Montana, Oregon, and Washington.[1] In Alaska, Montana, Oregon, and Washington, corporate members with reserved canonical powers are members of the leadership team of the Sisters of Providence, Mother Joseph Province. In southern California, corporate members with reserved canonical powers are members of the leadership teams of the Sisters of Providence, Mother Joseph Province, and the Little Company of Mary.[2] In 2007, Providence Health and Services had 45,220 employees.[3] Its corporate offices are located in Seattle, Washington.[4] The mission of Providence Health and Services is stated as follows: "As People of Providence we reveal God's love for all, especially the poor and vulnerable, through our compassionate service." [5]

A Brief History of the Sisters of Providence in the Pacific Northwest

Providence Health System traces its origins back to the ministry of the Sisters of Providence, a Catholic women's order founded in Canada in 1843 by Mother Emilie Gamelin, a French Canadian.[6] The Sisters' ministry in the Pacific Northwest began when Mother Joseph, a member of the Sisters of Providence community in Montreal, Canada, came to Fort Vancouver, Washington Territory, in 1856, along with four other sisters.[7] Mother Joseph is a truly mythic figure in the history of the Pacific Northwest. Each state is entitled to two statues in the National Statuary Hall Collection in the United States Capitol. Washington State's two statues represent Marcus Whitman, a Protestant missionary who was killed by members of the Cayuse tribe, and Mother Joseph.[8]

Mother Joseph was born Esther Pariseau, in St. Elzear, Quebec, in 1823.[9] In 1856, thirteen years after joining the Sisters of Providence, she traveled to Vancouver, Washington Territory, by way of the Isthmus of Panama.[10] During her forty-six years in the Pacific Northwest, until her death in 1902,

PART THREE: *The Struggle to Maintain Catholic Identity . . .*

she established numerous hospitals, schools, and social service agencies.[11] She served as an architect for the sisters' projects and traveled with her sisters to mines in order to raise money for their charities.[12]

In 1858, Mother Joseph and her sisters opened St. Joseph's Hospital in Vancouver, Washington Territory, the first permanent hospital in the Pacific Northwest.[13] In 1859, the Sisters of Charity of the House of Providence in the Territory of Washington was formally incorporated.[14] It is "the parent corporation of the sisters' current ministries and one of the oldest existing corporations in the region."[15] In 1895, the board of directors of this corporation was expanded to include "not only Provincial Council members but also . . . the mayor of each city where we [the Sisters of Providence] had a school, hospital, orphanage, or infirmaries and the Chairman of the Board of County Commissioners."[16]

Apparently, the sisters believed that the properties held by this corporation should not be considered as property subject to disposal by the Church under the 1917 *Code of Canon Law*.[17] This view was reinforced by the laws of the state of Washington by virtue of the fact that, as a Washington nonprofit corporation, its corporate assets were subject to control by the Secretary of State in the event of the dissolution of the corporation.[18] Over the years, several additional nonprofit corporations, directly under the management of the Provincial Superior and Council, were formed under the laws of Washington, Oregon, and California, as the sisters expanded their ministries.[19]

Throughout their existence, the Sisters of Providence have reorganized and consolidated their provincial administration and health care systems. In 1891, the sisters established three administrative provinces in the west: Sacred Heart Province, based in Vancouver, Washington; St. Ignatius Province, based in Missoula, Montana; and St. Vincent de Paul Province, based in Portland, Oregon.[20] In 1912, the St. Vincent de Paul Province was closed, its institutions in the western United States becoming part of the Sacred Heart Province.[21] In 1926, the provincial administration of St. Ignatius Province was moved to Sacred Heart Hospital in Spokane, Washington, from Missoula, Montana.[22] In January of 2001, St. Ignatius and Sacred Heart Provinces were consolidated into Mother Joseph Province, the sponsor of Providence Health System and Providence Services.[23]

In the 1970s, the sisters began a process of reorganizing the governance structure of their hospitals, resulting in a separation of hospital governance from the governance of the religious congregation.[24] By 1973, the Sisters had established four civil corporations in Sacred Heart Province: the Sisters of

Providence of Washington, Sisters of Providence of Oregon, Sisters of Providence of California, and the Pariseau Association.[25] The provincial council served as the board of directors of each of the corporations.[26] These three state corporations held the assets of the hospitals in their respective states; the Washington State corporation also held the assets in Alaska.[27] The Pariseau Association held the assets required for support of the sisters.[28] By 1975, loans relating to the hospitals were no longer secured by assets necessary for the sisters' support.[29]

During this time, a debate continued within the congregation over the nature of the health care assets held by their civil corporations and whether they were subject to ecclesial control under canon law. Sr. Beverly Dunn has observed that in the 1970s, before the revision of the Code of Canon Law, Sacred Heart Province, "at least in practice," followed the approach taken by McGrath (discussed *supra*) in treating these civil corporations holding health care assets as being subject only to civil law. But with the promulgation of the revised *Code of Canon Law* in 1983 came a general agreement that these assets were subject to both civil and canon law, an approach closer to Maida's than McGrath's position.[30]

In 1991, there was a reorganization of the governance of the health care corporations in Sacred Heart Province with the appointment of a board of directors separate from the sisters' Provincial Council.[31] At that time, it was announced that the Provincial Superior would not only no longer be the chairperson of the board but wouldn't even serve on the board.[32] The sisters still had a majority of the new board, however, with six of the eleven members.[33] At least initially, the chairperson of the board of directors was still required to be a member of the Sisters of Providence and was to be appointed by the Provincial Superior and Provincial Council.[34] The same board of directors served for all three of the health care corporations created in 1973.[35] Under the new governance system, the Provincial Superior and members of the Provincial Council were to serve as corporate members of all sponsored health care corporations in Sacred Heart Province, with certain reserved powers. These included the power "to adopt or change the mission and values of the Corporations"; "to amend or repeal the Articles of Incorporation or Bylaws of the Corporations"; to appoint and remove the chairperson of the board of directors "with or without cause"; to appoint and remove the CEOs of the corporations "with or without cause"; and "to approve the closure of any institution or major ministry or work within the Corporations."[36]

In 1993, the health care corporations in Sacred Heart Province became Sis-

PART THREE: *The Struggle to Maintain Catholic Identity . . .*

ters of Providence Health System, later to be known as Providence Health System.[37]

A somewhat different approach was taken to reorganization in St. Ignatius Province within the context of its strong tradition of decentralized management.[38] In this province were two health care corporations: The Sisters of Charity of Providence in Eastern Washington and the Sisters of Charity of Providence in Montana.[39] In addition, many hospitals were separately incorporated.[40] "The Provincial Superior and her council served as the board of directors of the various corporations, while one of the members of the council acted as director of health care ministries."[41] In 1992, the hospitals and other services in St. Ignatius were incorporated into a new holding company, Providence Services.[42] The Provincial Superior and her council were designated as the corporate members of Providence Services, with reserved powers.[43] The religious community of the province was separately incorporated.[44] There was also a second tier of corporations for the local institutions with local boards of directors, and the board of directors for Providence Services served as the corporate members for those local boards.[45] The majority of members of the Providence Services Board of Directors were not part of the Sisters of Providence.[46] In addition, the president of the Sisters of Providence Health System was a member of the board of directors for Providence Services.[47]

Thus, at the time of the consolidation of the provinces in 2001, two holding companies oversaw the sisters' operations within Mother Joseph Province: Providence Health System operated in Alaska, western Washington, Oregon, and California; and a separate holding company, Providence Services, operated in eastern Washington and Montana.[48] In September 2005, these two entities began to explore the possibility of formally integrating their operations.[49] On January 1, 2006, the formal integration took place, thus creating Providence Health and Services.[50] Its corporate headquarters are now in Seattle, with operations in the states of Alaska, California, Montana, Oregon, and Washington.[51]

By the end of 1902, the sisters operated seventeen hospitals and eight schools in Alaska, California, Idaho, Montana, Oregon, and Washington.[52] By the end of 1960, the sisters operated 22 hospitals,[53] but only six of those twenty-two hospitals had been built after 1925.[54] Accordingly, during the 1960s and '70s, the sisters undertook a massive rebuilding program, eventually accumulating over $100 million of debt in Sacred Heart Province alone.[55] This rebuilding was financed by "a combination of borrowing, local and state fund-raising, and Hill-Burton funds."[56] This approach worked well as long as there was significant community support; if that support was not forthcoming, then the Sisters "withdrew from the hospital" and turned it over to the community.[57] By the mid-1970s, they had withdrawn from eight hospitals.[58]

Beginning in the late 1970s and into the '80s, the sisters took over the sponsorship of existing community hospitals in Newberg, Oregon (1979); Seaside, Oregon (1983); Toppenish, Washington (1985); Milwaukie, Oregon (1986); Centralia, Washington (1988); and Polson, Montana (1990).[59] Their health care operations also expanded by assuming sponsorship or co-sponsorship of other Catholic hospitals. In 1993, they assumed sponsorship of the Dominican Network in eastern Washington,[60] followed by another in Toluca, California, in 1996.[61] In 1999, they assumed cosponsorship with the Little Company of Mary of several hospitals in southern California.[62]

The early years of the new century saw some divestitures, most significantly the transfer of Providence Hospital in Seattle, its flagship institution, from Providence Health System to Swedish Health Services in 2000.[63] In 2003, the Yakima and Toppenish hospitals in Washington State were sold to Health Management Associates, a for-profit company out of Naples, Florida.[64] The reason given for the sale of these hospitals in the Yakima valley was that Providence had lost money on them the past several years and was not able to invest the millions of dollars required for upgrades to the facilities.[65] By the time of its creation in January 2006, Providence Health and Services operated "27 hospitals, about 35 non-acute facilities, a health plan, a liberal arts university, and [had] 45,000 employees."[66]

The scale of operations of Providence Health and Services, as set out in their 2006 annual report, would have astonished Mother Joseph. In 2006, the net operating revenues for Providence Health and Services were $5,821,293,000.[67] Total operating expenses were $5,553,873,000.[68] Total philanthropic revenue raised was $96.2 million. Community benefits provided (not including unpaid Medicare) were $370.8 million.[69] The unpaid cost of Medicaid and the cost of charity care was the largest portion of community benefits, at $280.4 million. The percentage of revenue from Medicare was 27%, and from Medicaid, 8%.[70] Total acute admissions were 242,984.[71] Providence health plans had 228,450 members, including privately insured and self-funded, Medicare and Medicaid, and there were 438,533 PPO eligibles.[72]

Part Three: *The Struggle to Maintain Catholic Identity . . .*

The Shift to Lay Management and the Focus on Education and Planning for the Continuation of the Mission of the Sisters

The first lay administrator of a hospital in Sacred Heart Province was hired in 1969,[73] and in 1973, Jack Brown was appointed as executive vice president — the first layperson to serve as the director — of health care operations in Sacred Heart Province.[74] In 1979, Brown was named president of the health care corporations in Sacred Heart Province and, in 1980, Donald A. Brennan, also a layperson, succeeded him.[75]

Currently, in addition to the corporate members who are members of the Sisters of Providence and the Little Company of Mary, the fifteen members of the Providence Health and Services Board of Directors include only one member each from the Sisters of Providence and Little Company of Mary.[76] The current chief executive officer and other members of the senior leadership team are all laypersons;[77] a list of current administrators at Providence Health System facilities reveals that none are members of the Sisters of Providence.[78]

By the early 1980s, it had become clear that in the future, the mission of the Sisters of Providence health care organizations would have to be carried on primarily by laypeople — many of whom were not Catholic — in an environment where Catholics were a minority (less than 15% in most of their service areas).[79] Initially, the sisters developed an educational program to inculcate their lay employees in their mission.[80] Then, in the early 1980s, St. Ignatius Province — where there was not as yet centralized control of the hospitals — directed its facilities to evaluate their Catholic identity with the *Evaluative Criteria for Health Care Facilities*, an instrument developed by the CHA.[81] This instrument covered nine areas: "philosophy, relations with the Church, Christian management, patient care, pastoral care, medical-moral guidance, social justice, education, and relations with other institutions."[82]

Each of the hospitals in St. Ignatius Province came up with its own approach to the process. For example, at Sacred Heart Hospital in Spokane, the process was referred to as a Values Enrichment Process, viewed as a means of assisting employees in identifying and implementing "its own ecclesial values and mission."[83] After Providence Services was created in 1992, thereby centralizing health care administration in St. Ignatius Province, the board of directors initiated "a mission development process with a regional focus" to strengthen the "regional presence as value-based Providence Services organizations reflecting the call of God's love in the mission of healing."[84]

In the Sacred Heart Province, Sr. Beverly Dunn has traced the mission development program to the appointment of "sister representatives" in the early 1970s who served on the administrative councils of hospitals that were administered by laypersons.[85] In 1983, as the numbers of sisters working in hospitals continued to decline, it was realized that this approach was not sufficient and an Office of Mission Development was created at the province level.[86] There were also offices of mission effectiveness created in each hospital.[87] Sr. Beverly Dunn has characterized the shift in thinking that occurred in the 1990s concerning the mission as a movement "from expressing itself primarily in terms of its relationship to the Sisters of Providence to one more focused on its relationship to the mission of the Catholic Church."[88]

The Sisters of Providence in Sacred Heart Province promulgated *Mission Effectiveness Principles and Guidelines* in 1986 and revised it in 1990.[89] This document is divided into eight sections: "Compassionate Love for the Poor"; "Articulating and Integrating the Mission, Philosophy, and Values;" "Catholic Heritage and Traditions"; "Representing and Respecting the Moral Values of the Catholic Church"; "Providing Spiritual Care"; "The Continuing Presence of the Sisters of Providence in the Institutions and Associated Works"; "Respect for Colleagues;" and "Relating Gospel Values to Quality Care."[90]

The first section on "Compassionate Love for the Poor" commits Sisters of Providence institutions to providing "quality care . . . for all persons served . . . regardless of economic status or other considerations, including age, sex, race, religion, or disability."[91] The section dealing with mission requires Sisters of Providence institutions to provide an orientation on their mission to administrative staff, board members, and medical staff.[92] It also requires that all institutions are to be operated in accordance with the *Mission Effectiveness Principles and Guidelines*.[93]

The section on "Catholic Heritage and Traditions" requires that institutions "maintain open communications and collaboration with the bishops, priests, sisters, and Catholic agencies in its service area."[94] "A visible Eucharistic chapel is to be found in each hospital."[95] "Traditional symbols of the Catholic Church and the Sisters of Providence are to [be] displayed at each sponsored institution."[96] And, perhaps most significantly, it requires that those collaborating with the Sisters of Providence be made aware that Providence institutions are operated in accordance with "Gospel values, the Code of Canon Law . . . the teachings of the Catholic Church . . . [and] the *Ethical and Religious Directives for Catholic Health Care Facilities*."[97] Further, in the section on the moral values of the Catholic Church, it is expressly stated that abortion, euthanasia, and sterilization solely for contraceptive purposes are forbidden in Providence institutions.[98]

The section on spiritual matters requires Sisters of Providence institutions to be "supportive of the individual's growth in personal faith."[99] The section dealing with the continuing presence of Sisters of Providence in the hospitals requires the hospital administrators to include Sisters of Providence in policy review and consult regularly with sisters serving at the institution.[100] The administrative council, community advisory board, and the foundation board at each institution should include sisters.[101]

The section on "Respect for Colleagues" provides that employees are to be paid a "just wage" and recognizes the right of employees to unionize.[102] And finally, the section on "Relating Gospel Values to Quality Care" requires that institutions should "continually seek to provide appropriate care according to the needs of the patient, while offering the same level of care regardless of level of payment."[103]

The Role of the *ERDs* in Defining the Mission

As with many large Catholic systems, at Providence Health and Services there has been a constant tension among competing goals — i.e., service to the community, generating sufficient net revenues to remain competitive, and maintaining adherence to the *ERDs*. And it is becoming increasingly difficult for these health systems to carry out their religious mission while remaining competitive in a health care marketplace that can be volatile.[104] While Providence Health and Services acknowledges its adherence to the *ERDs*, it does not highlight the *ERDs* or its distinctively Catholic character. Instead it strives to be broadly acceptable to all persons of good will. This approach may be due to a confluence of various factors including a desire to strike a lower profile on controversial issues in order to blunt or avoid the virulent attacks by "pro-choice" activists, the pervasive influence of the secular bioethics movement, and the recognition that it is operating in an environment where practicing Catholics are a small minority. It may also be due to the fact that many of its key employees are not Catholic.

When the U.S. Supreme Court decision in *Roe v. Wade* was handed down on January 22, 1973, there was an almost immediate response to that decision by Catholic hospitals in the form of a press release from the Washington State Catholic Hospital & Health Care Organization stating that "none of the Catholic Hospitals in Washington State will admit patients for the purpose of terminating pregnancies by abortion."[105] All nineteen Catholic hospitals in Washington State are listed in this press release, including those hospitals sponsored by the Sisters of Providence. The press release continued by quoting Sr. Virginia Pearson, O.P., president of the association:

> The dignity of human life and our responsibility to respect and conserve it ... underlies the very reason for existence of Catholic sponsored health care facilities. We who sponsor and manage these institutions believe that life given by God has intrinsic value and cannot be taken at will. This respect for life is the basis of any civilized society and not merely a sectarian morality. It is the basis of our stand against abortion. As concerned citizens, we protest our right to speak in defense of life in all its stages and from the moment of conception. The decision of the U.S. Supreme Court on abortion does not change our commitment to these values.[106]

In contrast with this press release from the 1970s, the current approach taken by Providence Health and Services as set forth in its Web site is much more nuanced. Its Web site statement of mission and values does not mention the *ERD*s.[107] Although its Web site generally avoids mention of such controversial topics as abortion, contraception, or sterilization, it is noteworthy that the Providence Health Plans do not provide insurance coverage for abortion, sterilization, or contraception.[108] The only explicit reference to the *ERD*s on the Providence Health and Services Web site is in the form of a global disclaimer:

> Providence Health & Services, as a ministry of the Roman Catholic Church, does not recommend, endorse, or promote those medical procedures and interventions that are discussed on this site but which are prohibited by the *Ethical and Religious Directives for Catholic Health Care Services*.[109]

This disclaimer is apparently offered in connection with an online health information library, linked to the Providence Health Plan Web site, that discusses contraception[110] and sterilization,[111] but not abortion. Under the heading "abortion" it is stated: "Please note that this is a customized version of the Healthwise Knowledgebase. This topic is not among those selected by Providence Health System."[112]

Controversy over Emergency Contraception, Contraceptive Coverage, and the Early Induction of Labor

There has been some controversy over the availability of emergency contraception at Providence hospitals, contraceptive coverage for Providence employees, and the availability of early induction of labor in Providence hospitals. As to emergency contraception, in the Providence Health System's 2002 *Annual Report to the Community* it was noted that Providence Health System emergency departments offered emergency contraception to rape victims "after testing for pregnancy,"[113] but there is no mention of it in the 2006 Report.[114] The health library available on the current Providence Web site provides no information on emergency contraception.[115] In a 2002 article in the *Everett Herald*, it was noted that Providence Everett was providing emergency contraceptives to victims of sexual assault. Jan Heller, identified in the article as working in the office of ethics and theology of Providence Health Systems, was quoted as stating: "It is permissible under church teachings under these circumstances to give emergency contraception to victims of sexual assault."[116]

Subsequently, however, a 2003 article in *The Spokesman-Review,* focused on emergency contraception policies in hospitals operated by Providence Services of Eastern Washington, claimed that their hospitals were not providing emergency contraception to rape victims.[117] The article reviewed a portion of the Catholics for a Free Choice study, discussed *infra* in Chapter 13, claiming that six hospitals in Washington State, including Sacred Heart Medical Center in Spokane, were in violation of a Washington state law mandating provision of emergency contraception to sexual assault victims.[118] The article reports that the study claimed that triage nurses at some hospitals in the Providence Services system, including Sacred Heart, told "mystery callers" posing as rape victims that they did not provide emergency contraception.[119] A spokeswoman for Sacred Heart, however, denied that this was the hospital's policy, saying: "Sacred Heart has a written policy on this issue which explicitly states that in cases of sexual assault, we provide emergency contraception after tests indicate the patient is not currently pregnant."[120] According to the article:

> Other hospitals in the Providence Services Eastern Washington System gave callers differing information. Holy Family Hospital, Deer Park Hospital, and St. Mary Medical Center in Walla Walla told the survey callers that emergency contraception would be provided only in rape cases in which the victim was not pregnant. But Mt. Carmel Hospital in Colville said the pill was available to rape victims with no restrictions. And St. Joseph Hospital in Chewelah said it was available on request.[121]

There has also been controversy over the provision of contraceptive coverage to Providence employees. In an article in *The Spokesman-Review,* a Spokane, Washington newspaper, a spokeswoman for the state insurance commissioner's office stated that under an opinion issued by the Washington State Attorney General's Office, discussed *infra* in Chapter 12, Sacred Heart Medical Center was required to provide prescription birth control coverage for its employees. The article went on to note that the "ruling did provide a bit of a fig leaf for employers who find contraceptives objectionable: They can ask their insurer to wrap the costs of such coverage into overall policy costs, perhaps as an administrative or overhead cost."[122] In a subsequent editorial, *The Spokesman-Review* commented favorably on the new ruling:

> Surely, when the Sisters of Providence founded the hospital in the 19th century, they saw their mission as repairing body and soul. But Sacred Heart has become a modern health care conglomerate, forging partnerships with for-profit companies, accepting government money, hiring employees without a Catholic litmus test and taking all patients regardless of creed. Its makeup and mission are largely secular. Therefore, its employees have the same rights as anyone else.[123]

Finally, there has been controversy over the use of the early induction of labor procedure in Providence hospitals. In 2003, Providence Health system acknowledged that its hospitals were "performing a procedure known as early induction for fetuses with anomalies incompatible with life."[124] This procedure is made available in Providence Health System hospitals where a pregnant woman is carrying a baby who has been diagnosed as having a condition that would significantly shorten its life such as anencephaly or renal agenesis.[125] In these cases, labor could be induced at or after twenty-four weeks of pregnancy.[126]

The first acknowledgment of the policy came in a meeting between representatives of Alaska Right to Life and members of the management team for the Providence Alaska System.[127] At a second meeting, representatives of Alaska Right to Life met with a former vicar general of the Archdiocese of Anchorage and Jan Heller, System Ethicist for Providence Health System, who participated by speakerphone.[128] Ed Wassell, president of Alaska Right to Life, stated that his purpose in meeting with Providence officials was to convince them to "end the use of the procedure."[129] He further claimed that the only "therapeutic reason" given by them for performing the procedure was "to relieve familial distress."[130] Providence officials also told Wassell that they would stop performing the procedure if directed to do so by the archbishop.[131] After the meeting, on September 29, 2003, Providence Health System and the Archdiocese of Anchorage issued the following statement:

Earlier this year, Ed Wassell, president of Alaska Right to Life, approached Al Parrish, executive of Providence Health System in Alaska, requesting clarification on the early induction practices and guidelines of Providence Alaska Medical Center in Anchorage.

After further consultation with ethicists, Providence Health System, in collaboration with Anchorage Archbishop Roger Schwietz, determined that the practices are consistent with the *Ethical and Religious Directives for Catholic Health Care Services*. Providence leadership continues to be in dialogue with Archbishop Schwietz to assure that guidelines in development reflect Catholic teachings.[132]

In an interview with the *National Catholic Register*, the archbishop of Anchorage provided the Providence policy to the paper.[133] He also noted that he had received advice from the National Catholic Bioethics Center (NCBC) regarding the policy.[134] Experts from NCBC had advised the bishop that the policy was "problematic." He then asked Providence to provide him with a more detailed policy, particularly focusing on *ERD*s nos. 45, 47, and 49.

After receiving the new guidelines, the archbishop again authorized the system to perform the procedure.[135] The guidelines were apparently revised in accord with the suggestions made by the experts from NCBC.[136] Although the new guidelines approved by the archbishop are not available, an article by Fr. Norman Ford in *Ethics & Medics* (a commentary published by the NCBC) argues that early induction is morally permissible beginning at thirty-three weeks in order to relieve maternal distress.[137] This article opines that "[t]he withdrawal of pregnancy support by early induction would not be direct abortion since the normal fetus would also have reasonable prospects of long-term survival at this stage."[138] Accordingly, it concludes that "the cause of death would be the lethal defect, not the induction."[139] A March 2004 statement by NCBC, however, provides more stringent guidelines indicating that early induction of labor would be morally permissible under the *ERD*s only for the purpose of curing a serious pathology in the mother.[140] And Kevin O'Rourke and Ashley Benedict, have opined that early induction is not morally licit for "anencephalic and genetically deprived infants" because the "proximate purpose" of this procedure would be to cause the death of the infant.[141]

The Application of the *ERD*s in Mergers, Sales, and Acquisitions

Providence Health and Services has been involved in merger, sale, and acquisition transactions that have raised ethical issues. A major development occurred in 2000 when it was announced that Providence Hospital and its nine clinics located in the environs of Seattle, Washington would be taken over and operated by Swedish Hospital, Washington state's largest hospital.[142] Under the terms of the agreement, and subject to approval by the Vatican, Swedish was to "own and operate Providence Seattle Medical Center, the Jefferson Medical Tower on the Providence Seattle campus, and Providence Medical Group in King County . . . [and] Providence in Washington will form a new company that will be jointly owned and operated . . . [and] might pursue other new health care ventures."[143] While the parties characterized the Swedish transaction as a "strategic alliance," a spokesman for the Seattle Archdiocese described it as a sale.[144] Providence Health System was given two seats on Swedish's board, and would continue to operate its other health care facilities independently of Swedish.[145] The strategic alliance consisted primarily in of a continuing collaborative arrangement to provide centralized billing for both Swedish and Providence facilities.[146]

The Swedish merger came after the resignation of Derrick Pasternak, the chief executive officer of Providence Seattle Medical Center, and the closure and sale of several clinics following a $16 million operating loss in 1999.[147] Previously, Providence had to close a HMO-style health plan in 1998 because of financial problems.[148] In the early 1990s, under the leadership of Donald Brennan, Providence had established a network of clinics and a health plan in anticipation of the Clinton health care reform proposal. Brennan left Providence to serve as the Director of Washington state's new health care plan, enacted in 1993. The Washington state plan was patterned after the Clinton Administration's health care reform proposal. Providence had positioned itself in the market under Brennan's leadership to take advantage of the shift to universal health care. This involved establishing a HMO-type plan and several clinics. Brennan then signed on to oversee the new state program. Subsequently, however, the Washington state legislation was repealed, and the Clinton plan was never enacted.[149]

In order to obtain approval of the transfer from Church officials, Swedish agreed to stop providing "elective abortions" at any of its facilities.[150] Swedish had been providing approximately fifty elective abortions a year at its facilities.[151] The agreement by Swedish Hospital, a secular institution, to stop providing elective abortions raised the ire of groups such as NARAL.[152] Although Swedish would no longer provide elective abortions, it would continue to provide sterilizations and contraception, including the morning-after pill.[153] And there was no mention of any agreement to refrain from providing therapeutic abortions. Moreover, neither the definition of elective abortions nor the party that determines whether an abortion is elective is made clear under those terms of the agreement made public. It is possible that elective abortions may only include those abortions that physicians on the Swedish medical staff would not consider to have any therapeutic benefit. And if that is the case, then the agreement places no significant constraints on Swedish Hospital's provision of abortions because therapeutic could be broadly interpreted to include mental health concerns. Nonetheless, Frances Kissling, president of Catholics for a Free Choice, wrote a letter to *The Seattle Times* protesting the sale, stating: "The elimination of these medically indicated and necessary abortions by a Catholic entity goes against the grain of all understanding of what compassion as well as a commitment to women's health should mean for a Catholic institution."[154]

In 2002, after Swedish took over the Providence Campus, the 1910 Providence Hospital building was sold to the Sabey Corporation, a large real estate development company, with plans to turn it into a biotech-research center.[155] This building had been damaged by an earthquake and had held only administrative offices while Swedish utilized the remaining Providence Campus buildings to provide patient care.[156] Under the agreement with the Sabey Corporation, Swedish retained most of the campus and planned to continue to operate an acute care facility on the site, providing a broad range of outpatient and inpatient services.[157] And Sabey planned to invest approximately $40 million in redevelopment costs in addition to the purchase price of $37 million.[158] Originally, the campus was to retain the name Providence,[159] but eventually, Swedish renamed the Providence campus; it is now known as the Cherry Hill Campus.[160]

Providence Health System has also run into some controversy and opposition when it has taken over the operation of non-Catholic facilities and discontinued the provision of reproductive health services. Abortion rights activists have been concerned that the expansion of Providence in some communities could decrease access to abortions.[161] In 1994, Providence Health System merged with General Hospital Medical Center, a community hospital in Everett, Washington.[162] Prior to the merger, Everett was a two-hospital town.[163] The merger was necessitated by the patterns of decreasing utilization of both hospitals and the significant cost savings that could be realized by combining operations.[164] Under the terms of the agreement, General Hospital was to be absorbed into Providence Health System and stop performing elective abortions and most tubal ligations.[165] It was announced that General Hospital would, however, continue to perform abortions when the mother's life was in danger and tubal ligations "when deemed medically necessary."[166] A Planned Parenthood official voiced concern about the merger and its effect on access to abortions.[167] To assuage those concerns, and prior to the merger, General Hospital's board donated $500,000 to Planned Parenthood to provide "reproductive health services" at other facilities.[168]

In 2000, Providence Health System abandoned an affiliation arrangement under which it would manage a public health district consisting of a community hospital and five clinics in Lincoln County, Oregon, after opponents claimed that the affiliation would result in the discontinuation of sterilizations and abortions.[169] The partners in the affiliation, Pacific Communities Health District and Providence Health system, had gone to court to obtain a ruling on the validity of the affiliation agreement. Although the affiliation had broad support in the local community and was favored by officials at the health district, opponents, consisting primarily of activists from outside the community, viewed the affiliation as posing "a threat to women's reproductive rights and Lincoln County residents ability to participate in Oregon's Death with Dignity Act [authorizing physician-assisted suicide]."[170] Opponents also objected to the fact that under the affiliation agreement, Providence would continue to receive public funds amounting to approximately $450,000 annually.[171]

One issue in court proceeding was whether the hospital would become a "pervasively religious institution" under Providence's management.[172] In this regard, the health district administrator acknowledged that providers at the hospital would be required to conform to the *ERDs*.[173] The health district's attorney argued that the entity was not pervasively religious,[174] relying in part on *Wisconsin Health Facilities Authority v. Lindner*,[175] a 1979 Wisconsin Supreme Court decision that held that following the *ERDs* did not make a hospital pervasively religious. The Oregon court never ruled on this question because the affiliation was terminated.[176]

PART THREE: *The Struggle to Maintain Catholic Identity* ...

CHAPTER NINE

Ascension Health

Four Provinces of the Daughters of Charity, the Sisters of Saint Joseph of Nazareth, and the Sisters of St. Joseph of Carondelet sponsor Ascension Health.[1] It was formed in November of 1999 by the merger of two systems — the Daughters of Charity National Health System based in St. Louis, Missouri, and the Sisters of St. Joseph Health System, based in Ann Arbor, Michigan.[2] In 2002, the hospitals and health facilities of the Carondelet Health System, also based in St. Louis, Missouri, were added to the system.[3] Together, they form the largest nonprofit health care system in the United States.[4] As of February 2008, the Ascension system consisted of sixty general acute care hospitals as well as twelve long-term care, rehabilitation, or psychiatric facilities.[5] It operated in nineteen states, and its facilities had more than 16,700 licensed beds.[6] In 2007, it provided more $800 million in community benefits.[7]

At the time of the initial merger, the Daughters of Charity Health System had operations in fifteen states, and St. Joseph's operations were all in Michigan.[8] Post-merger, the members of the two religious orders were to hold a majority of the seats on Ascension Health's board.[9] At the time of the merger, the Daughters of Charity Health System's annual net revenues were in excess of $4 billion, and the Sisters of St. Joseph System had net revenues of $1.8 billion.[10] Ascension planned to sell $2.4 billion of bonds to finance the merger.[11] In May of 2000, however, the Internal Revenue Service announced it was auditing the bond issue. This, in turn, caused the yield on bonds to increase due to investor fears that the bonds might lose their tax-exempt status.[12] This was part of a more aggressive oversight posture of the Internal Revenue Service in the tax-exempt bond market.[13]

The year following the merger, the acquisition profits from the former St. Joseph facilities "added to Ascension's Bottom line."[14] Nonetheless, "Ascension lost $31 million on total operating revenue of $6.2 billion in its first fiscal year."[15] This was attributed to $41 million in restructuring costs and "other one-time charges."[16] In its first fiscal year "[o]verall, Ascension enjoyed profits of $199 million on total revenue of $6.4 billion."[17] Subsequently, in

June of 2002, Ascension announced that it would take over another smaller Catholic health care system, Carondelet Health System, which was also based in St. Louis.[18] The deal did not include a Carondelet facility in Newport Beach, California.[19] The merger was motivated, at least in part, by Ascension's higher bond ratings and the need for capital improvements at Carondelet facilities.[20] With the Carondelet acquisition, the combined system included sixty-seven acute care hospitals in twenty states.[21] By June 2003, Ascension was the nation's largest private, nonprofit health care system, and was ranked fourth in net revenue among both for-profit and nonprofit systems.[22]

Since its inception, Ascension has followed an "aggressive and entrepreneurial approach, getting rid of underperforming hospitals while acquiring new facilities and expanding market share in profitable markets."[23] Its adaptability has been illustrated by its willingness to continually restructure its operations in response to current market conditions. For example, in 2005, in Pasco, Washington, it successfully converted an underperforming 132-bed acute care hospital into a 25-bed critical access hospital with an additional 10 PPS rehabilitation beds and 13 observation beds.[24] In June 2006, it sold DeKalb Community Hospital in Smithville, Tennessee, to Cannon County Hospital in Nashville.[25] In November 2006, it sold its unprofitable St. Joseph Hospital in Augusta, Georgia, to Triad Hospitals, a for-profit chain.[26] In April 2007, it announced that it would sell St. John Detroit Riverview Hospital, an underperforming hospital in Detroit that had lost $9 million in 2006, to a cancer hospital.[27] And in April 2008, Ascension announced it was seeking a purchaser for St. Anthony's, a money-losing hospital on the west side of Chicago.[28]

Ascension has continued to be actively involved in merger, acquisition, and other affiliation and consolidation activities. In November 2006, it was announced that Ascension would become half-owner of Wichita, Kansas-based Via Christi Health System.[29] This was a non-cash transaction brought about by the Sisters of St. Joseph (a cosponsor of Via Christi) being merged into the Congregation of St. Joseph (one of the cosponsors of Ascension).[30] Via Christi is the largest health care system in Kansas and the owner of four acute care hospitals, an insurer, a rehabilitation hospital, and several long-term care and rehabilitation facilities.[31]

In late 2007, Ascension-owned St. Agnes Hospital in Baltimore announced it would work jointly on business clinical opportunities with St. Joseph Medical Center, another Baltimore hospital owned by Catholic Health Initiatives.[32] In July 2007, Ascension acquired Eastern Health System, a group of three hospitals in Alabama, and consolidated it with its St. Vincent's Hospital located in Birmingham, Alabama.[33] In April 2008, Ascension announced that in Schuylkill County, Pennsylvania, its Good Samaritan Regional Medical Center would be merged with the slightly-better-performing Pottsville Community Hospital.[34] And in early 2008, it was announced that Ascension's Columbia St. Mary's had entered into a joint operating agreement with Froedtert & Community Health — a system that includes the Academic Medical Center for Medical College of Wisconsin and three other hospitals — to make it the second largest provider in the Milwaukee market.[35]

Ascension has also passed on some deals. In 2007, Ascension considered, but then ultimately rejected, a deal that would have led to the acquisition of six chronically underperforming hospitals from the Archdiocese of Boston.[36]

Ascension has also been involved in innovative arrangements in its charitable activities. In 2007, Ascension announced that it would open a new permanent health clinic in the Ninth Ward of New Orleans, an area ravaged by Hurricane Katrina, in a vacant school building next to St. Cecilia's Church on Rampart Street.[37] The Daughters of Charity had been operating a temporary clinic out of St. Cecilia's since the storm and had treated more than 14,000 people at that location.[38] A second clinic was planned on Carrollton Avenue in New Orleans, to replace a clinic also destroyed by Katrina.[39] It was contemplated that both clinics would primarily serve the indigent and uninsured,[40] and it was hoped that a focus on providing primary care in the clinic setting, including the management of chronic conditions such as diabetes, could substantially reduce reliance on hospital emergency room visits.[41]

Due to its success in the marketplace, Ascension has been recognized as "a financial and commercial powerhouse within health care."[42] By 2006, in only its seventh year of operation, "Ascension's operating margin had increased fivefold, while its unrestricted investments . . . doubled, to $5.6 billion [and its] operating revenue doubled to $11.4 billion."[43] In 2007, there were only two health care systems larger than Ascension: HCA and the VA.[44] Ascension started a venture capital fund in 2001 to provide seed money for startup companies engaged in the development of emerging technologies that have a potential to improve health care delivery, such as information technology and medical devices.[45] In 2007, a second venture capital fund was started in conjunction with Catholic Health Initiatives and Catholic Health East.[46]

A Brief History of the Daughters of Charity

The Daughters of Charity Order dates back to seventeenth-century France, when a French priest (later to become known as St. Vincent de Paul) recruited Louise de Marillac, a widow from an aristocratic family, to assist him in caring for the sick poor.[47] The pair cofounded the Daughters of Charity in 1633.[48] The founding of the Daughters of Charity provided an alternative for women religious to the strict convent life: it was established "as a secular institution (confraternity) in order to avoid cloister and practice their active ministries."[49] The founding of the Daughters of Charity was an outgrowth of the Catholic Reformation in France, "manifested in a widespread proliferation of charitable works for the poor including hospitals, home-relief institutions, and schools."[50]

Although involved in providing nursing care, the early Daughters of Charity viewed their primary mission as providing "spiritual balm to the sick."[51] The early members of the Daughters, drawn primarily from the peasant class, were involved in providing care for the sick poor.[52] In 1639, the Daughters of Charity took over its first hospital in France,[53] and over time, took over several more there.[54] "By 1699, 163 institutions were identified with this burgeoning community, which — by episcopal permission in 1655, and papal decree in 1668 — was authorized to "live in the world . . ."[55] In 1792, during the French Revolution, the Daughters were disbanded, then were reconstituted in 1801.[56] Professor Kauffman notes:

> Since the Daughters were apothecaries and apprentice-like surgeons who dealt with physicians on almost a daily basis, the role of medical treatment of natural illness permeated their hospitals by late eighteenth century.[57]

"Elizabeth Seton founded the Sisters of Charity in 1809 in Baltimore, but soon moved it to Emmitsburg, Maryland, and adopted the rule of the Daughters of Charity."[58] The Sisters of Charity began their hospital ministry in the Baltimore infirmary in 1823.[59] In 1828, the Sisters of Charity opened the first Catholic hospital in the United States in St. Louis, Missouri, to serve those journeying to the West.[60] This hospital was founded through the efforts of the Female Charitable Society — an organization of Catholic and Protestant women — the local bishop, and the generosity of a wealthy Catholic businessman.[61] In 1840, the Sisters of Charity opened a mental hospital, Mt. St. Vincent's, near Baltimore.[62] During the frequent cholera epidemics in American cities in the nineteenth century, the Sisters of Charity performed heroically in providing nursing services to the victims of the disease.[63] In 1850, the French Daughters of Charity merged with the Sisters of Charity.[64] By the time of the merger, the Daughters of Charity were operating in several nations.[65] By 1909, health care had emerged as an important ministry for the

PART THREE: *The Struggle to Maintain Catholic Identity . . .*

American Daughters of Charity.[66] A 1998 *Wall Street Journal* article on the Daughters of Charity notes:

> The American Daughters, who wore distinctive coronets with wings, quickly mastered St. Vincent's legacy of "responsible stewardship," creating in the late 1800s what were then bold financing projects, very much like today's managed care contracts: in 1874, to finance their hospital in Saginaw, Mich., the sisters visited lumber camps and sold all-inclusive hospital service tickets for $5. They also negotiated with Texas railroads and Louisiana steamship companies for similar "exclusive provider" arrangements.[67]

In addition to being known for their humility, the Daughters of Charity are also known for the financial acumen; even earning the nickname "Daughters of Currency."[68] The Daughters of Charity became renowned on Wall Street for their willingness to "make tough decisions, like selling unprofitable hospitals or investing enough money to make them profitable."[69] From 1993 to 1998, the order divested itself of eleven unprofitable hospitals.[70] At the time of the creation of Ascension Health, the Daughters system had long held one of the highest credit ratings in the health care industry, but their partner in the merger, the Sisters of St. Joseph, had lower ratings.[71] By 1998, the Daughters had a reserve of cash and investments totaling approximately $2 billion.[72] At this time, the Daughters were spending 86 cents on charity care for every $1 of profit.[73]

The Shift to Lay Leadership

Donald Brennan, the first lay chief executive officer for the Daughters, was hired in 1995.[74] Brennan had previously served as CEO of Group Health Cooperative of Puget Sound,[75] and as CEO of the Sisters of Providence Health System in Seattle.[76] Brennan was part of a generation of health care managers that had to make a transition from an industry "dominated by freestanding hospitals to one populated by large integrated delivery systems."[77] This was also the generation that started their careers with the beginning of the Medicare program, "when reimbursement money flowed, and they hunkered down when government and private payers tightened the purse strings."[78] During this time, management style in health care systems shifted from a "rugged individualist" approach to a team strategy.[79]

As the management operations at Ascension have been increasingly taken over by laypersons, the sisters have become "adamant about training the lay staff in the teaching of St. Vincent and the order's values."[80] A 1998 *Wall Street Journal* article notes:

> Today, the sisters still think of themselves first as missionaries. Business cards and employee badges list their "core values," including respect, simplicity, and advocacy for the poor. Their 70,000 employees are evaluated on, among other things, "value-based behavior." Meetings begin with prayers and reflection time. Hospital executives attend spiritual retreats. The sisters practice humility by moving back and forth from top leadership jobs to lesser positions . . . About 250 nuns work in the system.[81]

In November of 2000, Ascension announced that Douglas French, another layman, would replace Donald Brennan as CEO,[82] as Brennan planned to retire at the end of the year.[83] His successor had served as executive vice president and chief operating officer under Brennan.[84]

Two months after French took over, Ascension announced an organizational restructuring[85] that divided management into five teams: clinical excellence, innovation, operations improvement, "voice for the voiceless," and "work-life community."[86] (The latter two teams were focused on mission-related activities.)[87] The "voice for the voiceless" team included "advocacy, governmental relations, and public policy executives."[88] "The work-life community team" was to include executives "from the mission, ethics, and public relations departments."[89] Anthony Tersigni became president and CEO of Ascension in June of 2004.[90]

Ethical Challenges in Mergers, Acquisitions, and Other Affiliation Agreements

Ascension and its predecessor, the Daughters of Charity Health System, have struggled with balancing adherence to the *ERDs* with the need to adapt to market conditions through entering into mergers, acquisitions, and joint operating agreements with non-Catholic facilities. At times, they've encountered vigorous opposition to such activities by "pro-choice" groups concerned about the potential impact on the availability of reproductive services.

For example, in 1998, prior to the formation of Ascension, the Daughters announced that they were considering merging Niagara Falls Memorial Hospital, a community hospital located in Niagara Falls, New York, with Mount St. Mary's, a nearby facility owned by the Daughters.[91] The local chapter of Planned Parenthood opposed the merger.[92] In order to defuse the opposition, the Daughters agreed to allow Niagara Falls Memorial to continue to provide surgical sterilizations, Depo-Provera shots, and even abortion referrals.[93] The local bishop approved this arrangement, at least on a temporary basis.[94]

That merger never took place; several years later, however, a New York state hospital commission pressured the parties to revisit it.[95] Ultimately, a full-asset merger between Niagara Falls Memorial and Mount St. Mary's was not pursued, but in 2007, the parties agreed to share some services.[96] The major impasse in the renewed merger negotiations was a disagreement over reproductive services. Niagara had proposed a full asset merger, which would have created an entity that provided a full range of reproductive services at the Niagara Falls campus but followed the *ERDs* at the St. Mary's campus.[97] That approach was rejected by Ascension.[98] On the other hand, Niagara rejected a proposal by Ascension that would have made Ascension the corporate sponsor of the merged entity, with provision for continuing reproductive services outside the combined hospitals through an unrelated entity.[99]

The Daughters' approach in the initial merger negotiations between Niagara Falls and Mount St. Mary's was influenced by advice from Dr. Gerald Magill, a priest and paid consultant for the Daughters, who at the time directed the Center for Health Care Ethics at St. Louis University.[100] Apparently, their long-term plan was to move the provision of reproductive health services to an offsite facility.[101] Professor Magill notes that the offsite strategy is key in resolving ethical dilemmas at Catholic hospitals.[102] "Offsite" may refer to either physical separation or, in some circumstances, separate bank accounts.[103]

The Daughters' flexibility in arriving at what Professor Magill characterizes as "practical solutions to complicated problems" may be seen in several transactions.[104] Naturally, any partnership between a Catholic health care provider and an entity providing sterilizations or other prohibited reproductive services must comply with the *ERDs* and is subject to the approval of the local bishop.[105] And the obvious problem of scandal that will result from any affiliation — however complex and nuanced — between a Catholic hospital system and a system that provides prohibited reproductive service has to be addressed.[106] Thus, the Daughters system, and now Ascension, have struggled to find ways to continue their entrepreneurial activity while maintaining adherence to the *ERDs*.

For example, at Middle Tennessee Medical Center in Murfreesboro, Tennessee — a facility at the time jointly owned by the Daughters and a Baptist hospital — "sterilizations ... [were] performed in the ground floor of the medical center."[107] It was considered separate because it has "its own sign, its own logo, and its own private driveway."[108] In addition, "two corporations were formed to operate the facilities separately, and the women's pavilion . . . [paid] rent to the main hospital."[109]

In Jacksonville, Florida, the Daughters entered into a joint venture that operated five hospitals.[110] Contraceptives, sterilizations, and even abortions were provided in all of these except the Catholic hospital.[111] Accounting was done so that the Daughters did not share in the revenues from these procedures.[112]

Reproductive services have continued to be a roadblock in merger and acquisition activities engaged in by Ascension. In 2002, Ascension called off a proposed merger of St. Mary's Hospital in Amsterdam, New York (a facility acquired by Ascension when it took over Carondelet Health Systems), with Nathan Littauer Hospital and Nursing Home in Gloversville, New York.[113] Under the terms of the proposed merger, Littauer would stop performing abortions but continue to perform tubal ligations.[114] The Merger Watch Project of the Family Planning Advocates of New York State opposed this merger.[115] Ascension called off the merger after the hospitals had overcome a legal challenge from the New York attorney general, who had argued that the merger needed court review to ensure the protection of charitable assets.[116]

Subsequently, however, in August 2008, a merger was announced between St. Mary's Hospital and Amsterdam Memorial Hospital that would result in the discontinuation of some reproductive services at Amsterdam.[117] The merger was subject to regulatory approval by the State Department of Health.[118] Amsterdam apparently did not provide abortions, but had been participating in a state-funded program to provide tubal ligations and contraceptive education.[119] But this program was set to expire, and the utilization of family-planning services at the hospital had been in decline.[120]

In 2003, Ascension ran into additional controversy when its affiliate, St. Thomas Health Services, asked state regulators to block construction of a new surgery center in DeKalb County, Tennessee, that would perform sterilizations.[121] Elective sterilizations had been available at Baptist Dekalb Hospital since 1969, but in 2001 Baptist Dekalb was taken over by St. Thomas and sterilizations were discontinued.[122] St. Thomas had explored plans for a joint venture with the doctors or a sale of the facility.[123] The Dekalb County executive wrote a letter to state regulators accusing St. Thomas of practicing "religious dictatorship."[124] He also claimed that Ascension violated "the constitutional separation of church and state" because it had issued $350 million in tax-exempt bonds to finance the acquisition of Baptist DeKalb and other hospitals in Tennessee.[125]

PART THREE: *The Struggle to Maintain Catholic Identity . . .*

In some more recent activities, Ascension has been able to defuse any controversy over the discontinuation of reproductive services. In July 2007, St. Vincent's Hospital completed a merger with Eastern Health System, the owner of Medical Center East in Huffman, Alabama, as well as hospitals in Blount and St. Clair Counties, Alabama.[126] It was noteworthy that crucifixes were being placed in the newly-acquired hospitals, and copies of the New Testament were being handed out at the time of the merger.[127] There was no significant opposition to this merger, despite the fact that it would result in the discontinuation of sterilizations in the hospital.[128]

There was, however, some discussion concerning the continuation of sterilizations in the acquired facilities. It was announced that physicians at Eastern Urology Associates would continue to perform vasectomies in their offices or at an outpatient surgery center located on the campus of Medical Center East.[129] This policy was justified by the fact that Ascension did not own the medical office buildings on the campus and owned only a small percentage of the ambulatory surgery center.[130] No abortions were performed on the Medical Center East campus prior to the acquisition, and that policy was to continue in force, regardless of building ownership.

With respect to tubal ligations following Cesarean section, Curtis James, the CEO of St. Vincent's, indicated that the patients might be taken to Trinity Medical Center, an unrelated nearby hospital.[131] This was consistent with the approach taken at the main St. Vincent's campus in Birmingham, where patients were taken across the street to an ambulatory surgery center owned by an unrelated company for vasectomies and tubal ligations.[132] This discussion over the availability of sterilizations at Medical Center East resulted in the issuance of a statement by Most Reverend David Foley (the former bishop and at-the-time diocesan administrator of Birmingham) indicating that no sterilizations would be permitted in Catholic hospitals; and that, while he could not control the "contraceptive conversations or practices in a physician's office," he was asking physicians practicing in buildings adjacent to Catholic hospitals to follow the *ERDs*.[133]

Recently, there has been an upsurge in hospitals and systems exploring new cooperative arrangements short of full asset mergers due to "greater cost pressures driving interest in economies of scale."[134] In some instances, these arrangements have also been motivated by the desire to avoid some of the issues related to the discontinuation of reproductive services that would arise in a full-asset merger between a Catholic and non-Catholic system.[135]

For example, in December 2007, it was announced that under a consolidation agreement between Columbia St. Mary's — a system cosponsored by

Ascension — and Froedtert & Community Health in Milwaukee, Froedtert Hospital, an academic medical center affiliated with the Medical College of Wisconsin, would continue to provide abortion training for residents and abortions for patients.[136] Columbia St. Mary's is not wholly owned by Ascension: it is cosponsored by Ascension and Columbia Health System, "a nonsectarian health system."[137] Although the details of the consolidation had not yet been announced, it was contemplated that the consolidation would involve "a financially integrated entity with a single board."[138] A representative of the local Planned Parenthood affiliate indicated it had no problem with the arrangement.[139]

In January 2008, word came that the boards of both Columbia St. Mary's and Froedtert had approved a joint operating agreement integrating the operations of the two systems under an entity to be known as Progressive Health.[140] The current presidents of the two systems would serve as co-presidents of the new entity, which would be governed by a 16-member community board.[141] Each system was entitled to half of the members of the board.[142] The potential economic efficiencies and increased leverage in negotiations with health plans seemed to be the primary motivations behind the merger,[143] but the deal has been characterized as "complicated" and the resulting entity not at "the top of the list of preferred health care affiliations."[144] Under the joint operating agreement, there was to be "separate borrowing and balance sheets but joint investment of profits."[145] There would be a "single integrated strategic and financial plan and a single governing board," but the assets of the two entities would "remain separate."[146] In December 2008, it was announced that the proposed partnership of the two systems had been deferred because of the economic downturn.[147]

It was not clear from press accounts whether the Froedtert-Columbia St. Mary's joint operating agreement had been approved by the Archbishop of Milwaukee. Nor was it clear how the potential ethical problems under the *ERDs* would be avoided. Mark Johnson, a professor of moral theology at Marquette University, acknowledged that "a health care system's purchase of supplies used for procedures that Catholics consider immoral . . . could be considered material cooperation," but merely concluded, "that's where the issue gets more difficult."[148]

The Brackenridge Case: A "Hospital within a Hospital"

Perhaps one of the most contentious and highly publicized ethical controversies involving Ascension resulted from the continuation of sterilization

PART THREE: *The Struggle to Maintain Catholic Identity* . . .

services at Brackenridge Hospital, a city-owned hospital in Austin, Texas, operated by Ascension.

In 1995, the City of Austin entered into a thirty-year lease to Seton Health Care, a Catholic health care system owned by the Daughters of Charity that later became part of Ascension.[149] At the time the lease was entered into, Seton agreed to continue to provide sterilizations, contraception (including emergency contraception), and abortion referrals at the facility.[150] Seton personnel did not provide the services; a separate company provided them, under contract with the city, within the leased hospital.[151] At the time of the lease, Brackenridge Hospital had been suffering significant operating losses, but Seton was operating the facility in the black and providing significant charity care to patients.[152]

However, in 2000, the local bishop coadjutor, Gregory Aymond, stated that the Vatican was dissatisfied with the arrangements at Brackenridge regarding reproductive health services and that Seton and the City of Austin were discussing modification of the lease provisions.[153] In June of 2001, Ascension Health notified the city that it would no longer provide sterilizations at Brackenridge.[154] (There had been about 400 sterilizations performed annually at the hospital.[155]) This announcement came shortly before the United States Catholic Bishops tightened up the Directives to prohibit arrangements like the Brackenridge lease.[156]

In August of 2001, the City of Austin announced that it had developed a plan for the continuation of the provision of sterilizations and other contraceptive services at Brackenridge. Under the plan, a separate licensed "hospital" would be created, on the fifth floor of the existing hospital, to provide services that could not be provided by Seton because of the *ERDs*.[157] The fifth floor would be remodeled to provide contraceptive services, including sterilizations, and childbirth facilities to "400 low-income women a year."[158] "[F]amily planning counseling" and twenty-four-hour urgent care would also be offered on that floor for those in the City-County indigent care program.[159] Under this plan, Seton was to pay $5 million to remodel the fifth floor.[160] The remodeled floor would include a pharmacy, medical records storage, a nursing unit, and housekeeping services.[161] The city would pay $2 million less annually to Seton for taking care of indigent patients, and Seton would pay $500,000 less on its lease.[162]

According to Bishop Aymond, "The Vatican has no problem with the 'hospital within a hospital.'"[163] Although both the Women's Health and Family Planning Association of Texas and the local chapter of the National Organization for Women seemed satisfied with the plan, others were opposed to operation of a city hospital by a religious group.¹⁶⁴ But an editorial in the *Austin American-Statesman* endorsed the plan:

> Providing them [sterilization and contraceptive services] on a separate floor of the hospital is a seamless way to offer reproductive services and still satisfy the more stringent directives from Rome.¹⁶⁵

In October of 2001, the plan ran into some additional difficulty when Seton announced that it would not provide emergency contraception to women who were ovulating.¹⁶⁶ After this announcement, the city announced that it was postponing action on the revised Brackenridge lease agreement.¹⁶⁷ Under the plan, as initially formulated, that service was to be provided in Brackenridge's emergency department.¹⁶⁸ Approximately sixty victims of sexual assault came to Brackenridge each year.¹⁶⁹

Ultimately, however, in February of 2002, the city and Seton finalized a revised lease agreement.¹⁷⁰ The terms of the revised agreement read:

> Starting in July 2003, women who visit Brackenridge for sterilizations or emergency contraception [in cases of rape or sexual assault] will be referred to the fifth floor, a legally separate, city-run hospital that will not be bound by the same directives as Seton.¹⁷¹

"[F]amily planning counseling" would also be provided on the fifth floor,¹⁷² which would be converted at a cost of $3 million to Seton.¹⁷³

In response to revised agreement, the executive director of the Women's Health and Family Planning Association of Texas commented, "It is disappointing that our City has let Catholic religious directives decide what women's health care is in a public hospital."¹⁷⁴ She was primarily concerned about the fact that under the final agreement, emergency contraception would only be available to victims of sexual assault, rather than to any woman upon request.¹⁷⁵ The CEO of the Austin/Travis County Community Health Centers, however, noted that most women seeking emergency contraception who were not victims of sexual assault "will go to a clinic [rather than a hospital], and that's what they should do."¹⁷⁶

A "hospital within a hospital" approach has also been utilized at Columbia Hospital in Milwaukee, a hospital in the Columbia St. Mary's System (discussed *supra*).¹⁷⁷ The Columbia St. Mary's Health System was formed in 1995, under a joint operating agreement between Ascension and Columbia Health System, a nonprofit, nonsectarian community organization.¹⁷⁸ Two of the hospitals in the new system, Columbia Hospital (operated by Columbia Health System) and St. Mary's Hospital (operated by Ascension) were both located on Milwaukee's east side, only about a mile apart, but continued to maintain separate physician staffs following the agreement.[179] Columbia hospital continued to allow its physicians to perform sterilizations (tubal ligations and vasectomies) in the hospital, but St. Mary's hospital did not permit them, in accordance with the *ERDs*.[180]

In August 2000, it was announced that the two hospitals would consolidate cardiac care at Columbia and OB/GYN at St. Mary's.[181] The reason for consolidating the OB/GYN services at St. Mary's was that the hospital had a neonatal intensive care unit and delivered 3,000 babies a year, compared to only 800 at Columbia.[182] Despite this persuasive economic rationale, however, the announcement of consolidation led to a protest by physicians at Columbia, who were concerned that they would not be permitted to perform sterilizations following Cesarean sections at St. Mary's Hospital.[183] The consolidation plans were subsequently placed on hold in anticipation of the 2001 revision of the *ERDs*.[184] A Columbia St. Mary's spokesman indicated that if the revisions by the bishops were too strict, then the consolidation of services might be called off.[185]

Ultimately, Ascension eventually proposed the creation of a 45-bed "independent birthing hospital" within Columbia Hospital.[186] The birthing center would do elective sterilizations, but not abortions.[187] Columbia Health System, the cosponsor with Ascension of the Columbia St. Mary's system, would own and operate the center and proceeds from it would "not be commingled with revenue" from the Ascension-owned facility.[188] The new entity, named Columbia Center, opened on the third floor of Columbia Hospital in 2001.[189] It was separately licensed with its own staff.[190] In 2005, it was announced that St. Mary's and Columbia hospitals would be merged into a single new facility.[191] As a result of the merger of the two campuses, in 2007, it was announced that the Columbia Center would be moved to the Columbia St. Mary's Hospital Ozaukee in Mequon.[192]

PART FOUR

Catholic Health Care and the Right of Conscientious Objection

Catholic hospitals may come under increasing governmental pressures to provide a full range of reproductive services, including sterilizations and abortions, in violation of the *ERD*s. These pressures may result from new conditions being placed on access to government funding, limitations on participation in government programs, or mandates to provide a full range of reproductive services. In the 1970s, after *Roe v. Wade* was decided, it was feared that Catholic hospitals would be forced to provide abortions and sterilizations because of their receipt of federal funding under various programs. Fortunately, shortly after *Roe* was decided, Congress adopted the Church Amendments (discussed *infra*), legislation that protects institutions with a conscientious objection from being forced to provide these procedures even though they receive federal funds.[1]

The enactment of the Church Amendments, in turn, facilitated the widespread adoption of the 1971 *ERD*s by United States bishops; in order to take advantage of their protections, Catholic hospitals had to clearly articulate their moral objections to abortion and sterilization.[2] Over the years, additional state and federal laws have been enacted to protect institutions and individuals from being coerced to participate in abortion and sterilization.[3]

Traditionally, the law has been more solicitous of protecting individual conscience and less protective of institutional conscience. The continuation of a distinctively Catholic health care system in the United States, however, requires legal protection for institutions that refuse to provide abortions and sterilizations. We live in an age where moral objection to sterilization and abortion is countercultural. We are already seeing an erosion of conscience protection for individuals with regard to pharmacists who object to dispensing Plan B (see discussion *infra*). If legal protection for individual conscience erodes, then this also endangers legal protection for institutions that refuse to perform sterilizations and abortions. Currently, there seems to be a concerted attack on conscience protection for Catholic hospitals.[4] Possible enactment of the Freedom of Choice Act (FOCA) and the Prevention First Act (PFA) (discussed *infra*) poses a significant threat to the continuation of Catholic health care, as it could override existing conscience-clause laws.

Moreover, under U.S. Supreme Court precedents, it has become increasingly difficult for Catholic institutions to claim exemption from laws mandating all hospitals to provide a full range of reproductive services. At one time, the Supreme Court used the strict scrutiny test in reviewing the constitutionality of general state laws impinging on the free exercise of religion. Under this test, the law had to serve a compelling state interest and be the least restrictive alternative available to achieve that state interest.[5]

In 1990, however, in *Employment Division, Department of Human Resources of Oregon v. Smith*,[6] the Supreme Court "formally rejected the strict scrutiny test of free exercise and adopted a lower-level scrutiny test."[7] Under *Smith*, the court will not apply strict scrutiny to neutral laws of general applicability, even if those laws have the incidental effect of burdening a particular religious practice, unless there is evidence that the law in question targeted a particular religion.[8] Accordingly, under *Smith*, governmental entities are no longer required to establish a compelling interest in support of general laws that result in incidental burdens on religious practices.

Subsequently, Congress adopted the Religious Freedom Restoration Act of 1993[9] (RFRA) to overrule *Smith* and restore the compelling state interest test. But in *City of Boerne v. Flores*,[10] the U.S. Supreme Court held RFRA unconstitutional as applied to state and local legislation. The gutting of RFRA by the Court removes a potentially significant shield against generally applicable state laws that arguably violate religious liberties. Fortunately, however, some states have adopted their own RFRA-type laws that impose a higher burden on justification for government.[11] And RFRA is still valid with respect to federal laws; it may require the federal government to satisfy the compelling state interest test.[12] But, of course, RFRA could be repealed or modified in an Obama administration — and this in turn would facilitate the enactment of a federal mandate requiring all hospitals to provide abortions.

It is possible that a state could pass a law requiring all hospitals to provide reproductive services, in violation of the *ERDs*, as a condition of licensure.

Indeed, as discussed *infra*, some states have already passed laws requiring Catholic hospitals to provide emergency contraception without regard to limitations set out in the *ERD*s, while other states have passed laws requiring Catholic organizations to provide contraceptive coverage to their employees if they provide them with prescription drug coverage. Under *Smith*, it may be very difficult to convince a court that such laws violate the First Amendment. On the other hand, if the law in question was clearly motivated by animus toward Catholics, or appears to single out Catholic institutions, then perhaps an argument could be made under *Church of Lukumi v. Hialeah*[13] that such a law is subject to strict scrutiny and violates the First Amendment. Otherwise, these laws would most likely be upheld.

Similarly, the federal government could pass a law requiring all hospitals receiving Medicare funds to provide a full range of reproductive services. Generally, this sort of conditional funding restriction has been upheld. For example, in *Rust v. Sullivan*,[14] the court upheld restrictions on the activities of Title X grantees with respect to promoting abortion as a family-planning method. On the other hand, a requirement that Catholic hospitals provide reproductive services, in violation of the *ERD*s, in order to receive Medicare funds could be viewed as a more substantial intrusion into the activities of the grantee than the restrictions on grantee activities upheld by the court in *Rust*. In *Rust*, the grantee could effectively avoid the impact of the law by segregating its abortion activities from its other activities. In the case of Catholic hospitals, the principles concerning material cooperation would still make such a mandate morally problematic, and might even force closure of the institution.

The Embrace of the Sexual Revolution by the U.S. Supreme Court

During the past forty years, state laws based on teachings concerning human sexuality and reproduction advocated by the Catholic Church have not fared well before the U.S. Supreme Court. Indeed, it is possible to view precedents dealing with issues such as contraception and abortion as motivated by an eagerness by some justices to endorse the sexual revolution and limit Catholic power in state legislatures. By the early 1950s, Connecticut and Massachusetts were the only states that continued to enforce laws banning the sale and distribution of contraceptives.[15] Not coincidentally, both states had significant Catholic populations and an active lobby in the state legislature on behalf of Catholic interests on these issues.

PART FOUR

Indeed, in *Griswold v. Connecticut*,[16] rather than allowing the state legislature to continue to deal with the issue of access to contraceptives, the court even invented a new federal constitutional "right of privacy" to strike down Connecticut's ban on the sale of contraceptives to married persons. Likewise, in *Eisenstadt v. Baird*,[17] the court, relying on the Equal Protection clause, struck down a Massachusetts law that had been modified to reflect the *Griswold* decision so as to restrict the ban on sale and distribution of contraceptives to apply only to married persons. Similarly, at the time of *Roe v. Wade*,[18] support for restrictions on access to abortion was viewed as a Catholic issue. Although many states had already liberalized their abortion laws, the court was impatient with the rate of change and, in a sweeping decision, struck down all existing state abortion laws as being too restrictive. *Roe* may be viewed primarily as a decision that removed the abortion issue from the state legislatures because of concern that there was still too much Catholic influence in those bodies.

Of course, the influence of Catholic interests in legislatures has sharply declined since the time of *Griswold*, *Eisenstadt*, and *Roe*, while the influence of the "pro-choice" lobby has significantly increased. And with the shift of cultural attitudes among elites, the current U.S. Supreme Court is unlikely to be receptive to arguments that state or federal laws requiring Catholic hospitals to provide reproductive services, in violation of Catholic teachings, violate the First Amendment. In this context, the Court will more than likely defer to the legislative branch, because the outcomes will embrace values shared by members of the Court. Indeed, sexual autonomy seems to have a preferred constitutional status in the eyes of the current Court.[19]

The combination of judicial commitment to sexual autonomy as a favored right, coupled with the de-emphasis of religious free exercise rights, does not bode well for Catholic institutions. It is clear that under *Smith*, the Free Exercise Clause has been substantially diluted. The states are free to pass neutral laws restricting religious activity by individuals and groups. Religion is now treated much like free speech, with religiously-based conduct being fully subject to state regulation. It is also clear that many members of the Court regard traditional Catholic views on human sexuality to be hopelessly primitive and perhaps even malicious.[20] At the same time, a majority of the justices have shown their high regard for claims based on sexual autonomy by their embrace of the famous mystery passage from *Planned Parenthood v. Casey*[21]:

> These matters, involving the most intimate and personal choices a person may make in a lifetime, choices central to personal dignity

and autonomy, are central to the liberty protected by the Fourteenth Amendment. At the heart of liberty is the right to define one's own concept of existence, of meaning, of the universe, and of the mystery of human life. Beliefs about these matters could not define the attributes of personhood were they formed under compulsion of the State.[22] [citations omitted]

This same passage was later invoked in *Lawrence v. Texas*,[23] the case striking down a Texas law banning homosexual sodomy.

Thus, in any conflict between religious groups supporting traditional attitudes toward human sexuality and persons advocating personal autonomy in sexual matters, it is probable that a majority of the current justices on the U.S. Supreme Court will favor advocates of sexual autonomy. Similarly, they will probably favor patients' rights in matters pertaining to sexuality — i.e., access to reproductive services — over the interests of Catholic health care institutions in continuing to observe the religiously-based restrictions found in the *ERD*s. Accordingly, it would not be surprising for the Court to uphold laws requiring Catholic hospitals to provide reproductive services that are contrary to the *ERD*s. And, unfortunately, it is now clear that "pro-choice" groups, including the American Civil Liberties Union, are seeking to narrow conscience-clause laws in order to mandate the provision of abortion by Catholic hospitals.[24]

Attacks on Conscientious Objection

Dr. Edmund Pellegrino has noted, "In the last fifty years, secularism has come to dominate much of medical ethics."[25] And the trend in medical ethics has been toward increasing emphasis on the physician's obligation to provide the care demanded by the patient and society, rather than on the care that the physician deems morally and medically indicated.[26] The effects of this trend have been compounded by the commercialization and "de-professionalization of medicine."[27] "In such a society, such profoundly religious issues as the morality of abortion, euthanasia, human cloning, and stem cell research are determined on grounds of utility, general consensus, or freedom of choice."[28]

The difficulty that both institutional and individual health care providers face in successfully seeking exemption from laws mandating the provision of reproductive services is exacerbated by the contemporary view of conscience as a judgment that is based on one's own life experiences rather than on objective moral truth. In discussing conscientious objection, James Childress has stated:

> Conscience is personal and subjective; it is a person's consciousness of and reflection on his own acts in relation to his standards of judgment. It is a first person claim, deriving from standards that he may or may not apply to the conduct of others.[29]

In contrast, the Catholic view of the exercise of conscience, as developed by John Paul II in *Veritatis Splendor,* is that of a practical judgment involving the application of the precepts of the natural law to a particular situation.[30] A claim of conscientious objection based on a personal, idiosyncratic reaction should not be entitled to the same level of deference as a judgment of conscience based on objective moral truth.[31] Unfortunately, however, in a contemporary, secular liberal democracy like the United States, where ethical relativism has become the prevailing public philosophy, an appeal to conscience based on objective moral truth is likely to be met with skepticism and even hostility. Indeed, in this society, ethical relativism is viewed as "an essential condition of democracy, inasmuch as it alone is held to guarantee tolerance, mutual respect between people and acceptance of the decisions of the majority, whereas moral norms considered to be objective and binding are held to lead to authoritarianism and intolerance."[32] And the influence of Sigmund Freud has also had a significant impact on attitudes toward conscience: "[t]hough Freud may not have intended it, Freudianism has made conscience suspect."[33]

John Paul II noted that the alliance between ethical relativism and liberal democracy has the potential "to remove any sure moral reference point from political and social life, and on a deeper level make the acknowledgment of truth impossible."[34] This is particularly the case when in comparison or opposition to claims of sexual or reproductive autonomy, perhaps the most cherished of contemporary rights in our highly individualistic culture. And, as Fr. Robert Araujo has prophesied, it may be that the liberal democracies of the twenty-first century will mandate compliance with their beliefs on abortion, euthanasia, and emergency contraception.[35]

John Paul II called upon Christians to not participate in such acts.[36] He characterized the right to refuse to participate in such procedures a "basic human right" and called for governments to provide "those who have recourse to conscientious objection . . . [with protection] not only from legal penalties but also from any negative effects on the legal, disciplinary, financial and professional plane."[37] But he also recognized that the refusal to cooperate in these procedures "may require the sacrifice of prestigious professional positions or the relinquishing of reasonable hopes of career advancement."[38]

At the institutional level, conscientious objection is even more problematic, particularly where the hospital purports to be a community hospital and receives governmental monies.[39] "Pro-choice" advocates argue that permitting Catholic hospitals to refuse to provide sterilizations or abortions limits those services to women. Thus there is a conflict: the right of a Catholic institution to refuse to provide immoral services conflicts with the right of access to those services now recognized as legal. And any argument in favor of exemption from laws requiring a hospital to provide those services may be substantially undermined by the fact that the Catholic hospital is already, in some fashion, involved in either providing those services — as in the case of sterilizations — or involved in partnerships with entities providing such services.

CHAPTER TEN

Protection of Conscientious Objection

Currently, under federal and state conscience-clause legislation, individuals and institutions are protected from having to perform medical procedures that they object to, such as abortion. According to Professor Bassett, the legacy of *Bradfield v. Roberts*[1] is one of governments treating Catholic health care as an essentially secular enterprise that is eligible for the receipt of government funding and fully subject to employment discrimination laws without a religious exemption.[2] It is this view of Catholic health care that necessitated the enactment of conscience-clause legislation in the aftermath of *Roe v. Wade*.[3]

In the 1970s, responding to *Roe v. Wade*, Congress passed the Church Amendments, the original federal conscience-clause legislation.[4] This legislation, named for its sponsor, the late Senator Frank Church (D-ID), is still in effect as of 2008 and prohibits courts and public officials from requiring recipients of federal funds under three specific programs to perform abortions or sterilizations if that would be contrary to their religious or moral beliefs.[5] It prohibits entities that receive funds under these federal programs from discriminating against employees who refuse to participate in the lawful performance of lawful sterilizations or abortion.[6] It prohibits research grantees under certain federal programs from discriminating in employment or the granting of staff privileges against health care providers who refuse to participate in research or health service programs because of religious and moral objections.[7] It prohibits requiring individuals to participate in certain federally funded health service programs or research where participation "would be contrary to his religious beliefs or moral convictions."[8] And it prohibits federal grantees under certain statutes from discriminating against applicants for training (including residents and interns) unwilling to participate in abortions or sterilizations.[9] Its constitutionality has been upheld against an Establishment clause claim.[10]

In the immediate aftermath of *Roe*, most states enacted conscience-clause legislation "in one form or another."[11] There was also sporadic activity at the federal level. In 1988, Congress adopted the Danforth Amendment.[12] This legislation provided that the prohibition of sex discrimination in Title IX could "not be construed to . . . require any individual or entity to provide or pay for abortion-related services."[13] In 1996, Congress passed the Coats Amendment, prohibiting governments from discriminating against medical residency programs that lose their accreditation because of their failure to provide abortion training.[14] And in 1997, Congress expanded conscience-clause protection to Medicaid-managed plans so that they could refuse to provide services or referrals for services they objected to on moral and religious grounds.[15]

The Controversy over the Abortion Non-Discrimination Act

By the early 2000s, it had become clear that existing conscience-clause legislation was inadequate to protect Catholic institutions. Dr. Edmund Pellegrino noted that under some existing laws, Catholic institutions might not be deemed sufficiently religious to qualify for protection unless they served only Catholics.[16] As Maureen Kramlich observed:

> Some federal laws limit the [conscience] protections to specific funding programs. Some state laws do not cover the full range of health care professionals. Others are unclear about whether the protections extend to all forms of objectionable participation (e.g., referrals).[17]

And in testimony before Congress, Professor Lynn Wardle of BYU asserted:

> Existing conscience clause laws are inadequate as drafted for at least five major reasons. First, most are narrow in terms of the practices, procedures or contexts in which they apply — most were drafted with abortion and sterilization in mind and go no further. Second, many of them are very narrow and restrictive, covering only a small group of health care providers, not workers in the health care industry generally. Third, the scope of protection (the discrimination forbidden) is limited. Fourth, the remedies and procedures for vindicating the rights are undeveloped and restricted. Fifth, most of the laws are outdated, having been written before many of the medical developments occurred that have created some of the most difficult moral dilemmas.[18]

The concern about the inadequacy of protection provided by existing conscience-clause laws was heightened by a 1997 case in which the Supreme

Court of Alaska held that a private nonprofit, non-sectarian hospital was required to provide abortions.[19] Groups such as the ACLU, however, contended that conscience-clause legislation had given institutions too much protection and this has resulted in restrictions in the availability of reproductive services.[20] In September of 2002, in anticipation of attempts to narrow the conscience-clause exemptions in order to force Catholic hospitals to provide abortion, the House passed legislation to expand the Coats Amendment.[21] The proposed 2002 legislation, H.R. 4691, referred to as the Abortion Non-Discrimination Amendment (ANDA), was supported by the United States Conference of Catholic Bishops (USCCB) in order to make it clear "that the term 'health care entity' in existing law includes the full range of participants involved in providing health care, such as health care professionals, health plans, hospitals and other health facilities."[22] ANDA did not pass the Senate in 2002; it was reintroduced in both houses in 2003, but once again failed to pass.[23]

In testifying against H.R. 4691, Catherine Weiss, Director of the ACLU's Reproductive Freedom Project, noted that the legislation "could thwart" the enforcement of state and local laws requiring entities certified or licensed by the state to address the full range of health care needs in the communities they serve."[24] She continued by providing an example: "A state might be prevented . . . from denying a 'certificate of need' . . . to a newly merged hospital that refused to provide even lifesaving abortions."[25]

In an attempt to refute this argument, the United States Conference of Catholic Bishops issued a fact sheet noting that only about 14 percent of hospitals currently provided a full range of abortion services; thus, "If states denied licenses and certification to all hospitals that fail to provide the 'full range' of abortions, our health care system would disappear."[26] The fact sheet further noted that "the vast majority of states already have their own conscience laws that would prevent the enforcement of such a coercive and harmful policy."[27] Weiss, however, further argued, "Because it does not define the term 'abortion,' H.R. 4691 could permit health care entities to refuse to provide emergency contraception, even to victims of rape."[28] Again, the Bishops' Conference fact sheet attempted to refute this argument: "Because H.R. 4691 does not provide its own definition of 'abortion' or 'contraception,' it does not change the current federal policy of classifying the morning-after pill as 'postcoital emergency *contraception.*'"[29]

ANDA was deemed by the USCCB to be necessary in order to strengthen "existing law by providing that health care entities should not be forced by government to pay for abortions."[30] Despite the failure to pass this legislation in 2002 and 2003, a coalition of forces — including the Southern Baptist Convention, the Catholic Health Association, the Family Research Council, and the United States Conference of Catholic Bishops — continued to press Congress for expanded conscience protection for institutional providers.[31] And, in support of these efforts, a 2003 memo from the Secretariat for Pro-Life Activities of the United States Conference of Catholic Bishops noted the existence of a widespread campaign to force hospitals to perform abortions.[32]

Finally, in December 2004, an appropriations bill for the Departments of Labor and Health and Human Services, that included the Weldon Amendment, was approved by Congress and signed by President Bush.[33] This legislation prohibits discrimination by the federal, state, and local governments against health care providers who decline to "provide, pay for, provide coverage of, or refer for abortions."[34] The bill enacted was substantially the same as ANDA, with two distinctions. Instead of denying all federal funding to those who engaged in abortion-related discrimination, it only denied funds available under the particular appropriation bill. And, as part of an appropriation bill, it only remained in effect for one year.[35] Nonetheless, this legislation enhanced conscience protection by increasing "both the number and type of health care providers and professionals who may refuse to provide abortion training or services without reprisal."[36] Thus, for example, it permits health insurers and HMOs to refuse to provide coverage or payment for abortions.[37]

Despite attempts to prevent it,[38] the Weldon Amendment was reenacted again the next year.[39] It was also included in appropriations bills in 2007 and 2008.[40] In 2008, a constitutional challenge to this legislation by the California attorney general Bill Lockyer was dismissed on summary judgment by a U.S. District Court in Northern California.[41] This constitutional attack was based on the argument that there was a conflict between the Weldon Amendment and provisions in California state law that required hospitals with emergency services to provide medically necessary abortions, but the court held that this claim was not ripe for review:

> Here, Plaintiffs' claims will not be ripe until a woman needs but is refused emergency abortion-related services, California then attempts to enforce its law requiring the provision of such services, and the federal government denies or threatens to deny California federal funds as a result.[42]

In 2006, the U.S. Court of Appeals for the D.C. Circuit also upheld the dismissal of a constitutional challenge to the Weldon amendment.[43] In this case, the focus was on a potential conflict between the duty under Title X to distribute funds only to sub-grantees that provide abortion counseling and the Weldon amendment, but the court found that the plaintiffs had failed to show the "imminence of any serious dilemma."[44] Removal of the Weldon Amendment from future appropriations bills will, however, be more likely in an Obama administration.

Conscience Protection for Pharmacists

While in general, a pharmacist may refuse to fill a particular prescription for a good reason, state laws vary as to whether a pharmacist may refuse to fill a prescription based upon a conscientious objection.[45] The refusal of some pharmacists to fill emergency contraception and contraception prescriptions has resulted in a flurry of state legislative activity regarding conscience-clause laws.[46] Although in August 2006, the FDA approved over-the-counter distribution of Plan B, the emergency contraceptive sold in the United States to women over eighteen years old, this has apparently not mooted the controversy, because pharmacists still act as gatekeepers for access to the drug.[47]

Although some states have provided pharmacists with a right to refuse to dispense emergency contraceptives, other states have limited this right of refusal.[48] And federal legislation has been proposed that would require pharmacies to fill prescriptions for contraceptives.[49] Although the current debate has focused on contraception, similar ethical concerns have also been raised with respect to the compulsion of a pharmacist to provide drugs to be used in an assisted suicide or legalized direct euthanasia.[50]

Some have argued that pharmacists should not be permitted to refuse to fill prescriptions for Plan B, because this could lead to a situation where emergency contraceptives were not readily available. In an editorial, the *New York Times* has argued that a pharmacist's right of conscientious objection cannot be accommodated, because otherwise it would be possible for pro-life groups to pressure pharmacies to not offer the drug — or in rural areas, there simply may not be a pharmacy available where it could be readily dispensed.[51]

Typically, it is argued that pharmacists or other health care providers who object on moral or religious grounds to performing procedures or providing medications that have become the standard of care should find another line of work.[52] On the other hand, a position paper issued by the ACLU is somewhat more willing to accommodate the religious beliefs of individual providers, but not institutional providers. The ACLU paper states:

A doctor, nurse, or pharmacist who cannot in good conscience participate in abortions or contraceptive services should be allowed to opt out, so long as the patient is ensured safe, timely, and financially feasible alternative access to treatment.[53]

There are now some reported cases dealing with the constitutionality of state rules requiring pharmacists to dispense contraceptives, notwithstanding their conscientious objection. In April 2005, Governor Rod Blagojevich (D-IL) issued an emergency rule requiring pharmacies to fill prescriptions for contraceptives.[54] The governor indicated that the rule was being issued in response to reports that, in February 2005, pharmacists at an Osco Pharmacy had refused to fill prescriptions for emergency contraceptives.[55] In 2007, the Illinois Court of Appeals upheld the dismissal of an action challenging this regulation brought by two individual pharmacists and three corporations that operated pharmacies. The plaintiffs in this action claimed that they believed that life begins at conception, and that the emergency contraceptive can prevent a fertilized egg from implanting.[56]

The Illinois appellate court, however, held that the plaintiffs' claim was not ripe for consideration because it was "extremely unlikely that one of the individual plaintiffs in this case will ever be placed in a position where he will either have to violate his conscience or the letter of the Rule."[57] It also held that the corporate plaintiffs failed to allege that the regulation had any impact on their business.[58] In a dissenting opinion, Justice Turner found that the plaintiffs had stated a claim under a state conscience-clause law, noting that Governor Blagojevich had specifically threatened pharmacists who failed to fill prescriptions because of their religious beliefs.[59]

Plaintiff pharmacists, however, fared somewhat better in a federal court action involving a constitutional challenge to the same regulation. In 2006, in *Menges v. Blagojevich*,[60] a judge in the U.S. District Court for the Central District of Illinois refused to dismiss a constitutional challenge to the regulations by individual pharmacists. In regard to this claim, the court held that plaintiffs' allegation of targeting religious conduct for distinctive treatment could be sufficient to subject the regulations to strict scrutiny:

> The alleged statements by Governor Blagojevich indicate that the objective of the Rule was to force individuals who have religious objections to Emergency Contraceptives to compromise their beliefs or to leave the practice of pharmacy. Governor Blagojevich allegedly stated that the Rule was prompted by pharmacists who declined to fill prescriptions for Emergency Contraceptives because of their religious and

moral opposition to Emergency Contraceptives. He later allegedly stated that the Rule was directed at individual pharmacists who object to dispensing certain drugs on moral grounds and that such individuals should find another profession.[61]

In November 2007, in *Stormans, Inc. v. Selecky*,[62] a federal judge issued a preliminary injunction preventing the State of Washington from enforcing regulations adopted by Washington State Pharmacy Board (the Board) that prohibited pharmacies from permitting pharmacists to refuse to fill a prescription on religious or moral grounds and refer the patient (known as "refuse and refer"). The order specifically focused on refusal to fill prescriptions for Plan B. Plaintiffs were individual pharmacists and pharmacies who claimed that they believe that life begins at conception and that Plan B could operate to prevent implantation of a fertilized egg, so that requiring them to dispense the medication would violate their consciences.[63] The plaintiffs sought the right to refuse to fill the prescription and refer the patient to another nearby pharmacy. The defendants were members of the Board and the Washington State Human Rights Commission (HRC).

Washington state laws provide a right of conscientious refusal, as long as the patient is not denied timely access to services.[64] Initially, the Board had proposed a regulation embracing the "refuse and refer" approach — even though an April 2006 letter from the HRC informed the board that a "refuse and refer" approach would violate Washington antidiscrimination laws and subject violators to prosecution — and that the Board itself would be in violation of these laws if it adopted the proposed regulation.[65] But then Governor Christine Gregoire (D.-WA) intervened and threatened board members with retaliation unless they adopted a regulation that provided no right of conscientious refusal.[66]

After the governor's intervention, the Board adopted a regulation that imposed a duty to fill, disallowed an exemption for conscientious objectors, and largely excluded the "refuse and refer" approach.[67] In a subsequent letter interpreting the regulations for pharmacy owners, however, the Board opined that the rule excluded a "refuse and refer" approach, but further commented that a pharmacist could refuse to fill a prescription if another pharmacist was available on the same shift to dispense the medication.[68] Under this approach, the pharmacy had no right of conscientious objection, but individual pharmacists did have a very narrow right to object.

Plaintiffs in *Stormans* claimed that the regulations adopted by the board violated their rights under the free exercise clause, the equal protection clause, and federal antidiscrimination laws.[69] The court found that the controversy was ripe for adjudication in light of the threat to prosecute contained in the April 2006 letter from the HRC to the Board (which had been posted on the HRC Web site), and the fact that the individual pharmacists' rights would primarily be affected by pressuring pharmacies to employ additional pharmacists if they were to adopt a "refuse and refer" policy.[70]

The court then reviewed the background of the regulations and determined that there was evidence that the defendants had deliberately targeted those who refused to dispense Plan B for religious reasons.[71] On that basis, it applied strict scrutiny to the regulations and determined that, at this point in the litigation, it did not appear that there was a compelling state interest.[72] Accordingly, it determined that the plaintiffs had established a substantial likelihood of success on the merits, and enjoined the enforcement of the regulation as to pharmacists and pharmacies that refused to dispense Plan B and instead referred the customer to another nearby source.[73]

Subsequently, the Ninth Circuit refused to issue a stay pending appeal of the preliminary injunction issued in *Stormans*, holding that the defendants had failed to show irreparable harm would result from allowing the injunction to continue in effect.[74] The Ninth Circuit panel noted that the district court had found that there were no problems with access to Plan B and concluded that the defendants had failed to establish the possibility of irreparable harm.[75] In addition, in 2008, the Wisconsin Court of Appeals upheld an order by the state pharmacy board reprimanding and placing limitations on the license of a Roman Catholic pharmacist employed by K-Mart who had refused to fill or transfer a birth control prescription, and also rejected his free exercise claim under the Wisconsin constitution.[76]

The HHS Provider Conscience Regulations

Although the Church Amendments went into effect in the 1970s, there were not any regulations determining how it and other conscience-clause legislation were to be applied.[77] In December 2008, however, "provider conscience regulations" were issued by the Department of Health and Human Services in the waning days of the Bush Administration. The issuance of these regulations was prompted in part by an opinion issued in November 2007 by the American College of Obstetricians and Gynecologists (ACOG) requiring doctors who refuse to perform abortions to refer patients to abortion providers.[78] This was followed by regulations issued by the American

Board of Obstetricians and Gynecologists (ABOG) that appeared to link board recertification to compliance with the ACOG referral requirement.[79]

The ABOG regulations were objected to by the American Association of Pro-Life Obstetricians and Gynecologists.[80] Michael Leavitt, Secretary of Health and Human Services, wrote to ABOG advising that denial of board certification for failure to make abortion referrals would violate existing federal conscience legislation.[81] An ABOG official responded that it did not have a policy that required abortion referrals and that it was not a requirement of recertification.[82] Secretary Leavitt was apparently not satisfied with this response, and the department reacted by preparing draft regulations to strengthen the right of conscientious refusal.[83] These regulations were issued for notice and comment in August 2008.[84]

The proposed provider conscience regulations were issued out of a concern that the health care field was "intolerant of individual conscience, certain religious beliefs, ethnic and cultural traditions, and moral convictions."[85] It was thought that this environment could discourage persons from "diverse backgrounds from entering health care professions" and promote "mistaken beliefs" that conscience protections did not apply to health care providers.[86] The Department believed that the rules were necessary to increase awareness of conscience-clause laws and ensure compliance with their antidiscrimination provisions.[87]

The proposed regulations clarified the application of existing laws to individuals and institutions, and required recipients of federal funds to certify compliance with these laws.[88] The Office of Civil Rights was designated to receive complaints of noncompliance.[89] Not surprisingly, the Catholic Health Association supported the proposed regulations. It did, however, request that the regulations be clarified to extend conscience protection "to those who understand abortion to include the destruction of an embryo prior to implantation."[90] Also predictably, Catholics for Choice submitted comments opposing the regulations, even contending they would violate Catholic teaching by "imposing the beliefs of conscientious objectors on those seeking abortions."[91]

In the last days of the 110th Congress, Senators Murray and Clinton introduced legislation to prevent the promulgation of the regulations.[92] The final regulations were issued in December 2008 without any significant revisions except as to the compliance certification requirements.[93] The department declined to add a definition of abortion so as to clarify it to encompass drugs that could prevent implantation of an embryo. It is probable that the Obama administration will attempt to rescind the regulations.[94]

The Freedom of Choice Act

Identical versions of the Freedom of Choice Act (FOCA) were introduced in both the House and Senate in the 110th Congress, but never passed.[95] After declaring that access to abortion is "a fundamental right," the proposed act prohibits governments from interfering with "a woman's right" to an abortion "prior to viability" and post-viability "where termination is necessary to protect the life or health of the mother."[96] It prohibits governmental discrimination against women who choose to have an abortion.[97] And it provides a private right of action for violation of the Act.[98] If enacted, FOCA would apply retroactively to every state or federal law enacted prior to its adoption.[99]

Although proponents of FOCA claim that it would merely codify *Roe v. Wade*,[100] a fact sheet issued by the Secretariat for Pro-Life Activities of the United States Conference of Catholic Bishops claims that "FOCA goes far beyond even *Roe*."[101] The fact sheet asserts that FOCA would require that abortion be treated no differently than live birth, thereby overriding a number of state and federal laws.[102] For example, FOCA would require governments to pay for abortions in publicly funded programs, displace the federal ban on partial-birth abortions, and "bar laws protecting a right of conscientious objection to abortion."[103]

An analysis of FOCA by the Office of General Counsel of the USCCB opines that FOCA would render *Planned Parenthood v. Casey*[104] — a 1992 Supreme Court decision that had given states somewhat more leeway in regulating abortion than *Roe* — "superfluous," insofar as it creates "a statutory abortion right that goes beyond what *Casey* and even *Roe* require."[105] Moreover, it opines that "[b]y outlawing *any* interference with the abortion decision, FOCA would bar a broad range of abortion regulations, however slight or *de minimis* their impact on the woman's decision whether to have an abortion."[106] The opinion also notes that the version of FOCA introduced in the 110th Congress does not include language included in earlier versions that would have saved conscience protection clause legislation, and concludes that it is intended to preclude such laws.[107] It states that FOCA "would impose an abortion regime far worse . . . than *Roe*," invite legal challenges to existing federal and state abortion laws, and "put these laws in jeopardy."[108]

In September 2008, this opinion was sent to members of Congress, along with a letter from Cardinal Justin Rigali, Chairman, Committee on Pro-Life Activities, United States Conference of Catholic Bishops, urging members of Congress to "pledge their opposition to FOCA."[109] The letter noted that "[n]o

PART FOUR: *Catholic Health Care and the Right of Conscientious Objection*

one who sponsors or supports legislation like FOCA can credibly claim to be part of a good faith discussion on how to reduce abortions."[110]

On November 25, 2008, a document titled *Advancing Reproductive Rights in a New Administration* was posted on the Obama-Biden transition Web site, with a notation that it had been submitted to the transition team by an outside group.[111] The document lists among its supporting groups the ACLU, ACOG, the Religious Coalition for Abortion Rights, Planned Parenthood, and Catholics for Choice.[112] It lists a number of priority measures for the first hundred days of the new administration, plus additional recommended measures beyond this initial period. The passage of FOCA is mentioned as a longer-term goal, but not as a priority.[113] At this writing, it is not clear how quickly FOCA will advance in the 111th Congress.[114] Although President Obama promised to sign FOCA during his campaign, abortion-rights advocates in Washington may have concluded that there are not sufficient votes to pass it, and that it would not be wise to push such a divisive measure.[115]

In stark contrast with the concerns voiced by the USCCB over the possible impact of FOCA on Catholic hospitals, the headline of an article published by the Catholic News Service on January, 28, 2009, proclaimed: "Rumors Aside, FOCA No Threat to Catholic Health Care."[116] The article contends that there is "no threat" because FOCA is unlikely to pass; and even if it does pass, it will have no impact on Catholic health care.[117] Nancy Frazier O'Brien, the author of the article, blames the "confusion over FOCA" on the commencement of USCCB's postcard campaign against FOCA, and "misinformation" and "false internet rumors" spread by bloggers and Web sites as to what FOCA "would do."[118]

O'Brien quotes Bishop Robert Lynch of St. Petersburg, Florida, a member of the board of trustees of the Catholic Health Association (CHA), as saying that the CHA is opposed to the passage of FOCA, "[b]ut there is no plan to shut down any hospital if it passes" and "[t]here is no sense of ominous danger threatening Catholic health care institutions."[119] CHA president Sr. Carol Keehan is quoted as saying that FOCA "has never contained anything that would force Catholic hospitals or Catholic personnel to do abortions or to participate in them."[120] Keehan further states: "I want to make it very clear that Catholic health care will not close and we will not compromise our principles."[121] Professor Ron Rychlak of the University of Mississippi Law School has noted that Sr. Carol Keehan's and Bishop Lynch's comments could be construed as indicating that if FOCA passes, there will be some sort of civil disobedience to it, but that is not clear from the context.[122] The article appears to be designed to blunt Catholic opposition to FOCA and undercut the USCCB's postcard campaign.[123]

There has been some disagreement among scholars over the possible impact of FOCA. Cathleen Kaveny, a professor at the University of Notre Dame School of Law and a supporter of President Obama, criticizes FOCA because of its divisiveness, but otherwise downplays its impact.[124] She argues that although the text of FOCA is unclear, it is unlikely that it will be construed to override existing state abortion regulations heretofore deemed permissible under U.S. Supreme Court precedents (e.g., informed consent regulations, waiting periods, etc), conscience-clause protection, or restrictions on abortion funding. She also questions the constitutionality of FOCA.[125] On the other hand, Professor Michael Stokes Paulsen of the University of St. Thomas disagrees with Kaveny's analysis of the FOCA text and its constitutionality. Paulsen states:

> Professor Kaveny's essential argument is that FOCA's legal consequences are unclear. With all due respect, this position is simply indefensible under a straightforward reading of FOCA's language and any realistic assessment of how that language would be interpreted and applied. While there is room for uncertainty or disagreement concerning *a few* issues, in the main, FOCA's legal effects are clear. FOCA would invalidate nearly every state and federal law bearing on, or attempting to influence, the exercise of a choice of abortion. FOCA would invalidate nearly every state or federal law substantively disfavoring abortion in the provision of benefits, services, and information. FOCA would invalidate nearly every state or federal law protecting the conscience of medical workers or religious hospitals from participating in abortion. FOCA would likely invalidate nearly any state law prohibiting partial-birth abortion. And FOCA would entrench abortion rights against further meaningful legal challenge.[126]

The potential impact of FOCA on existing conscience legislation is particularly troubling. If FOCA is interpreted to implicitly repeal state and federal conscience protections, then it is possible that individuals and institutions could be forced into performing abortions despite moral objection. Moreover, it would be prelude to changes in federal law that would require Catholic hospitals, as a condition of participation in the Medicaid and Medicare programs, to perform abortions notwithstanding moral objections. It could also set the stage for lawsuits claiming that Catholic hospitals are state actors because of their receipt of federal funds, and thus required to provide abortions.[127] It promises a future of continuing litigation over these matters as it threatens the continued existence of a distinctively Catholic health care system.[128]

e. The Prevention First Act

In January 2009, the Prevention First Act (PFA) was introduced in both the Senate and the House.[129] This legislation would require health insurers that provide coverage for group health plans and health plans that provide prescription drug coverage to include contraceptive coverage.[130] This contraceptive coverage mandate would also apply in the individual market.[131] PFA would also require hospitals that receive federal funds to provide emergency contraception to rape victims.[132] And hospitals would be required to inform sexual assault victims that "emergency contraception does not cause an abortion."[133] There are no conscience-clause protections in this legislation. Judie Brown, the president of the American Life League, has referred to PFA as FOCA's "evil twin."[134] At this time, the passage of PFA seems more likely than the passage of FOCA.

CHAPTER ELEVEN

Mandated Contraceptive Coverage

Legislation has been proposed in Congress to force employers that provide prescription drug coverage for their employees to include coverage for contraceptives, and this legislation does not provide a religious exemption that would cover Catholic institutions.[1] In a letter to the Senate Health, Education, Labor, and Pensions Committee, Gail Quinn, Executive Director of the United States Conference of Catholic Bishops' Secretariat for Pro-life Activities, stated that such a bill would "force church entities to end all prescription drug benefits if they are to avoid violating their fundamental moral and religious teaching on the dignity of human procreation."[2]

A number of states have passed statutes or adopted regulations requiring employers and insurers to provide contraceptive coverage when they provide prescription drug coverage for their employees.[3] Some states have adopted mandates without any conscience-clause limitations, thereby potentially requiring religious employers to provide coverage notwithstanding their religious objections.[4] Other states have provided "broad exemptions" covering all religious organizations.[5] (Naturally, these laws are not problematic for Catholic organizations.) And a few states have passed legislation requiring employer health plans to provide coverage for prescription contraceptives with more narrowly drawn conscience clauses.[6] In some instances, the application of these laws to Catholic institutions is based upon a narrowing of protection under conscience-clause legislation by drawing a distinction between activities that are essentially secular and activities that are essentially religious.[7] While a Catholic parish could satisfy these requirements, a Catholic hospital would not.

One way to avoid complying with these laws is to stop providing health insurance for employees, or at least to cut out prescription drug coverage, but most Catholic entities don't want to drop prescription drug coverage for their employees.[8] Under the Employee Retirement Income Security Act (ERISA), a federal law that preempts most state laws regulating employee benefits, states can mandate that insurers provide certain types of coverage in health insurance policies.[9] Thus, if an employer provides insurance coverage for its employees by purchasing an insurance policy, the contraceptive coverage mandate will apply.[10] On the other hand, under ERISA, states cannot impose coverage mandates on self-insured employer plans.[11] Accordingly, some of the larger Catholic health care systems that self-insure for employee health coverage would not be subject to these state law contraceptive coverage mandates. Smaller Catholic employers, however, cannot afford to self-insure.[12]

Peter J. Cataldo has argued that it is morally licit for Catholic organizations to comply with contraceptive coverage mandates if they have exhausted all attempts to obtain an exemption, and if they provide a disclaimer in any contracts with health insurers or health plan literature to the effect that the benefits are being provided under legal compulsion, and that contraception is contrary to Catholic moral teaching.[13] Cataldo further argues that it could also be morally licit to comply with such laws even if there is a possibility that oral contraceptives provided under the health plan could have an abortifacient effect.[14] And he contends that, as long as these conditions are met, compliance with the law would not seem to create scandal in violation of Directive 45 of the *ERDs*,[15] but he acknowledges that this is a matter for determination by the local bishop.[16]

Clearly, however, it would not be morally licit for Catholic institutions to comply with such laws if the mandate includes RU-486 or any emergency contraceptives known with moral certitude to have an abortifacient effect.[17] Indeed, if such mandates were to be construed to include coverage for emergency contraceptives that could act as abortifacients, or perhaps even RU-486, then the line between abortion and contraception is illusory. Moreover, if Catholic hospitals can be forced to provide contraceptive coverage for employees under their health plans, it's then easier to argue that they ought to be required to provide a full range of reproductive health services to the community.

In this chapter, I will review legal authorities concerning conscientious objection to mandated contraceptive coverage, including a Washington state attorney general's opinion and decisions from California and New York.

a. The Washington State Attorney General's Opinion

On December 14, 2001, the Equal Employment Opportunity Commission interpreted the federal Pregnancy Discrimination Act to require employers to provide contraceptive coverage when they provide prescription drug coverage.[18] Subsequently, in *Erickson v. Bartell Drug Co.*,[19] a federal district court in Washington state held that the exclusion of prescription contraceptives from a prescription drug plan provided by an employer violated the Pregnancy Discrimination Act. This decision was appealed to the Ninth Circuit, but the case later settled and the appeal was dropped.[20] Neither the EEOC ruling nor the *Erickson* case, however, considered claims for exemption on the basis of religion.

In a Washington state attorney general's opinion, however, Washington State's conscience-clause statute was narrowly interpreted as applied to employers with a religious or moral objection to providing contraceptive coverage.[21] The opinion assumed that the employer would otherwise be required to provide such coverage under Washington State's Basic Health Plan.[22] Moreover, it noted that under Washington law, it would be an "unfair practice" for an employer who provides generally comprehensive coverage of prescription drugs to exclude coverage for prescription contraceptive drugs.[23] The Insurance Commissioner requested the attorney general opinion to clarify whether this rule applied to employers with a religious objection to providing contraceptive coverage. The statute mandating contraceptive coverage contained a conscience clause, providing:

> (3)(a) No individual with a religious or moral tenet opposed to a specific service may be required to purchase coverage for the service or services if they object to doing so for reason of conscience or religion.
>
> (b) The provisions of this section shall not result in an enrollee being denied coverage of, and timely access to, any service or services excluded from their benefits package as a result of their employer's or another individual's exercise of the conscience clause in (a) of this subsection.[24]

The Washington state attorney general opinion concluded that notwithstanding the conscience-clause statute, a religiously affiliated employer would commit an "unfair practice," in violation of state law, if it provided prescription drug coverage without contraceptive coverage.[25] The opinion noted that the conscience clause would protect the employer from being coerced into purchasing coverage to which it objected, but the employer could not lawfully charge the employee for such coverage.[26] It then concluded:

> Inclusion of the cost of prescription drug coverage as a component (such as administrative, overhead, contingency, or other expense allowance) in the actuarial analysis of a carrier's rates is therefore permissible under RCW 48.43.065 if it does not require employers to directly purchase the health service that is objected to; ensures enrollees will

not be denied coverage of, and timely access to, any service or services excluded from their benefits package; does not require extra payments by the enrollee to receive coverage; and does not require carriers to provide services without 'appropriate payment of premium or fee.'[27]

b. The California Mandated Contraceptive Coverage Case

In *Catholic Charities of Sacramento, Inc. v. Superior Court*,[28] the Supreme Court of California upheld the constitutionality of the Women's Contraception Equity Act (WCEA), a law requiring most Catholic institutions, including Catholic hospitals, to provide their employees with contraceptive coverage. The WCEA required health and disability insurance policies providing coverage for prescription drugs to cover prescription contraceptive drugs.[29] The act includes a narrowly drawn religious exemption that permits a "religious employer" to avoid the mandate, but distinguishes between Church activities that are essentially secular and those that are religious.[30] In order to qualify for the "religious employer" exemption, these laws require organizations to have as their purpose "the inculcation of religious values," to employ persons primarily of the sponsoring faith, to serve primarily persons of the sponsoring faith, and to be incorporated under the particular provisions of the Internal Revenue Code referenced in the statute.[31] Catholic Charities candidly acknowledged that it did not meet any of these criteria.[32] In addition, the mandate could be avoided by simply not providing any prescription drug coverage for employees, but Catholic Charities argued it had a moral obligation to provide such coverage.[33]

Catholic Charities primarily claimed that the state had violated its First Amendment rights by deliberately targeting Catholic institutions and imposing a mandate with a narrow religious exemption that interfered with the autonomy of the Church in attempting to distinguish between its religious and secular activities.[34] In rejecting these arguments, the California Supreme Court decision is illustrative of the difficulty a religious organization in the post-*Smith* era in mounting a constitutional attack on a supposedly neutral state law of general application that forces it to violate a core belief. The majority opinion of the Supreme Court of California was generally dismissive of Catholic Charities' constitutional arguments. It relied heavily on *Smith* in rejecting Catholic Charities' claims and focused on what it viewed as the benign purpose of the law — i.e., reducing gender discrimination and extending contraceptive coverage to the 10% of women not currently provided contraceptive coverage from commercial insurers.

In this case, the Superior Court denied Catholic Charities' motion for a preliminary injunction, rejecting its contention that the contraceptive mandate was unconstitutional.[35] The Court of Appeals denied a petition for writ of mandate, holding that the Superior Court properly denied the request for a preliminary injunction because plaintiff had failed to establish that it was likely to prevail on the merits.[36] The California Court of Appeals also held that the challenged law did not violate either the Free Exercise or Establishment clauses of the First Amendment.[37] It concluded that the contraceptive mandate was a general law of neutral application that did not violate the religious guarantees of either the United States or California constitutions.[38]

Subsequently, the California Supreme Court granted review in this case.[39] Catholic Charities raised several issues in its Petition for Review, including Free Exercise and Establishment Clause claims under the United States Constitution, as well as a claim under the California State Constitution.[40] Perhaps the most compelling argument made in the Petition for Review is that, in crafting this legislation and its narrow conscience clause, the California legislature deliberately targeted the Catholic Church based on general antipathy toward the Church and contempt for its position on contraception.[41]

The Petition for Review to the California Supreme Court focused primarily on the legislative history of the contraceptive coverage mandate to support its contention that, in enacting the contraceptive mandate, the legislature "deliberately" targeted the Catholic Church.[42] Although the Court of Appeals had rejected the claim that the mandate targeted religious conduct for distinctive treatment and was therefore invalid under *Church of Lukumi Babalu Aye, Inc. v. City of Hialeah*,[43] the Petition for Review contended that the legislative "process evidenced an obvious conflict between the policy interests of the Legislature and the religious freedom rights of the Catholic Church."[44] It further stated:

> Catholic Charities contests the refusal of the California Legislature to exempt Catholic institutions from the mandate and strenuously objects to the deliberate targeting of Catholic institutions by coercing institutions into making a choice between alternatives that are morally unacceptable according to Catholic belief.[45]

The Petition for Review filed by Catholic Charities referred to an extensive legislative history indicating the purpose of the contraception coverage mandate and its narrowly crafted religious exemption was to close "the Catholic gap."[46] For example, a consultant's study relied on by the legislature indicated that 90% of insured Californians already had contraceptive coverage,

PART FOUR: *Catholic Health Care and the Right of Conscientious Objection*

and at a legislative hearing on the proposed mandate, the CEO of Planned Parenthood of California argued that a broadly crafted religious exemption would undermine the purpose of the bill.[47] Thus, the sponsors and authors of the bill crafted an exemption specifically designed not to cover most Catholic institutions.[48] The Petition for Review summarized the legislative history as follows:

> The record establishes that the authors and sponsors of the bill principally wanted to "close the gap" left by Catholic religious institutions, which are a significant and easily identifiable group of employers with an institutional religious prohibition against offering contraceptive insurance coverage. For the authors and sponsors, Catholic religious institutional employers were viewed as the problem — a problem to be "dealt with" by imposing the contraceptive mandate upon them. If such an exemption were needed for constitutional or political reasons, the authors and sponsors posited, that exemption must be deliberately fashioned to exclude Catholic hospitals, universities, and social service agencies. Indeed, if closing the Catholic gap were not the problem, then "granting an exemption" to Catholic employers could hardly be said to "defeat the original purpose of the bill."[49]

Moreover, the Petition for Review contended that the legislative history was replete with evidence of antipathy to the Catholic Church and its position on contraception.[50] It notes that sponsors of the bill repeatedly stated that Catholic teaching on contraception was archaic and not followed by most Catholics and Catholic institutions.[51] It specifically referred to a floor statement by Senator Jackie Speier noting that 75% of Catholic hospitals in California already provide contraceptive coverage to their employees.[52] Senator Speier was also quoted as stating in a floor debate:

> Let me point out that 59 percent of all women of childbearing age practice contraception. 88 percent of Catholics believe in a New York Times poll that someone who practices artificial birth control can still be a good Catholic. I agree with that. I think it's time to do the right thing.[53]

The Petition also pointed to statements made by legislators comparing the Catholic Church to "a witches' coven, a 'new age' bakery, and a chinchilla ranch" as providing further evidence of hostility toward the Catholic Church.[54]

The Supreme Court of California rejected Catholic Charities Free Exercise argument, noting that under *Smith* such a claim would ordinarily be precluded.[55] Catholic Charities, however, argued that notwithstanding *Smith*, strict scrutiny was the appropriate standard for review of this law because the mandate was not a neutral or generally applicable law insofar as it specifically targets Catholic institutions.[56]

Catholic Charities argued that the law is the result of a "religious gerrymander" specifically designed to deny the exemption to Catholic organizations engaged in charitable works rather than purely spiritual works.[57] The court rejected this argument, noting that the law does not treat Catholic employers less favorably than other employers and applied equally to non-religious and religious organizations involved in social work.[58]

Catholic Charities also argued that the exemption was crafted for the purpose of including "as few Catholic organizations as possible and specifically to exclude Catholic hospitals and social service agencies."[59] In this regard, it relied on the legislative history indicating that the purpose of the mandate and the limited exemption was specifically designed "to close a 'Catholic gap' in insurance coverage for prescription contraceptives."[60]

Notwithstanding this legislative history, the California Supreme Court held there was no evidentiary basis for this claim.[61] Specifically, the court rejected Catholic Charities' reliance on the testimony of the Planned Parenthood representative, referring to the necessity of closing the "gap" in coverage.[62] The Court says the "gap" referred to here by the Planned Parenthood representative was the failure of some PPO and indemnity plans to provide contraceptive coverage, rather than the failure of Catholic organizations to provide such coverage.[63] This observation by the court, however, seems disingenuous in light of the fact that the representative refers to the "gap" in the context of opposing an exemption for religious employers.[64]

In affirming the Court of Appeals and upholding the constitutionality of the WCEA despite the extensive evidence of targeting, the Court adopted a very different reading of the legislative history than that put forward by Catholic Charities. And, unfortunately, although not expressly relied upon by the court and questioned by the appellant's brief, portions of the legislative history indicating that many Catholic institutions in California, including several hospitals and the Diocese of Sacramento, were already providing contraceptive coverage to their employees may have seriously undermined the claim that this legislation was a significant infringement on the religious freedom of Catholic institutions.[65] It is possible that, in light of the pattern of widespread dissent on the issue of contraception within the Church, neither the members of the majority in the Supreme Court nor the legislature believed that the objection to providing such benefits was sincere and well-founded.

PART FOUR: *Catholic Health Care and the Right of Conscientious Objection*

The California Supreme Court also rejected Catholic Charities' arguments that the law unconstitutionally interfered with "matters of religious doctrine and internal church governance."[66] In this regard, it found the church property and ministerial exception cases were inapposite.[67] In regard to the question of whether the law impermissibly interferes with matters of Church doctrine, the California Court rejected the contention by Catholic Charities that the legislature improperly took the side of Catholics who dissent from Church teaching on contraception. It specifically rejected Catholic Charities' reliance on the legislative history, particularly comments by Senator Speier, by simply noting "the Legislature's motive cannot reliably be inferred from a single senator's remarks."[68] While there may be some truth in this comment, it ignored the fact that Senator Speier was the moving force behind the bill in the California Senate.[69]

The California Supreme Court further rejected the contention that the exemption violated the First Amendment insofar as it distinguished between the religious and secular activities of the Church. It held that it was perfectly proper for the government to make such a distinction for the purpose of providing an exemption designed to accommodate religious exercise.[70] Similarly, it rejected the argument that the exemption to the mandate violated the Establishment Clause by requiring a governmental inquiry into religious beliefs by noting that here Catholic Charities acknowledged that it did not fit any of the criteria set forth in the exemption.[71]

Catholic Charities further argued that the exemption was vulnerable under the *Lukumi* exception.[72] Catholic Charities claimed that the law was not neutral on its face because of the use of religious terminology in the exemption, but the Supreme Court rejected the *Lukumi* analogy on the basis that the purpose of these references was to provide a religious exemption.[73] Accordingly, the court determines that *Lukumi* was distinguishable because it involved the use of religious language for the purpose of prohibiting religious activity.[74]

Finally, the California Supreme Court rejected Catholic Charities' arguments that the mandate was unconstitutional under the California State Constitution.[75] First, Catholic Charities argued that strict scrutiny applied under the California Constitution, but the court holds that even if strict scrutiny was applicable, the law served a compelling state interest — i.e., gender equity — and was narrowly tailored because a broader exemption would increase those affected by discrimination.[76] Catholic Charities then argued that the statute could not even survive the rational basis test because its criteria were arbitrary: i.e., its exclusion from the exemption of Church bodies providing service or employing persons of other religions was unrelated to any state interest.[77] The Court also rejected this argument, noting that the criterion requiring employment of persons of the same religion substantially overlapped with the constitutionally required ministerial exception.[78] While it acknowledged that the requirement that the organization primarily serve those of the same religion was problematic, it concluded that it was irrelevant because Catholic Charities failed to satisfy any of the other criteria set forth in the exemption.[79]

Justice Brown was the sole dissenter from the Court's opinion in *Catholic Charities*.[80] While the majority opinion found that the freedom of religious organizations to practice their religion was trumped by the demands of gender equity, Justice Brown would have invalidated the law in light of its restrictions on religious freedom. She stated the issue in the case as follows:

> May the government impose a mandate on a religiously affiliated employer that requires the employer to pay for contraceptives — in violation of an acknowledged religious tenet — or to redefine what constitutes religious conduct[?]"[81]

She questioned whether *Smith* was controlling in this case.[82] First, she noted that *Smith* involved "the denial of a benefit to an individual because of a violation of existing law."[83] On the other hand, this case involved a "law that requires a religious organization to provide a benefit despite its theological objections."[84] And Justice Brown's opinion took a much more positive view of the importance of religious liberty than did the majority opinion.[85] She noted that while the church property and ministerial cases were inapposite here, they were merely examples of cases within a broader category of constitutional protection for religious organizations and not exhaustive.[86] She stated, "Some courts have reasoned that religious institutions are exempted entirely from the *Smith* analysis."[87]

Justice Brown was also troubled by the exemption's distinction between religious and secular organizations within the Church and found it to be problematic under Establishment Clause precedents.[88] She observed that, in this case, the exemption provisions represented an "intentional, purposeful intrusion into a religious organization's expression of its religious tenets and sense of mission."[89] As compared with the majority opinion, Justice Brown gave more credence to the legislative history relied on by Catholic Charities indicating religious bias on the part of legislators. She referred to the tension between the traditional views of the Catholic Church on human sexuality and the predominant view that sexual autonomy was the preeminent value.[90]

In this regard, she questioned the religious neutrality of the contraceptive mandate, noting that during the debates over it, the remarks of several legislators indicated they believed that the Church's position was archaic.[91] Specifically, she referred to statements by Senator Speier that most Catholics believe that one can practice birth control and still be a good Catholic, and that she agreed with that position.[92] She also noted that the harm caused by the state's imposition of the contraceptive mandate could greatly outweigh the benefits of the law in light of the relatively small number of employees actually affected.[93] She concluded that the attempt to distinguish between the religious and secular activities of the Catholic Church was "an impermissible government entanglement in religion" and a violation of the Establishment Clause.[94]

Moreover, if the law was determined not to be neutral, Justice Brown questioned whether it would pass the federal strict scrutiny test, since the exemption took "such a crabbed and constricted view of religion that it would define the ministry of Jesus Christ as a secular activity."[95] She also found the narrow exemption "baffling," in light of the fact that religious employers can avoid the impact of the mandate by either dropping prescription drug coverage or self-insuring.[96] Finally, she would have invalidated the narrow exemption under the California State Constitution because of the lack of a compelling state interest; i.e., the evidence showed that 90% of commercially insured Californians already had contraceptive coverage, and only a small number of employees of Catholic organizations would be affected by the mandate.[97]

Justice Brown's views would, of course, be much more protective of religious institutions against state attempts to force them to violate their core religious beliefs. And this seems more in keeping with the values underlying the First Amendment. But in this day and age, if the views of the religious organization in question run counter to the prevailing orthodoxy on sexual autonomy, then they are likely to get short shrift in the courts.[98] It seems clear from the legislative history that the contraceptive mandate and its narrow conscience clause were deliberately aimed at forcing Catholic institutions such as hospitals to provide contraceptive coverage. This is particularly troubling in light of the fact that the mandate could be construed to also include coverage of RU-486, a drug used for the purpose of causing abortions.[99] Accordingly, under the approach taken by the majority in Catholic Charities, it is very likely that a state law requiring all hospitals, including Catholic hospitals, to provide sterilizations and abortions as a condition of licensure would be upheld as constitutional by the California Court.

The California Supreme Court was not particularly sympathetic to the plight of Catholic organizations that now must either drop prescription drug coverage for their employees or run afoul of the Catholic Church's traditional proscription on material cooperation with evil. Catholic Charities argued, under the hybrid rights doctrine, that the provision of contraceptive coverage by Catholic organizations could be viewed as an endorsement of the morality of contraception, and as such the law effectively forced them to engage in symbolic speech that they find objectionable.[100] The hybrid rights doctrine suggests that a free exercise claim could be strengthened if combined with a free speech claim. But the Supreme Court rejected this argument, noting that Catholic Charities was still free to voice its disapproval while providing contraceptive coverage.[101] But this may still be problematic for many Catholic organizations. For example, with respect to Catholic health care institutions, Directive 70 provides: "Catholic health care institutions are not permitted to engage in immediate material cooperation in actions that are intrinsically immoral."[102] And, of course, under the Catholic natural-law tradition, artificial contraception is judged to be intrinsically immoral.[103]

There is also the risk of scandal that would arise from a Catholic institution providing contraceptive coverage to its employees, and this, in and of itself, could be a basis for the moral condemnation of any institutional compliance with a contraceptive mandate.[104] This in turn presents Catholic organizations with a difficult dilemma: either cease providing coverage for outpatient prescriptions in its employee health plan — a possible violation of Catholic social teaching — or create the risk of scandal by complying with the state's mandate.

c. The New York Mandated Contraceptive Coverage Case

Catholic Charities v. Serio,[105] a 2006 decision by the New York Court of Appeals, upheld the New York contraceptive coverage mandate against Free Exercise Clause claims under the state and federal constitution, and Establishment Clause claims under the federal constitution. The New York law at issue in this case, the Women's Health and Wellness Act (WHWA), required employers that provide prescription drug coverage for their employees to provide contraceptive coverage, and contained a narrowly drawn conscience clause identical to the conscience clause in the California law.[106]

The Plaintiffs in this case were "10 faith-based social service organizations that object to the contraceptive coverage mandate in the WHWA."[107] Eight of these entities were affiliated with the Catholic Church, while the other two were affiliates of the Baptist Bible Fellowship International.[108] All organizations considered contraception sinful, and none of them qualified for the statutory exemption. The Court's rejection of the federal Free Exercise Clause substantially tracked the California Court's analysis insofar as it characterized the law as a neutral law of general application under *Smith*, but there was no discussion of any targeting claim by the plaintiffs.[109]

Under the New York Free Exercise Clause,[110] the court modified the *Smith* approach somewhat, opining that those claiming an exemption from a neutral law of general application could prevail by showing "that the State has interfered unreasonably with their right to practice their religion."[111] But the court concluded that the plaintiffs in this case had not made that showing.[112] In support of this holding, the court acknowledged that the WHWA had placed a serious burden on plaintiffs, but they could avoid its impact by simply refraining from providing prescription drug coverage to their employees.[113] It also emphasized that the plaintiffs also hired persons who do not share their religious beliefs and accordingly should "be prepared to accept neutral regulations imposed to protect those employees' legitimate interests in doing what their own beliefs permit."[114] But, of course, the law in question forced the plaintiffs to pay for contraceptive benefits in contravention of their beliefs, while their employees remained free to practice or not practice contraception.

Although the Free Exercise Clause test employed by *Serio* under the New York Constitution was an improvement over the *Smith* test, the court still did not give sufficient weight to the burden placed upon Catholic employers. As Susan Stabile has pointed out, the courts in both the California and New York, betrayed "a fundamental misunderstanding of, and therefore lack of respect for, what it means to be Catholic and what constitutes Catholic religious activity."[115] The narrow definition of the religious entity in the New York and California laws made an artificial distinction between religious inculcation and participation in acts of charity.[116] And the courts failed to recognize that Catholic organizations hire and serve non-Catholics as an aspect of evangelization.[117]

CHAPTER TWELVE
===

Emergency Contraception Laws

The administration of emergency contraception methods has become the standard of care for the treatment of female sexual assault victims.[1] The two most widely used methods "are the combined estrogen-progestin . . . and progestin only methods."[2] "Both regimes consist of two doses of contraceptive steroids taken 12 hours apart after intercourse."[3] In August 2006, the FDA approved the over the counter (OTC) sale of Plan B, the progestin (levonorgestrel)-only emergency contraceptive drug available in the United States, to women eighteen years of age and older.[4] Although combined estrogen-progestin daily birth control pills are still available in the United States, Preven, a single dose combined estrogen-progestin emergency contraceptive, is no longer available in the United States because its manufacturer quit selling it here.[5]

Plan B is supposed to prevent 89% of pregnancies that otherwise occur, while Preven was only 75% effective and had more side effects.[6] The proponents of Plan B contend it prevents fertilization by interfering with ability of sperm to fertilize the ova and by suppressing the LH surge, thereby preventing ovulation or making the ova more resistant to fertilization, but deny that it also works as an abortifacient post-fertilization by preventing implantation in the endometrial lining.[7] Nonetheless (as noted *infra*), controversy continues over whether Plan B can act as an abortifacient.

A 2000 statement issued by the Pontifical Academy of Life indicates that the administration of the "morning-after pill" (which presumably includes Plan B) would not be morally permissible because it could prevent implantation of a fertilized ovum into the uterine wall.[8] But Directive 36 of the 2001 *ERDs* permits the administration of emergency contraception by Catholic institutions where the woman is a victim of sexual assault and "if, after appropriate testing, there is no evidence that conception has occurred already."[9]

In effect, Directive 36 provides for an exception to the traditional prohibition on the use of artificial contraception: in accordance with Catholic teaching, a married woman who engaged in consensual sexual intercourse would not be permitted to resort to contraception to prevent pregnancy, but a sexual assault victim is permitted to prevent conception.[10] The basis for this exception is the right of the rape victim to self-defense.[11] The directive further provides, however, that it is not morally permissible "to initiate or recommend treatments that have as their purpose or direct effect the removal, destruction, or interference with the implantation of a fertilized ovum."[12]

The Prevention First Act (PFA), proposed federal legislation introduced in the 111th Congress, would cut off federal funds to hospitals that do not provide emergency contraception to female sexual assault victims, regardless of any moral objection on the part of a Catholic hospital.[13] In addition, there has been a flurry of state legislation concerning emergency contraceptives, and several states have passed legislation requiring health care providers to dispense emergency contraceptives to sexual assault victims.[14] For example, California has adopted legislation that requires physicians and other health care providers to provide female victims of sexual assaults with "postcoital contraception."[15] This legislation does not contain a conscience clause.

Similarly, Washington state law requires every hospital that treats rape victims, including Catholic hospitals, to: (1) provide the victim accurate and unbiased information about emergency contraception; (2) orally inform the victim that she has the option to receive emergency contraception at the hospital; and (3) provide emergency contraception to every victim who requests it, unless there is a medical reason not to do so.[16] This law also requires printed informational materials to be distributed and used in all emergency rooms in the state.[17] In addition, there is a specific requirement that the Washington State Department of Health respond to complaints about the failure of hospitals to comply with the emergency contraception mandate.[18]

New York has also adopted a law requiring all hospitals to provide emergency contraception to rape victims without any conscience-clause protection.[19] It does, however, provide that emergency contraception need not be provided to rape victims who are pregnant.[20] In 2007, Connecticut adopted a law requiring all hospitals to provide emergency contraception to victims of sexual assault, and this law does not contain a conscience clause.[21] The law does permit the administration of a pregnancy test and does not require that an emergency contraceptive be made available if the victim is already pregnant, but it does not permit the administration of an ovulation test or the right not to provide the medication if the victim has already ovulated.[22]

Initially, the Connecticut Catholic Conference and the Connecticut bishops opposed the legislation, but after its passage, the bishops issued a statement that Catholic hospitals in Connecticut would comply with the law.[23]

The bishops' statement noted that the teaching authority of the Church had not "authoritatively resolved" the morality of the administration of an emergency contraceptive to a victim of sexual assault without the prior administration of an ovulation test.[24] They further opined that such an act was not morally equivalent to an abortion because of uncertainty as to whether it could prevent implantation and thus could not be considered "intrinsically evil."[25] The National Catholic Bioethics Center subsequently issued a statement in response to the action by Connecticut bishops, indicating that while it understood the position of the Connecticut bishops that failure to administer an ovulation test was not "intrinsically evil," there was "virtual unanimity that an ovulation test should be administered before giving an anovulant medication."[26]

State laws mandating provision of emergency contraception without conscience-clause limitations may be problematic for Catholic hospitals. As discussed *infra*, some argue that it is not morally permissible for a Catholic hospital to provide emergency contraception to a rape victim who is ovulating because of the potential abortifacient effect of emergency contraceptive medications. But state laws mandating provision of emergency contraception to all rape victims, without any conscience-clause limitations, would not permit denial of emergency contraceptive based on moral considerations. Thus, laws of this type could require Catholic hospitals to disregard their local bishop's interpretation of the *ERD*s and may establish a dangerous precedent: if they go along with laws of this type without protest, policy makers may in turn assume that Catholic hospitals are not all that serious about maintaining compliance with the *ERD*s.

The adoption of these laws has been fostered by studies claiming many Catholic hospitals do not provide emergency contraception to rape victims, even within the parameters set forth in Directive 36. In a small pilot study of the actual practices of hospitals published in 2000, the authors telephoned the emergency departments of seventy-eight large hospitals located in urban areas to ask a series of questions on the availability of emergency contraception to rape victims.[27] The questions focused on whether the hospitals permitted the discussing or dispensing of emergency contraception, whether the hospital made referrals for emergency contraception, and the number of rape cases treated.[28] Staff members at nine of the hospitals refused to answer the questions; staff at another eleven indicated they did not provide treatment for rape victims.[29] The final pool for the study consisted of fifty-eight hospitals, twenty-seven of which were Catholic hospitals.[30] The study found that seven of the Catholic hospitals had policies prohibiting physicians from prescribing contraceptives, and five of these seven also prohibited physicians from discussing contraceptives with patients.[31] Twelve of the Catholic hospitals had policies prohibiting discussion of emergency contraception with rape victims.[32] Notwithstanding these policies, respondents at eight of the twelve hospitals indicated "that relevant information would likely be provided to rape victims."[33] Seventeen of the Catholic hospitals prohibited the dispensing of emergency contraception in their hospital pharmacies.[34] It was also noted that several Catholic hospitals had no restrictions on the availability of emergency contraception, but the issue was considered to be controversial even at these institutions.[35]

As to the morality of providing emergency contraception in Catholic hospitals, the study notes: "The proscription on the use of contraceptive does not apply in case of rape."[36] It also notes that provision of emergency contraception may be impermissible under Catholic teaching where it prevents implantation of an embryo in the endometrium.[37] But it states:

> Testing a rape victim to determine whether conception has occurred as a result of rape is not feasible, and the most that can be accomplished is an extremely rough judgment of probabilities.[38]

Nonetheless, it opines that under the principle of double effect, it is morally permissible for providers in Catholic hospitals to provide rape victims with emergency contraception where their intent is to prevent ovulation or conception, even though they realize that the effect could be abortifacient.[39]

A 2002 study conducted by Ibis Reproductive Health for Catholics for a Free Choice targeted the practices of Catholic hospitals with respect to Emergency Contraception (EC) and identified the *ERDs* as "a potential obstacle to the provision of EC in hospital emergency rooms."[40] Notwithstanding Directive 36, this study opines:

> In spite of ample medical evidence to the contrary, the dominant view among the US bishops is that EC can work to cause an abortion and, therefore, must be forbidden in all circumstances.[41]

The Catholics for a Free Choice study was conducted in late August 2002. Its surveyors called virtually all of the Catholic hospital emergency rooms in the United States to question "the triage nurse or whoever else answered the phone about the availability of emergency contraception in the emergency room."[42] The study concluded:

Only 5% of the emergency rooms provided EC on request. An additional 23% of Catholic emergency rooms provide EC to rape victims only. Thus, only 28% of Catholic ERs will provide women who have been raped with EC. Among those hospitals that do provide EC to rape victims, the majority set up unnecessary barriers, such as pregnancy tests or police reports. These hospitals also do not volunteer information over the phone, but admit to dispensing EC to rape victims only after repeated questioning, which could deter some victims. Some hospitals (6%) indicated that the decision about providing EC was left to the attending physician. Presumably, with good luck, a woman who had been raped might be seen by an attending physician who would provide EC, but there were no guarantees.[43]

The results of the Catholics for a Free Choice study have been widely reported and have been used both to promote popular support for legislation mandating the provision of emergency contraception and to place greater pressure on public agencies to enforce existing legislation.

Sexual Assault Protocols Developed by Catholic Hospitals

If Plan B does prevent implantation of the fertilized ovum in the endometrium, then state laws requiring Catholic hospitals to provide emergency contraception to rape victims could conflict with the *ERDs*. Bioethicists employed by Catholic hospitals differ in their approaches to the application of Directive 36, due to the uncertainty over whether emergency contraceptive medications could have an abortifacient effect. Some bioethicists working with Catholic hospitals are extremely skeptical as to whether emergency contraception treatments can have an abortifacient effect,[44] while others believe they may.[45]

Directive 36 seems to recognize the possibility of an abortifacient effect in that it prohibits any treatments that would interfere with implantation of a fertilized ovum.[46] Directive 36 permits the treatment with emergency contraception medications "[I]f, after appropriate testing, there is no evidence that conception has occurred already." But since Directive 36 "does not spell out precisely what constitutes 'appropriate testing' and 'evidence that conception has occurred,'" there is disagreement as to its application.[47]

Two approaches to the issue have emerged: the ovulation approach and the pregnancy approach.[48] The ovulation approach relies on testing to determine whether the victim is ovulating, in order to avoid providing emergency contraceptive medications that could have an abortifacient effect. The pregnancy approach discounts the possibility of an abortifacient effect and focuses on testing to determine whether the victim has some preexisting pregnancy.[49] If the victim is pregnant, then no emergency contraception would be provided. Of course, in this case, no emergency contraception would be needed — the pregnancy would not have resulted from the rape, and the medication would not interfere with an existing pregnancy.[50]

The arguments in favor of the pregnancy approach are based on the assumption that emergency contraceptive medications do not have an abortifacient effect.[51] But proponents of the pregnancy method may "have overstated the case against the abortifacient effects of high-dose estrogen-progestin pills."[52] Some studies indicate that emergency contraception methods "may impair endometrial receptivity to the implantation of a fertilized egg."[53] In a 2001 article reviewing the literature on the mechanism of action for various emergency contraception medications, the authors conclude there is "no clearcut answer to the question" of how emergency contraception medications prevent pregnancy.[54] And here is what the manufacturer says about Plan B:

> How does Plan B® work?
>
> Plan B® contains a dose of the hormone levonorgestrel that is higher than in a single birth control pill. Levonorgestrel has been used in birth control pills for over 35 years. Plan B® works like a birth control pill to prevent pregnancy mainly by stopping the release of an egg from the ovary. It is possible that Plan B® may also work by preventing fertilization of an egg (the uniting of sperm with the egg) or by preventing attachment (implantation) to the uterus (womb), which usually occurs beginning 7 days after release of an egg from the ovary. Plan B® will not do anything to a fertilized egg already attached to the uterus. The pregnancy will continue. [55]

But a recent article in the *National Catholic Bioethics Quarterly* discounts both the significance of earlier studies indicating that Plan B could be an abortifacient and the manufacturer's labeling information. It cites recent studies undermining claims that Plan B could act as an abortifacient and asserts that "[l]abels mean nothing without the scientific data to back up their claims."[56]

Proponents of the ovulation approach point to the possibility of an abortifacient effect as the basis for their concerns. Some physicians argue that since it potentially prevents implantation, emergency contraception should be regarded as an abortifacient.[57] And Kevin O'Rourke, a Catholic moral theologian who favors the ovulation approach, argues:

> Although impregnating a woman through rape would be a great injustice, it would not be so great an injustice as killing an infant whom rape had brought into being.[58]

So, although science has not at this time authoritatively determined that emergency contraceptives have an abortifacient effect, neither has that possibility been authoritatively rejected. Accordingly, proponents of the ovulation approach use the analogy of the hunter in the woods who sees movement behind a bush but cannot discern whether it is a deer or a human. Under these circumstances, it would not be morally permissible for the hunter to shoot whatever is behind the bush.[59]

Proponents of the pregnancy approach reject this analogy as inapposite; while the hunter's intention is to kill what is behind the bush, the intention of the provider administering emergency contraceptive medication is to prevent conception.[60] While intention can be hard to prove, the more likely intention may often be to prevent pregnancy by whatever means necessary. Proponents of the pregnancy approach also point to the lack of absolute proof of an abortifacient effect, but this merely increases the level of uncertainty. Certainly, it would still be morally impermissible for the hunter to shoot, even if he was some distance from the target and a poor shot.

The most prominent example of the ovulation approach is what is now known as the "Peoria Protocol," developed in 1995 by Joseph Piccione and Gerard McShane for use at St. Francis Hospital in Peoria, Illinois.[61] Directive 36 requires the hospital to conduct tests to determine whether conception has already occurred and permits administration of emergency contraception if the test is negative.[62] But, as noted by Fr. Kevin O'Rourke, the requirement of pregnancy testing seems a bit peculiar — any detectable conception would have had to result prior to the rape, in light of the fact that such tests are not reliable until ten days after conception has occurred.[63] In addition, according to O'Rourke, the second requirement is also problematic: Ovral, an oral contraceptive medication provided to suppress ovulation, will also act as an abortifacient by preventing implantation.[64] O'Rourke concludes, therefore, that the timing of ovulation is the critical determination in preventing a possible abortion induced by taking Ovral.[65] Thus, the Peoria Protocol uses a progesterone test and a urine dipstick test to ascertain the presence of luteinizing hormones (LH).[66] O'Rourke summarizes:

PART FOUR: *Catholic Health Care and the Right of Conscientious Objection*

If the LH test is negative and supported by progesterone level findings, ovulation is not occurring and Ovral may be used. If the LH test is positive, the process of ovulation is under way and Ovral should not be used. The method seems to obviate the quandary that occurs when a rape victim is unsure whether she has ovulated.[67]

The Peoria Protocol specifically notes that it provides for "contraceptive intervention" only where "there is a clinical indication that the effect of the intervention will be truly contraceptive and not abortifacient."[68] The clinical determination that the contraceptive intervention would not be abortifacient is based on the following: (1) the menstrual history of the victim; (2) a blood test to determine hormone levels in order to determine the timing of the ovulatory cycle; and (3) an OvuKit urine test to determine whether ovulation has begun[69] By requiring both the urine dipstick test and the progesterone level test, the Peoria Protocol goes beyond other ovulation approach protocols.[70]

The Peoria Protocol has been approved by the Illinois State Department of Public Health.[71] Under Illinois law, hospitals that care for sexual assault victims are required to develop a protocol to ensure that victims will receive information on emergency contraception.[72] The protocol must be submitted to the state Department of Public Health for approval.[73] Under the Illinois law, the information provided to sexual assault victims must include:

> ... medically and factually accurate and written and oral information about emergency contraception; the indications and counter-indications and risks associated with the use of emergency contraception; and a description of how and when victims may be provided emergency contraception upon the written order of a physician licensed to practice medicine in all its branches.[74]

The implementing regulations adopted by the Illinois Department of Public Health also set forth sample protocols, including one developed by the Catholic Hospital Association.[75] Under the Catholic Hospital Association protocol, a sexual assault victim who tests negative for pregnancy on the blood test and also has a negative result on the urine dipstick test is to be offered Ovral, but if she tests positive on either of the tests, she will be told that the emergency department will not provide Ovral.[76] Moreover, if the woman is determined to be in her midcycle LH surge or in the early post-ovulatory stage, then Ovral or its equivalent will not be provided.[77]

Another example of the ovulatory approach is seen in the *Guidelines for Catholic Hospitals Treating Victims of Sexual Assault*, as approved by the

Board of Governors of the Pennsylvania Catholic Conference.[78] These guidelines provide that no antiovulant drugs may be used if the pregnancy test is positive.[79] They emphasize that medical interventions are permitted "as long as there is no anticipated effect of an abortifacient."[80] Thus it is permissible to "use medications which prevent ovulation, sperm capacitation, or fertilization."[81] If the pregnancy test is negative, then clinical determinations would be based on: "a menstrual history provided by the victim;" "hormonal levels as determined by a blood test to categorize the timing of a woman's ovulatory cycle;" and "results of a urine test which is a reliable guide to the prediction of ovulation."[82] The Pennsylvania guidelines go on to state: "If the urine test is positive, this would indicate the hormonal shift to ovulation has begun. The use of a contraceptive steroid intervention could be abortifacient and is therefore not permitted, even though there might be no evidence that conception has occurred."[83]

The ovulatory approach has been criticized as imposing unacceptable limitations on the moral options available under Directive 36, insofar as the directive itself does not explicitly prohibit the use of emergency contraceptive medications in women who have recently ovulated or are about to ovulate.[84] This criticism, however, seems a bit disingenuous; Directive 36 does prohibit use of treatments that have as "their purpose or direct effect . . . interference with the implantation of a fertilized ovum."[85] And in addition, Directive 45 clearly prohibits "[e]very procedure whose sole immediate effect is the termination of pregnancy before viability . . . which . . . includes the interval between conception and implantation of the embryo."[86]

Perhaps more persuasively, critics of the ovulatory approach also point out that conception only occurs when fertilization is complete, and fertilization is a process that occurs over a twenty-four-hour period.[87] Accordingly, they argue that it is morally permissible to administer emergency contraception to any sexual assault victim who comes to the emergency treatment within that twenty-four-hour-period.[88] They bolster their argument by noting that it is very unlikely that a conception will occur as a result of rape.[89] They further argue that the weight of medical evidence at this time does not support the notion that emergency contraception medications act as an abortifacient by preventing implantation.[90] And they criticize the Peoria Protocol as seeking absolute certainty, emphasizing "the extremely small risk of destruction of a conceptus."[91] Finally, they argue that proponents of the ovulation approach have distorted the moral object of administering the emergency contraception medication to a woman who is ovulating in light of the small risk of preventing implantation.[92]

PART FOUR: *Catholic Health Care and the Right of Conscientious Objection*

In contrast to the ovulation approach, the pregnancy approach tests only for an existing pregnancy. If the test result is negative, then the victim would be offered emergency contraception.[93] Of course, as noted by O'Rourke, the problem with this approach is that a pregnancy resulting from the rape would not show up for at least ten days following the incident.[94] Nonetheless, proponents of the pregnancy approach argue that it is morally preferable for several reasons. They argue that no tests can provide evidence of conception from recent sexual assault and prior pregnancy is ruled out so as to protect a developing embryo.[95] They argue that the ruling out of a prior pregnancy provides sufficient moral certainty in light of relatively unlikely chance of a conception occurring because of rape and the lack of scientific studies establishing an abortifacient effect for emergency contraceptive medications. In this regard, they characterize the moral object of the administration of the medication as being the preventing of conception rather than the prevention of implantation. They also refer to a proportionate justification for the act — i.e., "the prevention of pregnancy resulting from the sexual assault and its subsequent impact on the overall well-being of the woman."[96] Finally, they argue that the Catholic moral tradition does not always require taking the safest approach. In this regard, they point to the principle of double effect as applied in the cases of administering morphine to patients in severe pain, even if that may hasten death, and the allowance for the bombing of military targets in wartime, even if there is some risk of collateral damage to civilian targets.[97]

In September 2008, the Congregation for the Doctrine of the Faith issued an instruction dealing with certain bioethical issues, including emergency contraception, that seems to support the approach taken in the Peoria Protocol. In discussing "interceptive methods" of birth control, the instruction refers to "morning-after pills," noting:

> It is true that there is not always complete knowledge of the way that different pharmaceuticals operate, but scientific studies indicate that *the effect of inhibiting implantation is certainly present*, even if this does not mean that such interceptives cause an abortion every time they are used, also because conception does not occur after every act of sexual intercourse. It must be noted, however, that anyone who seeks to prevent the implantation of an embryo which may possibly have been conceived and who therefore either requests or prescribes such a pharmaceutical, generally intends abortion.[98]

On this basis, and in light of the CDF's recognition that emergency contraceptives can prevent implantation, thereby acting as an abortifacient,

Marie Hillard argues that, in order to avoid immediate material cooperation with evil, Catholic hospitals must have moral certainty that emergency contraceptives will not prevent implantation of a fertilized ovum before providing it in accordance with a government mandate or a patient's request.[99] And, she argues, "the ovulation test provides this certainty."[100] She further observes that emergency contraception cannot prevent ovulation once the LH surge has begun and cannot interfere with sperm capacitation so as to prevent fertilization.[101] Thus, the only reason that an emergency contraceptive can be given is to prevent ovulation, and "moral certitude can be achieved only through the administration of the LH test."[102] She concludes that Catholic health care providers should not capitulate to legislative mandates requiring them to provide emergency contraception to sexual assault victims without performing the LH test.[103]

PART FIVE

End-of-Life Care

Introduction

Unlike secular bioethics, individual autonomy is not the ultimate value in Catholic bioethics.[1] Indeed, the Catholic natural-law tradition has long condemned suicide and voluntary euthanasia.[2] It has also, however, been recognized that while patients are morally obligated to accept "ordinary" medical treatment, treatment that is considered "extraordinary" may be refused even if the result of non-treatment may be to hasten death.[3]

Under the *ERD*s, Catholic hospitals are morally obligated to follow Catholic teaching in withdrawing medical treatment notwithstanding the preferences of the patient or the patient's surrogate decision maker.[4] At times, however, this moral obligation may be in tension with the patient's legal right to refuse treatment.[5] Ordinarily, it is the patient or the patient's surrogate who makes the determination as to whether the proffered treatment is extraordinary and thus may be refused.[6]

Certainly, under Catholic teaching, a competent patient is the "primary decision maker," but the patient is morally "bound by norms that prohibit the directly intended causing of death through action or omission and by the distinction between ordinary and extraordinary means."[7] In the case of incompetent patients, it is appropriate that family members or a guardian who share "the patient's moral convictions" act as surrogate decision makers, but these surrogate decision makers are morally obligated to make decisions in accordance with these norms, even if they believe that the patient would have decided otherwise.[8] And a health care provider, while ordinarily required to accede to the wishes of the patient or the appropriate surrogate decision maker, is morally obligated to refuse to participate in a course of treatment "which he or she views as clearly immoral."[9]

When the availability of more advanced forms of artificial nutrition and hydration (ANH) made it possible to sustain the life of unconscious patients for several years, the question arose among ethicists working in the Catholic tradition as to whether it was morally permissible to withdraw ANH from a patient in a persistent vegetative state (PVS).[10] This issue has been debated among Catholic bioethicists over the past three decades with some arguing that continuing to provide ANH for PVS patients is not morally obligatory while others have argued that it is in most cases.[11] A 2004 statement by Pope John Paul II, and a more recent clarification of this statement by the Congregation for the Doctrine of the Faith, have, however, indicated that the continued administration of ANH and nutrition for PVS patients is morally obligatory in most cases.[12]

The disagreement of Catholic bioethicists on this issue was brought to the forefront by the case of Terri Schiavo, a young woman who has been diagnosed by some physicians as being in a persistent vegetative state. This case involved a dispute between the parents of Terri Schiavo, devout Catholics who wished to continue to provide their daughter with ANH, and her husband who wished to withdraw it. Both sides in the dispute were relying on statements by Catholic bioethicists to support their positions. After a lengthy legal dispute, the husband prevailed and ANH was withdrawn. Terri died shortly thereafter.

The labeling of patients as being in a PVS is controversial with some, including John Paul II, who has characterized the term "vegetative" as an adjective that deprives the patient of human dignity.[13] He has also questioned whether "persistent vegetative state" is a helpful diagnostic category, noting that "there are well-documented cases of at least partial recovery even after many years" of patients with this diagnosis.[14]

The socio-legal shift in favor of physician-assisted suicide and euthanasia is well under way in Europe[15] and is becoming more prevalent in the United States. No state at this time has legalized euthanasia, although it seems probable that it is being practiced in some hospitals in the United States.[16] Both Oregon[17] and Washington state[18] now have laws permitting physician-assisted suicide. Both the Oregon and the Washington laws contain exemption clauses for health care providers who conscientiously object to participation in physician-assisted suicide.[19] In addition, in December 2008, a trial court judge in Montana ruled that terminally ill patients had a right to physician-assisted suicide under the Montana Constitution.[20]

The recent clarification of Catholic teaching substantially limiting the withdrawal of ANH from PVS patients (discussed *infra*) will, if implemented in Catholic hospitals, put them at odds with what has become the prevailing practice. All of these developments suggest that in end-of-life care, increased pressure will be brought to bear on Catholic hospitals to provide care in conflict with the *ERD*s and Catholic teaching. At some point, there could even be mandates enforced by threatened withdrawals of federal funding.

Chapter Thirteen

Catholic Teaching on End-of-Life Care

In the Catholic natural-law tradition, certain specific moral norms are "absolute and exceptionless," while others, while being true, are not absolute.[1] An example of the former is the prohibition on the intentional taking of innocent human life.[2] Accordingly, the prohibitions on euthanasia and suicide are also considered absolute norms.[3] The principle of double effect also plays a significant role in the traditional Catholic natural-law approach to end-of-life issues. For example, the principle of double effect treats as morally licit the use of painkillers such as morphine for terminally ill persons, even if the effect of such painkillers may be to hasten death, if the intent is to relieve suffering rather than to cause death.[4]

The distinction between ordinary and extraordinary treatment dates back to the sixteenth century.[5] In recent years it has become more common to replace the terms "ordinary" and "extraordinary" with the terms "proportionate" and "disproportionate" care.[6] This focus on proportionality places less emphasis on the particular means of treatment and greater emphasis on the context and ends of treatment.[7] The methodology employed by some Catholic bioethicists in this area focuses on the relative benefits and burdens of treatments in determining whether a particular medical treatment is disproportionate and thus may be withdrawn or refused.[8] But others focus more on the quality of life to be sustained by the treatments.[9]

In a 1957 address to a group of anesthesiologists, Pope Pius XII explicitly drew the distinction between ordinary and extraordinary treatment in response to a specific question:

> Does the anesthesiologist have the right, or is he bound, in all cases of deep unconsciousness, even in those that are considered to be completely hopeless in the opinion of the competent doctor, to use modern artificial respiration apparatus, even against the will of the family?[10]

In answering the question, Pius XII opined that one is required to accept only "ordinary" treatments to preserve life — i.e., "means that do not involve a grave burden for oneself or another."[11]

In 1980, the Sacred Congregation for the Doctrine of the Faith, with the approval of Pope John Paul II, issued a *Declaration on Euthanasia*[12] that retained and expanded on the 1957 address and other papal statements in light of "new aspects of the question of euthanasia" that have been brought about "by the progress of medical science."[13] The *Declaration* rejects both suicide[14] and euthanasia, i.e., intentionally causing another's death in order to eliminate suffering.[15] In discussing the "Value of Human Life," the *Declaration* notes that "Everyone has the duty to lead his or her life in accordance with God's plan."[16] Accordingly, because our lives were "entrusted" to us by God, suicide is equated with murder and "considered as a rejection of God's sovereignty and loving plan."[17] Similarly, with respect to euthanasia, "the killing of an innocent human being," including those "suffering from an incurable disease, or a person who is dying," is impermissible.[18] It is also morally impermissible for a person to ask to be killed, to request it for others, or to "consent to it, either explicitly or implicitly."

In the section titled "Due Proportion In the Use of Remedies," the *Declaration on Euthanasia* focuses on the moral obligations of the sick person or those charged with that person's care, whether family members or health care providers, to accept or provide various modes of treatment. It acknowledges the potential complexity of these decisions and the difficulty in applying ethical principles in a given case.[19] While reiterating the traditional principle that no one is obligated to use "'extraordinary' means," the *Declaration* acknowledges that the obligation "is perhaps less clear today, by reason of the imprecision of the term and the rapid progress made in the treatment of sickness."[20] It notes that "some people prefer to speak of 'proportionate' and 'disproportionate' means rather than 'ordinary' and 'extraordinary'"[21] Kevin O'Rourke observes that this reference to the change in terminology may have been motivated by a prior tendency to determine whether a particular means of treatment was "ordinary" without reference to the condition of the patient.[22] The *Declaration* continues:

> In any case, it will be possible to make a correct judgment as to the means of studying the type of treatment to be used, its degree of complexity or risk, its cost and the possibilities of using it, and comparing these elements with the result that can be expected, taking into

PART FIVE: *End-of-Life Care*

account the state of the sick person and his or her physical and moral resources.[23]

In applying this approach, the *Declaration* notes that it is morally permissible to refuse to accept even readily available, established modes of treatment that are risky or burdensome, and that such refusal is not to be equated with suicide where the refusal is motivated by desire to avoid burdens of the treatment that are "disproportionate to the results to be expected" or the treatment is excessively expensive to "the family or community."[24]

The *Catechism of the Catholic Church* discusses end-of-life issues within its discourse on the Fifth Commandment.[25] Paragraph 2276 states: "Those who lives are diminished or weakened deserve special respect. Sick or handicapped persons should be helped to lead lives as normal as possible."[26] Paragraph 227 defines "direct Euthanasia" as "an act or omission which of itself, or by intention, causes death in order to eliminate suffering," and deems it morally unacceptable.[27] Paragraph 2278, however, further recognizes that the withdrawal of "medical procedures that are burdensome, dangerous, extraordinary, or disproportionate to the expected outcome can be legitimate."[28] This approval of withdrawal of treatment is premised on the notion that in these circumstances the intent is not to cause death, but merely the acceptance of the inability to impede it.[29] Either the patient or those authorized by law to speak for the patient may make this decision, as long as the patient's "reasonable will" and "legitimate interests" are respected.[30]

In *Evangelium Vitae*, John Paul II explicitly condemns euthanasia as "a grave violation of the law of God."[31] This condemnation "is based upon the natural law and the written word of God" as taught by the "ordinary and universal Magisterium."[32] The encyclical notes that the situation of those who are "incurably ill" or "dying" is exacerbated "by a cultural climate which fails to perceive any meaning or value in suffering, but rather considers suffering the epitome of evil, to be eliminated at all costs."[33] It observes that euthanasia is frequently justified by "a utilitarian motive of avoiding costs which bring no return and which weigh heavily on society."[34]

Although *Evangelium Vitae* condemns euthanasia, i.e., "an act or omission which of itself and by intention causes death, with the purpose of eliminating all suffering,"[35] it further distinguishes euthanasia from the refusal of "aggressive medical treatment" where the burdens imposed by treatment are disproportionate to the expected benefits or "impose an excessive burden on the patient and his family."[36] In such cases, where death is "imminent and inevitable," it is permissible to refuse excessively burdensome treatment so long as normal care is continued.[37] At this point, the encyclical seems to suggest that it may be appropriate to take into account quality-of-life concerns by stating: "Certainly there is a moral obligation to care for oneself and to allow oneself to be cared for, but this duty must take account of concrete circumstances. It needs to be determined whether the means of treatment available are objectively proportionate to the prospects for improvement."[38] But this comment appears in the context of a discussion of cases where death is imminent and inevitable, and thus does not seem to be applicable to PVS patients.

In 1994, the Pontifical Council for Pastoral Assistance to Health Care Workers issued a *Charter for Health Care Workers*.[39] The preface refers to the document as a "deontological code for those engaged in health care."[40] The *Charter* admonishes health care workers to provide patients with all "'proportionate' remedies," but further states there is "no obligation to apply 'disproportionate' ones."[41] It further refers to the distinction between ordinary and extraordinary remedies, ordinary methods being those "where there is *due proportion* between the means used and the end intended."[42] The document also specifically addresses the withholding of ANH from a patient whose death is imminent. In a section titled "Death With Dignity," it states: "The administration of food and liquids, even artificially, is part of the normal treatment always due to the patient when this is not burdensome for him: their undue suspension could be real and properly called euthanasia."[43]

End-of-life care is also addressed in the *ERD*s.[44] The *ERD*s restate traditional Catholic teaching on the distinction between ordinary and extraordinary care. Thus persons are morally obligated "to use ordinary or proportionate means in preserving life,"[45] but "may forego extraordinary or disproportionate means."[46] The proportionality of treatment is to be determined by balancing the burdens imposed on the patient by the treatment and its expense for the patient's family and community against the expected benefits of the treatment for the patient.[47]

Chapter Fourteen

The Controversy over Withdrawing Artificial Nutrition and Hydration from Patients in a Persistent Vegetative State

The morality of withdrawing artificial nutrition and hydration (ANH) from patients in a persistent vegetative state (PVS) has been debated among Catholic bioethicists since the 1980s. In this chapter, I distinguish between Catholic bioethicists who focus on the sanctity of life and favor the provision of ANH to PVS patients in most cases, and other Catholic bioethicists who focus on quality-of-life concerns and argue that it is morally licit to withdraw ANH from PVS patients. In these cases, the former group has tended to focus on the burdens and benefits of ANH itself, rather than on quality-of-life concerns in the PVS patient.[1] Accordingly, they argue that in cases of PVS patients, continuation of ANH is morally obligatory where the patient can assimilate the nourishment and it does not cause additional pain or complications.[2]

On the other hand, other Catholic bioethicists have tended to focus on quality-of-life concerns.[3] They largely ignore the benefits of ANH in sustaining life and focus instead on the lack of cognitive function in PVS patients, and the costs to others, both emotional and financial, of keeping them alive. Accordingly, these theologians have argued that in PVS cases continuation of ANH is not morally obligatory.[4]

The approach taken by those focusing on the sanctity of life was set out by William May and others in a 1987 article.[5] Initially, they set out some basic presuppositions and principles: "the omission of nutrition is an act of killing by omission,"[6] and "remaining alive is never rightly regarded as a burden, and deliberately killing innocent human life is never rightly regarded as rendering a benefit."[7] Deliberately withholding ANH from PVS patients for the purpose of causing death should be viewed as homicide,[8] and the withholding of it from disabled persons should be considered "status based discrimination" when done because of quality-of-life concerns.[9] They also argue that the withholding of ANH from PVS patients could easily be extended to other disabled persons whose quality of life is deemed inadequate, and, since death by starvation is painful and slow, to the acceptance of lethal injection as the preferred means of causing death.[10] In effect, they characterize ANH as ordinary treatment that should be provided to PVS patients.[11]

May, *et al.*, also concede that there may be exceptional circumstances in individual cases where the continued feeding could be considered "useless or excessively burdensome" because of complications from the feeding itself rather than because of quality-of-life concerns.[12] But they reject arguments that continued feeding of PVS patients could "ordinarily impose excessive burdens by reason of pain or damage to bodily self, psychological repugnance, restrictions on physical liberty and preferred activities, or harm to the person's mental life."[13]

Likewise, they reject arguments that such care could be considered excessively costly, noting that the cost of the treatment itself is not expensive. They further assert that the cost of continuing the lives of disabled persons should be borne by society without respect to quality-of-life concerns.[14] Thus, they conclude "that, in the ordinary circumstances of life in our society today, it is not morally right, nor ought it to be legally permissible, to withhold or withdraw nutrition and hydration provided by artificial means to the permanently unconscious."[15]

Among Catholic bioethicists, one of the leading advocates for the morality of withdrawing ANH from PVS patients has been Kevin O'Rourke, who argues that allowing the withdrawal of ANH from PVS patients is in keeping with Magisterial teaching.[16] In a 1986 article, O'Rourke concludes that it is appropriate to withhold tube feeding from persons in an irreversible coma in order to allow a fatal pathology to take its course.[17] In support of this conclusion, he argues that there is no obligation to preserve life in one who no longer has the cognitive-affective ability to pursue the purpose of life.[18] O'Rourke does not consider the ability to preserve physiological function sufficient to justify continued feeding.[19] In this article, however, O'Rourke does not attempt to characterize the treatment as extraordinary based on a balancing of the burdens of the treatment against the benefits.[20] Instead, he holds that the sole criterion in determining the morality of withdrawing ANH from an irreversibly comatose patient is whether the treatment could be useful in restoring cognitive function.[21]

In a 1988 article, republished in book form by the Catholic Health Association, O'Rourke refined his arguments in favor of the morality of withdrawing ANH from PVS patients.[22] In this article, he focuses on the traditional distinction between ordinary and extraordinary treatment — but modifies those categories by focusing on spiritual goals as well as physical goals. He argues that modern technology has created a situation where a patient may be kept alive but unable to participate in spiritual activity.[23] He further argues that "any medical therapy that would make the attainment of the spiritual goals of life less secure or seriously difficulty could be judged a grave burden and could be considered an optional or extraordinary means of to prolong life."[24] Observing that only physiological function can be sustained in a PVS patient, he concludes that there is no moral obligation to preserve life where there is no cognitive function to support spiritual activity.[25] O'Rourke bases his argument on a statement by Pope Pius XII, who, in discussing the morality of refusing extraordinary treatment, opined:" Life, health, all temporal activities are in fact subordinated to spiritual ends."[26] O'Rourke thus reformulates the distinction between ordinary and extraordinary treatment as follows:

> Emphasizing the spiritual goal of human life specifies more clearly the terms "ordinary" and "extraordinary," a specification that was not required when life support systems were not as advanced as they are today. Contemporary life support systems may prolong a state of existence which not only involves grave burdens for the patient, but also precludes spiritual activity on the part of the patient. Thus a more adequate and contemporary explanation of "ordinary" means to prolong life would be: those means which are obligatory because they enable a person to strive for the spiritual purpose of life without grave burden. "Extraordinary" means would seem to be: those means which are optional because they are ineffective or a grave burden in helping a person strive for the spiritual purpose of life. One cannot judge what is effective or a grave burden without considering the physiological condition, as well as the social and spiritual circumstances of the patient.[27]

In a 2008 article, Kevin O'Rourke reviews the controversy over the removal of ANH from PVS patients, concluding: "There are no consistent teachings offered by theologians or the Magisterium indicating that the use of some forms of life support is an absolute necessity."[28] In this article, he criticizes the notion that life support can only be removed where the patient is in danger of imminent death as being inconsistent with traditional teaching.[29] He argues that the consistent teaching of the Church does allow for continuing reevaluation of the benefit and burden of treatment, in light of changing conditions, and rejects the assumption that once ANH has been commenced with a patient in a PVS, it cannot be discontinued.[30]

There have been several responses to Fr. O'Rourke's arguments. William May argues that "O'Rourke errs seriously when he claims that a means is 'ordinary' only if it *enables* a person to pursue . . . [a spiritual] goal and that it is 'extraordinary' and hence not obligatory if it is ineffective in helping a person strive for the spiritual goal of life."[31] May asserts that persons who are incapable of spiritual activity because they are cognitively impaired are still to be regarded as "persons" and are thereby entitled to medical treatments even if those treatments would not allow them to pursue spiritual goals.[32] He provides the example of an elderly person who is mentally incompetent cutting an artery; that person would be entitled to treatment to stanch the bleeding, even though that treatment would not enable them to pursue spiritual goals.[33] He further argues that a proper understanding of the 1957 statement by Pope Pius XII is that treatments that have the potential side effect of impairing cognitive function so as preclude the pursuit of spiritual goals could properly be refused as extraordinary treatments.[34]

A 1989 paper issued by Bishop James McHugh of Camden, New Jersey, also attempts to refute O'Rourke's arguments by focusing on the question of ANH being considered extraordinary medical treatment[35] and considering the situation of PVS patients who could live for many years if provided with ANH.[36] Referring to O'Rourke's argument that there is no obligation to continue feeding PVS patients because of their inability to pursue spiritual goals, Bishop McHugh argues that such patients could continue to pursue a spiritual purpose — i.e., union with God — "if that person has intended that all of his or her suffering or debilitation be offered to God in union with the suffering of Christ."[37] He also characterizes ANH as a "basic means of sustaining life" rather than as "forms of therapeutic medical treatment."[38]

Bishop McHugh further observes that continuing ANH is "not customarily burdensome because they are commonplace medical technologies, not overly expensive . . . [and] do not usually increase the suffering of the patient."[39] Obviously, there have been cases where PVS patients have regained consciousness;[40] therefore, he asserts that if those withdrawing feeding intend that the PVS patient die, their action amounts to euthanasia.[41] Finally, he concludes, "Absent any other indication of a definite burden for the patient, withdrawal of nutrition/hydration is not morally justifiable."[42]

In an open letter responding to Bishop McHugh's paper, Kevin O'Rourke reiterated his arguments that the use of ANH in PVS patients is "an ineffective means of treatment."[43] He argues that persons who are PVS are not capable of performing "human acts," so a previous intention — i.e., to offer up one's suffering to God — would not be spiritually efficacious.[44] He notes that McHugh and others would recognize that ANH need not be continued in persons whose death is imminent, and argued that this recognition implies that ANH is a medical treatment subject to ethical evaluation.[45] Accordingly, he specifies that the true basis for disagreement with McHugh revolves around the question of whether this care is ineffective.[46]

In terms of balancing the burdens and benefits of continued feeding in PVS patients, he takes issue with Bishop McHugh's statement that such treatment is not "overly expensive," noting that the relevant cost is the cost per day of continuing care in a hospital or long-term care facility, rather than simply the cost of the feeding.[47] He also counts as costs the psychological and social stresses on the family.[48] He analogizes the removal of ANH from PVS patients to the removal of a ventilator, which has been widely recognized as morally permissible.[49] Finally, he argues that the PVS patient has a fatal pathology — i.e., the inability to swallow — and thus should be treated as a dying patient.[50]

In a 1988 article, Thomas A. Shannon and James J. Walter also argued in favor of the morality of withdrawing ANH from PVS patients.[51] They explicitly endorse the use of quality-of-life considerations in arguing that the withdrawal of ANH is consistent with the Catholic ethical tradition.[52] They caution against treating the continuation of physical life as an absolute value and contend that "quality of life judgments properly supplement and enhance the Christian emphasis on the sanctity of life."[53] With reference to the traditional distinction between ordinary and extraordinary treatment, Shannon and Walter say, "the concepts of burden and quality of life should be linked."[54] On this basis, they conclude that continuing ANH in PVS patients may be considered extraordinary treatment precisely because of quality-of-life considerations, i.e., the burden of continuing the patient's life for the patient's family and the professionals who care for the patient.[55]

David Kelly has argued that permitting the withdrawal of ANH from PVS patients is consistent with the Catholic natural-law tradition because artificial nutrition has been traditionally regarded as an extraordinary means of treatment.[56] He notes that Gerald Kelly, S.J., the leading expert on medical ethical issues in the 1940s and '50s, had argued that intravenous feeding may be discontinued in some cases.[57]

But Gerald Kelly focused on their discontinuation in "hopeless cases"— i.e., cases where the patient is diagnosed as terminal and near death.[58] In a 1950 article, he states that even if the continuation of intravenous feeding could be considered an ordinary means in such cases, it would not necessarily be obligatory because of its lack of utility; i.e., it may be "relatively useless."[59] He also discusses several scenarios: Where a terminal patient is calm and conscious while receiving intravenous feeding, then it should be presumed that the patient would want it to continue.[60] Where the terminal patient is conscious and suffering from pain, then it would be reasonable to discontinue it.[61] And where the patient is in a terminal coma, then it would be permissible to discontinue the intravenous feeding.[62] But none of these cases is analogous to the case of a patient with PVS who could live for years if provided with ANH.

David Kelly also notes the disagreement among bishops on this issue.[63] In 1988, Bishop Louis Gelineau, bishop of Providence, Rhode Island, issued a statement endorsing the removal of ANH from a PVS patient.[64] In 1990, the Texas Conference of Catholic Bishops issued a statement opining that, in some cases, it is morally permissible for the family of PVS patients to discontinue ANH.[65]

On the other hand, in 1991, the Catholic bishops of Pennsylvania issued a statement concluding, "in almost every instance there is an obligation to continue supplying nutrition and hydration to the unconscious patient."[66] And in 1992, the Committee for Pro-Life Activities of the National Conference of Catholic Bishops issued a paper analyzing the ethics of withdrawing ANH [hereinafter referred to as NCCB paper] that argued for a strong presumption in favor of continuing ANH in PVS patients.[67] The NCCB paper begins by noting: "Catholic theologians may differ on how best to apply moral principles to some questions not explicitly resolved by the Church's teaching authority."[68] It then turns to a discussion of the traditional distinction between ordinary and extraordinary treatment,[69] and answers a series of questions posed concerning ANH.[70] The NCCB paper observes that the omission of treatment may be considered euthanasia "when the purpose of the omission is to kill the patient."[71] It further notes that ANH is sometimes withdrawn because a patient is not dying quickly enough, "and someone believes it would be better if he or she did, generally because the patient is perceived as having an unacceptably low 'quality of life' or as imposing burdens on others."[72]

As to the question of whether ANH is a form of medical treatment, the NCCB paper notes that as of 1992, the Magisterium had not resolved this question,[73] but further observes that "even medical 'treatments' are morally obligatory when they are 'ordinary' means."[74] The paper then applies the traditional approach of balancing the benefits and burdens of the treatment in order to determine whether ANH could be considered ordinary or extraordinary treatment. The paper's discussion of the benefits and burdens of ANH is primarily focuses on the feeding itself rather than on the benefits and burdens of continued life for the patient. Nonetheless, the paper notes that "the 'quality of life' of a seriously ill patient is relevant to treatment decisions."[75] But it further states that quality-of-life is only relevant to the extent that "a disabling condition may directly influence the benefits and burdens of a specific treatment for a particular patient."[76] Moreover, the paper states:

> It is one thing to withhold a procedure because it would impose new disabilities on a patient, and quite another thing to say that patients who already have such disabilities should not have their lives preserved. A means considered ordinary or proportionate for other patients should not be considered extraordinary or disproportionate for severely impaired patients solely because of a judgment that their lives are not worth living.[77]

In discussing the burdens of ANH, the NCCB paper acknowledges that Catholic teaching recognizes that it is morally legitimate to refuse life-prolonging measures that impose excessive burdens such as pain, emotional distress, restrictions on activities, suppression of mental life, or expense.[78] And in discussing physical burdens, it notes that in a particular case "a feeding procedure could become harmful or even life-threatening."[79] When assessing the burdens of feeding, however, the risks of the procedure should be "compared with the adverse effects of dehydration or malnutrition."[80] As to economic burdens, it recognizes that cost can be a factor that is taken into account in assessing burdens, but opines that individual treatment decisions should not be based on "macro-economic concerns such as national budget priorities and the high cost of health care."[81]

This analysis seems to reject an approach that would focus on the overall cost of maintaining the life of someone who is not economically productive, and suggests that rather the focus should be on the cost of the treatment itself. It further notes that "tube feeding alone is generally not very expensive and may cost no more than oral feeding."[82] It also notes that in PVS patients tube feeding may be employed not because the patient is unable to swallow food, but "because tube feeding is less costly and difficult for health care personnel."[83]

The paper also has a section focusing specifically on the debate among Catholic ethicists on withdrawing ANH from PVS patients.[84] It notes that those who argue in favor of the morality of withdrawal argue that in balancing the benefits and burdens of treatment, it is inappropriate to focus only on the prolongation of physical life, "since physical life is not an absolute good but is relative to the spiritual good of the person."[85] They further argue that because spiritual good can only be enhanced by "conscious, free acts," and since PVS patients are incapable of such acts, it is not morally obligatory to prolong their lives by continuing by "such interventions as a respirator, antibiotics, or medically assisted ANH and nutrition."[86] The NCCB paper, however, rejects this line of argument stating: "While this rationale is convincing to some, it is not theologically conclusive, and we are not persuaded by it."[87] Rather, it sides with those theologians who argue if the burden that is sought to be relieved by the withdrawal of ANH is the continuation of life, then "such a decision is unacceptable, because one's intent is only achieved by deliberately ensuring the patient's death from malnutrition or dehydration."[88] The paper further concurred with the arguments of theologians who have held that the PVS patient is not terminally ill in the sense that death is imminent, and accordingly, their "inherent dignity and worth . . . obligates us to provide this patient with care and support."[89]

The NCCB paper further rejects the argument, based on the tradition of probabilism in Catholic moral theology, that in light of disagreement on the issue among ethicists, individuals should be permitted to choose the approach they find most persuasive.[90] In this regard, the paper relies on a sort of slippery slope argument evincing concern "about current attitudes and policy trends in our society that would too easily dismiss patients without apparent mental faculties as non-persons or as undeserving of human concerns."[91] It then refers to the possibility that arguments in favor of withdrawal of ANH from PVS patients could be used to "erode respect for the lives of some of our society's most helpless members."[92] It also mentions medical uncertainty about the ability of PVS patients to experience pain and prognoses for such patients.[93] But despite these concerns, the paper stops short of explicitly ruling out the withdrawal of ANH and in all PVS cases. Instead, it opts for "a presumption in favor of medically assisted nutrition and hydration."[94] It does, however, explicitly "reject any omission of nutrition and hydration intended to cause a patient's death."[95]

The 1994 version of the *ERD*s directly addressed for the first time "the moral issues concerning medically assisted hydration and nutrition."[96] While noting that the Church's teaching prohibits euthanasia, the 1994 *ERD*s further notes "that hydration and nutrition are not morally obligatory either when they bring no comfort to a person who is imminently dying or when they cannot be assimilated by a person's body."[97] Directive 58 of the 1994 *ERD*s states: "There should be a presumption in favor of providing nutrition and hydration to all patients, including patients who require medically assisted nutrition and hydration, as long as this is of sufficient benefit to outweigh the burdens involved to the patient."[98] Identical language is used in the 2001 *ERDs*.[99] Both the 1994 and 2001 editions of the *ERDs* also specifically address the withdrawal of ANH from PVS patients by referring to a report of the NCCB Committee on Pro-Life Activities that "points out the necessary distinctions between questions already resolved by the Magisterium and those requiring further reflection."[100] Thus, the 2001 *ERDs* do not take a definitive position on the withdrawal of ANH from PVS patients.

On March 20, 2004, in a papal allocution delivered to an International Congress focusing on the treatment of PVS patients, John Paul II stated:

> I should like particularly to underline how the administration of water and food, even when provided by artificial means, always represents a *natural means* of preserving life, not a *medical act*. Its use, furthermore, should be considered, in principle, *ordinary* and *proportionate*, and as such morally obligatory, insofar as and until it is seen to have attained its proper finality, which in the present case consists in providing nourishment to the patient and alleviation of his suffering.[101]

In his allocution, John Paul II states: "The sick person in a vegetative state ... has the right to basic health care (nutrition, ANH, cleanliness, warmth, etc.)."[102] He characterizes PVS as a "conventional prognostic judgment," because it refers to the statistical unlikelihood of recovery, rather than a "diagnosis."[103] He also notes that there are "well-documented cases of at least partial recovery" from PVS.[104]

He continues:

> The evaluation of probabilities, founded on waning hopes of recovery when the vegetative state is prolonged beyond a year, cannot ethically justify the cessation or interruption of *minimal care* for the patient, including nutrition and hydration.[105]

Thus, he characterizes the withdrawal of ANH from PVS patients as "euthanasia by omission."[106] And he further rejects the use of "quality of life" considerations as "introducing into social relations a discriminatory and eugenic principle."[107]

The papal allocution garnered an immediate response. An article in *USA Today* notes:

> Until now, the 565 hospitals in the Catholic Health Association (CHA) considered feeding tubes for people in a persistent vegetative state

"medical treatments," which could be provided or discontinued, based on evaluating the benefits and burdens on patient and family.[108]

Michael Place, the president of the Catholic Health Association, was quoted as acknowledging the "significant ethical, legal, clinical implications" of the statement, and further observing: "This text has to be put in context with what the pope has said on euthanasia and on life. You can't read this in a vacuum."[109] There was also "a common theme" sounded in many reports to the effect that "no action will be taken, no changes to current practices will take place, until those who administer Catholic health care facilities receive instructions on how to interpret the allocution."[110]

On the other hand, Richard Doerflinger, Deputy Director for the Secretariat for Pro-Life Activities, United States Conference of Catholic Bishops, greeted the papal allocation with enthusiasm, characterizing it as "the culmination of a longstanding trend at the Vatican."[111] Doerflinger concluded:

> ... the Holy Father has not declared an absolute moral obligation to provide assisted feeding in all cases, regardless of whether it effectively provides nourishment or might in a given case impose grave suffering and other burdens on a patient. But he has established the provision of food and fluids as a general norm for all helpless patients, including those who seem completely unresponsive to the outside world.[112]

There was also a negative reaction to the papal allocution among some Catholic bioethicists. John F. Tuohey, the holder of an endowed chair in applied health care ethics at Providence St. Vincent Medical Center in Portland, Oregon, criticized the papal allocation in an article in *Commonweal* as if it was a thesis proposal submitted to an interdisciplinary committee for review at a Catholic university — then used this literary device to argue that its reasoning is inadequate and inconsistent with the Catholic ethical tradition.[113] He rejects the papal statement's emphasis on the importance of the distinction between prognosis and diagnosis.[114] He criticizes the papal allocution for requiring a diagnosis of a terminal disease in order to justify withdrawal of ANH, rather than allowing withdrawal because of a poor prognosis.[115]

Tuohey argues that the Catholic ethical tradition does take into account the patient's prognosis in determining whether care is ordinary and proportionate.[116] He also notes the failure of the papal statement to distinguish between "clinical certainty" and "moral certainty."[117] He argues that in the case of PVS patients, there may not be a clinical certainty that the patient

PART FIVE: *End-of-Life Care*

will not recover, but there is a moral certainty in most cases.[118] He also criticizes the argument that care should be continued where there is any doubt as to prognosis. He pejoratively characterizes this position as "tutiorism."[119] Instead, he states:

> If there is legitimate clinical doubt that a person in PVS will recover, or if it is unreasonable to expect the person will recover, it is ethical to make decisions with "moral certainty" the person will probably *not* recover — what the tradition has called probabilism.[120]

Thomas Shannon, a professor at Worcester Polytechnic Institute and longtime member of the Catholic Theological Society of America, also responded negatively to the Pope's address. In an article in the *National Catholic Reporter*, he argues:

> The analysis and conclusion drawn from it appear to represent a major reversal of the moral tradition of the Catholic Church in assessing whether a particular medical or other intervention is morally obligatory, particularly in the determination of whether this intervention is ordinary or extraordinary treatment.[121]

Shannon asserts that the papal statement departs from Catholic tradition in that it focuses on whether treatment is a "natural means," or normally used, rather than on the effect on the patient.[122]

Shannon also argues that classifying a treatment as extraordinary neither demeans the human dignity of the patient nor indicates that the intention of the family or physician is to end the life of the patient by withdrawing.[123] And he argues that since a PVS patient is incapable of eating on his/her own, and the condition is typically irreversible, using ANH may be "morally counter-indicated."[124] He also notes that this treatment may be expensive and, in particular cases, actually harmful to the patient. He accuses John Paul II of elevating "biological or physical life to an almost absolute value."[125] He further argues that the papal allocution is likely to be ignored by "many people" because it "contradicts their deepest moral instincts," and may encourage them to resort to active euthanasia.[126] He raised a number of questions about "the level of magisterial authority" of the statement and its application to non-PVS patients.[127] Finally, he concludes that the effect of the allocution was unlikely to "protect patients in a persistent vegetative state and to curb the movement toward euthanasia."[128]

Others tried to minimize the potential changes in Catholic hospitals that could follow from implementation of the principles in the papal allocution. In his 2004 book, David Kelly discounted the significance of the allocution, noting that it has "significantly less importance and authority than more formal addresses and written pronouncements like encyclicals, which are usually prepared with considerable care."[129] He also notes that, according to traditional Catholic teaching, feeding PVS patients is indeed morally extraordinary and may rightly be foregone.[130]

Kevin O'Rourke reacted by observing that the papal allocution "does not preclude the consideration of excessive burdens that might rule out the use of ANH therapy" noting particularly a statement by the Australian bishops stating that ANH could be withdrawn "if the patient is unable to assimilate the material provided or if the manner of the provision itself causes undue suffering to the patient, or involves an undue burden to others."[131] He then suggests that financial burdens should also be considered in determining whether to continue ANH for PVS patients noting that "the cost of nursing care for a PVS patient . . . may be excessive, even though the cost of nutrition might be minimal."[132] Later in his article, he suggests that the cost of a surgical procedure to install a gastrostomy tube in the vena cava of a PVS patient could be considered as a significant financial burden even if use of a nasogastric tube would not be.[133] In another article, O'Rourke argues that the teaching in the papal allocution was not authoritative because "the allocution's statements have not been repeated by the teaching authority of the Church."[134] He also criticizes attempts by some state Catholic conferences to develop policies on advance directives that would limit the withdrawal of ANH.[135]

There was also continuing controversy over the meaning of the papal allocution. An article coauthored by Ronald Hamel, senior director for ethics at the Catholic Health Association, criticized "recent revisions" in traditional teaching that would impose an obligation to provide nutrition and hydration in all cases, without a holistic consideration of benefits and burdens.[136] They noted that these changes had resulted in a more "restrictive standard" for withdrawal of ANH which they characterized as resulting from a "limited physical understanding" of the burdens imposed by the continued provision of ANH.[137] But as to the papal allocution they stated:

> He [John Paul II] does not radically and completely depart from traditional understandings or his own previous teachings by making their use an absolute requirement with no exceptions. If the pope's statement is read in light of the tradition, what he might be saying is that in principle nutrition and hydration are ordinary means of preserving life,

PART FIVE: *End-of-Life Care*

and hence morally obligatory for all patients. This appears just to be a continuation of what we have seen already in the U.S. bishops' Pro-Life Committee document of 1992 and in Directive 58, where we hear of a presumption in favor of providing nutrition and hydration.[138]

In August 2007, the Congregation for the Doctrine of the Faith (CDF) responded to two questions posed by the United States Conference of Catholic Bishops concerning the administration of ANH to PVS patients.[139] In these responses, the CDF clearly indicates that it is morally obligatory to continue providing ANH to PVS patients as long as they can assimilate the nourishment and it does not cause significant physical discomfort, and that ANH is to be considered ordinary and proportionate treatment.[140] Moreover, it opines that ANH cannot be withdrawn merely because the physicians determine that the patient will not regain consciousness.[141] In the commentary accompanying these responses, the CDF further states: "Its use should therefore be considered ordinary and proportionate, even when the 'vegetative state' is prolonged."[142]

There has been continuing controversy over whether the papal allocution, and the CDF response and commentary, represented a change in Church teaching. In some questions and answers concerning the CDF response and commentary, the USCCB Committee on Doctrine and Committee on Pro-Life Activities stated:

Does this represent a change in Church teaching?

No. These Responses reaffirm what was taught by Pope John Paul II in his 2004 Address, which is itself in continuity with the Holy See's Declaration of Euthanasia of 1980 and other documents regarding the right of patients to receive normal or basic care. As the Commentary points out, in developing this teaching, the Church's Magisterium has paid close attention to "the progress of medicine and the questions which this has raised."[143]

The U.S. bishops further noted that in "modern societies with advanced medical services," the provision of AHN to PVS patients could not be deemed extraordinary or disproportionate treatment.[144] And that since PVS patients are not as such cases where death is imminent, the reception of ANH would not be considered disproportionately burdensome for them.[145] Moreover, the costs directly attributable to ANH could not generally be deemed excessive "in technologically advanced societies."[146]

There were several reactions to the CDF's statement. Ron Hamel, Senior Director of Ethics at the Catholic Health Association, stated that it set standards that were "different from the general practice in the United States and in Catholic healthcare" and that Catholic hospitals "should examine the practice and develop a policy."[147] He also noted that this statement may require hospitals to notify "family members upfront . . . that a feeding tube could only be withdrawn under certain circumstances, certain limited circumstances."[148] John Allen noted that the CDF statement "closes a door in Catholic debate that had earlier remained open."[149] On the other hand, Thomas Kopfensteiner, senior vice president at Catholic Health Initiatives (CHI), the owner of seventy-one hospitals, said that the allocution would not alter any policies in place at CHI facilities because it was merely a "clarification" of existing teaching and did not represent any change.[150]

Sr. Carol Keehan, president and CEO of the Catholic Health Association, welcomed the statement and accompanying commentary, stating that they made it clear that "the provision of artificially administered nutrition and hydration to patients in a vegetative state is morally obligatory except when they cannot be assimilated by the patient's body (and, hence, don't achieve their purpose) or cause significant discomfort."[151] She also acknowledges that ANH for PVS patients must be continued "even when physicians have determined with reasonable certainty that the patient will never recover consciousness."[152] But she then emphasizes that the documents were merely a clarification of existing teaching and not "new doctrine."[153]

John Hardt and Kevin O'Rourke argued for a narrow construction of the CDF documents in light of European events and general provisions of canon law.[154] As to European events, they note that the growing acceptance of euthanasia in Europe suggests that the Holy See is being particularly vigilant and forceful in protecting human life.[155] But, of course, this could just as easily be a justification for a broad interpretation of the CDF documents. since there are similar developments in the United States. As to canon law, they argue that these statements should be deemed applicable only to PVS, but not to those suffering from Alzheimer's disease or acute dementia.[156] But it would seem that the same provisions for continuation of ANH should apply to persons who are actually conscious, although with diminished abilities, as would apply to those who appear to be permanently unconscious with no higher brain activity.

Chapter Fifteen

A Case Study in End-of-Life Care: Terri Schiavo

The case of Terri Schiavo brought intense media focus on a dispute within a family over the appropriate treatment of a PVS patient. And, since the parties involved were Catholics, it also brought into sharper focus the confusion over Catholic teaching on the morality of withdrawal of ANH from PVS patients.[1] Unfortunately, however, that confusion may have contributed to the final result. Terri Schiavo died on March 31, 2005, approximately two weeks after the removal of her feeding tube pursuant to a court order.[2]

Her death occurred after several years of legal wrangling between her parents, Robert and Mary Schindler, who opposed removal of the feeding tube, and her husband Michael Schiavo, who sought its removal.[3] The Vatican called her death a "violation of the sacred nature of life."[4] One priest, Fr. Frank Pavone, a spiritual advisor to the Schindlers, referred to Michael Schiavo's "heartless cruelty"; another priest, Monsignor Theodore Malanowski, who administered last rites to Terri, compared her to Jesus Christ and said "He was put on trial unjustly, just like Terri."[5]

A feeding tube was inserted into Terri after she had suffered extensive brain damage in 1990 due to a cardiac arrest that may have been caused by a potassium imbalance brought on by bulimia.[6] In 1998, her husband, Michael, asked a Florida state court for permission to remove the feeding tube. The court granted permission after determining that Terri was in a PVS, and that is what she would have wanted.[7] At the time removal of the feeding tube was sought, it was clear that with ANH, Terri Schiavo could continue to live for many years; if it was withdrawn, she would die from starvation in a few days.[8]

The Florida courts — based on some rather scant evidence and applying a substituted judgment standard — authorized the withdrawal of ANH from Terri, based on the assumption that she, if competent to make the decision, would have wanted it withdrawn.[9] Terri Schiavo and her family were Catholic, and so Catholic teaching was an important issue in the case, bearing on the question of what she would have wanted if competent to express her wishes. In the original proceedings before the trial court, Fr. Gerald Murphy, a Catholic priest from the Diocese of St. Petersburg, Florida, testified as to Church teaching on the withdrawal of ANH from PVS patients.[10] His testimony was offered by George Felos, the attorney for Michael Schiavo.[11] Although he did not have a degree in moral theology, Fr. Murphy was the diocesan and statewide chaplain for the Catholic Medical Association.[12]

Attorney Felos asked Fr. Murphy whether removal of ANH from Terri Schiavo would be consistent with the teaching of the Catholic Church.[13] He asked Fr. Murphy to assume, for purposes of this question, that Terri Schiavo had told her husband that she would not want to live "if she was dependent on the care of others."[14] And, further, that she "mentioned to her husband and to her brother and sister-in-law that she would not want to be kept alive artificially."[15] Fr. Murphy answered, "After all that has transpired, I believe, yes, it would be consistent with the teaching of the Catholic Church."[16] On cross examination, Fr. Murphy was asked specifically whether he was familiar with Directive 58 in the 1994 *ERDs*, which states that there should be a presumption in favor of providing ANH.[17] He stated that he was familiar with Directive 58, but characterized it as providing an ideal standard; further, "You have to go back and evaluate the proportion."[18]

The parents also attempted to convince the trial court that Terri was a practicing Catholic who was serious about her faith, but her husband testified that Terri was a lapsed Catholic. The appellate court, in a rather offhanded manner, sided with the husband on the question of Teresa's religiosity and affirmed the trial court order permitting the husband to order the withdrawal of treatment.[19]

The case has focused public attention on the confusion in Catholic teaching with regard to the morality of withdrawing ANH from PVS patients.[20] This confusion is illustrated by two statements on the Schiavo case emanating from the St. Petersburg Catholic Diocese. An official statement on the Schiavo case, issued by the Catholic Diocese of St. Petersburg on October 15, 2002, stated that Roman Catholic teaching would permit removal of ANH from a comatose person ". . . only if the natural projected path of the individual's medical condition will lead inevitably to death, sooner rather than later."[21] It then referred to a disagreement over whether or not Terri Schiavo's medical condition was "irreversible and inevitably deteriorating toward death."[22]

PART FIVE: *End-of-Life Care*

This seems to misrepresent the position of the parties in this case: Michael Schiavo contended that Terri's PVS was irreversible, but he did not contend that she was in a terminal condition.[23] Nonetheless, on this basis, the Diocese refused to take a position on the morality of withdrawing ANH, although the statement acknowledged that the case involved a "serious moral issue" that could not be adequately resolved in a court.[24]

A subsequent statement issued on August 12, 2003, by Bishop Robert J. Lynch of St. Petersburg, further muddied the waters. It recommended that Terri Schiavo's parents be permitted "to attempt a medical protocol which they feel would improve her condition," and referred to a presumption in favor of continuing ANH.[25] The bishop stated in this letter that removal of her feeding tube could be morally permissible if it was unreasonably burdensome for her or her family, but then stated that it would not be morally permissible if removed to hasten her death or because of the low quality of her life.[26] This statement also indicated that the source of the problem in the Schiavo case was "uncertainty about her actual physical state" and her failure to execute a living will clearly indicating her wishes.[27]

Unfortunately, this statement seems to further obfuscate the moral aspects of the Schiavo case. Michael Schiavo claimed he was seeking removal of the feeding tube to hasten Terri's death because he believed she would not have wanted to remain alive with such a low quality of life.[28] The court found, based on medical testimony, that Terri was in a PVS and would not regain consciousness.[29] Certainly, the presence of an advance directive from Terri would have made the case much easier legally, but the moral issue in the case was whether it was morally licit under Catholic teaching to remove ANH from a PVS patient in order to bring about the patient's death; Bishop Lynch never answered this question.

A subsequent statement of the Florida bishops added to the confusion by endorsing Bishop Lynch's statement, indicating that the Florida bishops "respect[ed] the need for finality of the court's decision," but called for "additional time to allow greater certainty as to her [Terri Schiavo's] true condition."[30] This could be interpreted to suggest that the problem in the Schiavo case was medical uncertainty about her condition, and that removal of the feeding tube would be morally permissible if she was in a PVS state.[31] But the bishops further stated: "If additional medical treatment can be shown to be helpful to her condition, we urge that all parties involved take the safer course and allow it to be used."[32] If the additional medical treatment that they are referring to is continuing ANH in order to sustain life, then their statement could be read to oppose withdrawal of ANH.

On the other hand, they could have been referring to additional therapy to improve her medical and physical condition, and may have therefore been suggesting that her feeding be continued to allow this therapy to be provided if it could be of benefit. This would suggest that if she would not benefit from additional therapy, then ANH could be withdrawn. But in an earlier statement, the Florida bishops opined, "As a general rule . . . artificial sustenance should not be withheld or withdrawn from these patients."[33]

In 2004, subsequent to the original proceedings, there was a papal allocution indicating that continuation of ANH in PVS patients would be morally obligatory, see discussion *supra*, Chapter 14.[34] The papal allocution may have been an attempt to clarify Church teaching with reference to the Schiavo case and other like cases.[35] After this allocution, the parents tried without success to reopen the case, arguing that under the substituted judgment standard, the court should assume that Terri, as a faithful Catholic, would want her treatment continued in accordance with the papal allocution.[36] In this motion, they argued that the withdrawal of ANH would require Terri Schiavo to violate her religious beliefs and that this type of coercion would violate the free exercise clause of the First Amendment.[37] They also provided affidavits from Terri's family arguing that Catholic was a practicing Catholic at the time of her collapse on February 25, 1990.[38] This was intended to counteract an earlier observation by the District Court of Appeals that she did not regularly attend Mass or have a religious advisor who could assist the court in weighing her religious attitudes about life-support methods."[39] On October 22, 2004, Judge Greer denied this motion. [40]

Even if it doesn't state an absolute norm that requires continuation of ANH in all PVS patients, the papal allocution states that such treatment is morally obligatory if the treatment itself imposes no disproportionate burdens on the patient (see discussion Chapter 14, *supra*). Ordinarily, in such cases the treatment itself is not burdensome; rather it is continued life that is considered burdensome. Under these circumstances, it would not be morally permissible to discontinue ANH. Perhaps an earlier papal statement clarifying the teaching of the Church, coupled with a clear statement from the local bishop on the issue, would have been sufficient to persuade the trial judge to continue feeding; if coupled with proof that Terri was a faithful practicing Catholic, this could have undermined other evidence that she would have wanted such treatment discontinued.

After Terri's death, a neuropathological consultant's report accompanying the autopsy report confirmed the severity of the injuries to Terri's brain, noting:

Brain Weight is an important index of its pathological state. Brain weight is correlated with height, weight, age and sex. The decedent's brain was grossly abnormal and weighed only 615 grams (1.35 lb.). That weight is less than half of the expected tabular weight for a decedent of her adult age of 41 years 3 months 28 days. By way of comparison, the brain of Karen Ann Quinlan weighed 835 grams at the time of her death, after 10 years in a similar persistent vegetative state.[41]

Nonetheless, the neurological consult report concluded that "[n]euro-pathological examination alone of the decedent's brain — or any brain for that matter — cannot prove or disprove a diagnosis of persistent vegetative state."[42] And notwithstanding whether Terri was accurately diagnosed as being in a PVS, the papal allocution and a subsequent clarification of the allocution by the CDF, discussed *supra* in Chapter 14, certainly supports the efforts by the Schindlers to provide ANH to keep their daughter alive.

Part Six

Social Justice and Health Care Reform

Introduction

The debate over health care reform in the United States was an important issue in the 2008 presidential campaign.[1] Public opinion polls suggest there is a consensus across the political spectrum on the desirability of achieving universal access to health care through legislative reforms,[2] and the primary focus of the debate has shifted to the means of achieving that goal. With the election of Barack Obama, it is possible that there will be significant health care reform in 2009.[3]

The Catholic Health Association and many Catholic health care systems have been advocates of reforms that could expand the role of the federal government in providing access to health care — but that expansion in the role of government could also result in a further erosion of the autonomy of Catholic hospitals and dilution of their distinctive identity.

Many Catholic hospitals originally began as community hospitals before there was a market for private health insurance. They were essentially religious ministries, with the principal function of giving spiritual support and medical treatment to the sick and dying. Many of their patients were unable to pay for the care they received, and so, their ministry was also charitable. With the advent of health insurance in the 1930s and its vast expansion during and following World War II, many of the patients treated in Catholic hospitals were adequately insured, although a substantial number of elderly and poor people were still without insurance.

Originally, nonprofit hospitals were granted tax-exempt status under state and federal laws in recognition of the substantial benefit that society received from the medical care that they provided to patients who were unable to pay for it. In fact, the provision of charitable care was required under federal law to retain nonprofit status.[4] The creation of the Medicare and Medicaid programs in 1965 brought about an assumption that most people would have either private health insurance or be covered by a governmental program, so federal law was changed so that hospitals were no longer required to provide care to indigents in order to retain their nonprofit status.[5]

Under current federal law, nonprofit hospitals are required to provide community benefit — a rather vague concept that includes indigent care — but hospitals are no longer required to provide care for indigents in order to be tax-exempt.[6] In 1969, the Internal Revenue Service (IRS) recognized the promotion of health as a charitable purpose.[7] Thus, to be entitled to tax-exempt status under Internal Revenue Code 501(c)(3), a health care provider must make its services available to all in the community plus provide additional community or public benefits. A totality-of-circumstances approach is taken by the IRS in ascertaining whether the "community benefit" standard is met. The IRS uses a multi-factorial test to determine qualification for tax-exempt status: (1) operation of a full-time emergency room open to the public; (2) governance by a community board; (3) an open medical staff; (4) providing non-emergent care to anyone in the community who is able to pay; and (5) providing benefits to the community through research and education or providing charity care.[8]

In recent years, nonprofit hospitals, including Catholic hospitals, have come under more intense scrutiny. An April 2008 article in the Wall Street Journal noted that "many nonprofit hospitals have seen earnings soar in recent years."[9] It cited a 2006 report by the Congressional Budget Office, finding that nonprofit hospitals had received $12.6 billion in tax exemptions.[10] The amount of community benefit reported by nonprofit hospitals, the article noted, could be inflated by the inclusion of bad debts and the use of list prices rather than actual charges.[11] And it noted complaints about excessive executive compensation: the *Wall Street Journal* reported the annual compensation package for the CEO of Catholic Health Care West in 2005 was $5.8 million.[12] Thus, there have been hearings in both the House and Senate concerning the conduct of nonprofit hospitals.[13]

Professor John Colombo has argued that, in light of similarity between the operations of for-profit and nonprofit hospitals, the current standard for tax-exempt status for nonprofit hospitals is unwarranted and should be changed so that only organizations that enhance access to services for underserved populations should be tax-exempt.[14] Legislation may be introduced in Congress in 2009 to require nonprofit hospitals to provide a minimum of charity care for the poor.[15] If this legislation is adopted, hospitals failing to provide this free care would be subject to penalties ranging from "taxes and fines to stripping a hospital of its federal tax exemption if it continues to misbehave."[16]

Catholic hospitals have also been denied exemption from state property taxes because of failing to provide adequate charity care. In August 2008, an Illinois appellate court upheld the denial of an application for exemption from Illinois property taxes by Provena Covenant Medical Center, a Catholic nonprofit hospital located in Urbana, Illinois, primarily based on its failure to provide adequate charity care.[17] And Catholic hospitals have been accused of an unethical behavior in their treatment of uninsured patients. In 2007, a California judge approved a $473 million settlement in a lawsuit against Catholic Health Care West brought on behalf of uninsured patients complaining about its hospitals overcharging them and using aggressive debt collection techniques against them.[18]

A controversy continues over whether nonprofit hospitals provide more charitable care than for-profit hospitals. Some studies claim that comparable nonprofit and for-profit hospitals provide similar amounts of uncompensated care.[19] On the other hand, one study claims that nonprofit hospitals offer more unprofitable services utilized by the poor,[20] and another concludes that Catholic hospitals offer more "access," "stigmatized," and "compassionate care services" than other private nonprofit and investor-owned hospitals.[21] These services may be linked to the Catholic identity of the hospitals and seem particularly appropriate in light of their religious sponsorship.[22]

If universal health care is adopted and virtually all Americans have adequate health insurance, then the effect on nonprofit hospitals is uncertain. It may substantially undermine the argument for continued tax-exempt status for hospitals. And it is possible that any universal health care program will be accompanied by a mandate that participating hospitals must provide health services not permissible under the *ERDs*. Despite these possibilities, Catholic organizations have continued to be strong advocates of a governmental system of universal health care.

Chapter Sixteen

The United States Health Care System

The United States is the only OECD country without a national health care system. By way of contrast, Britain[1] has adopted a system of socialized medicine where the government owns most of the hospitals, employs the specialists attached to the hospitals, and contracts with general practitioners to provide primary care.[2] Britain's National Health Service exists alongside an active private sector.[3] And in Canada, the financing of health care has been socialized at the Province level,[4] and until recently the sale of private insurance coverage for services covered by the provincial plans has been prohibited.[5] Nonetheless, there is a growing private sector in Canada.[6] In the United States, there is mixed private and public financing of health care, some government owned health care facilities and government employed physicians, and large numbers of persons without any health insurance coverage.

A typical critique of the health care system in the United States argues that we spend too much on health care, derive too little benefit from our expenditures, and that our health care system is not really a system at all[7] but instead a sort of Rube Goldberg machine.[8] The United States spends more on health care per capita than any other OECD country, and more as a percentage of GDP than any other country in the world.[9] And while the public spending as a percentage of GDP is about the same as the United Kingdom and slightly lower than Canada,[10] the United States. does not provide universal access as do Canada and Britain. Notwithstanding these expenditures, the United States ranks 12th of 13 developed countries for 16 available indicators.[11] For example, it ranks 13th for low birth weight babies, 13th for neonatal and infant mortality, and 10th for age-adjusted mortality.[12]

Comparison of the United States Health Care system with the British and Canadian Systems

The British, Canadian, and United States health care systems have all struggled with problems of cost, access, and quality in recent years. In all three countries there is a mix of government and private health care, but there are significant differences among all three countries with respect to the role of private markets. In all three countries, an aging population has naturally led to increased demand for health care.

While Canada and Britain have provided universal access, the deployment of newer technology has lagged in Canada and Britain as compared to its availability to insured patients in the United States. Technological innovations in imaging such as CT scans and MRIs are more widely available and readily accessible for insured persons in the United States than in Britain or Canada, and both also lag behind the United States in the rates of performance of coronary angioplasties and dialysis.[13]

In Britain and Canada the national health care systems have been supported and even expanded by their respective conservative parties. Perhaps, this is due to the fact that in both Canada and Britain the conservative parties tend to be more communitarian and less libertarian in outlook than the Republican Party in the United States which includes both communitarians and libertarians. In Britain, the creation of the NHS was first suggested under the wartime coalition government headed by Churchill, the Conservative Party Prime Minister.[14] And while the Conservative Party government under Margaret Thatcher later attempted to implement market-oriented reforms to the system, it never questioned the commitment to universal access and provision of free care at the point of delivery.[15]

Similarly, in Canada, the Progressive Conservative Party was instrumental in the creation of the Canadian health care system and the current Conservative government is committed to the preservation and improvement of the health care system albeit with a greater role for the private sector.[16] This is not particularly surprising in light of the fact that the first national health care system in Europe was created in Germany under the Bismarck government as a means of "preserving his power and calming the working population."[17] And in Germany, conservative elements continue to be very supportive of the health care system.[18] Indeed, conservative parties in Europe and Canada have traditionally viewed the creation of a comprehensive governmental health care system as a way to increase support for the nation and enhance community solidarity.[19]

The United States has a mixed system of public and private financing for the delivery of health care. In contrast with Britain and Canada, as of 2008, the United States did not provide universal access to health care through a governmental program. The Congressional Budget Office estimates that the average number of uninsured non-elderly (under sixty-five years old) "will rise from 45 million in 2009 to about 54 million in 2019."[20] In the United States, private health insurance is typically linked to employment.[21] Currently, approximately 160 million people are covered by employment-linked insurance.[22] Most insurance coverage in the private sector is through managed care plans.[23] These plans are subject to state laws regulating health insurance, but federal legislation known as ERISA preempts state laws regulating self-insured plans.[24] As a result, many larger employers now self-insure to avoid state mandated benefit laws.[25]

Employer-Provided Health Insurance in the United States

Melissa Thomasson has provided a summary of the development of private health insurance in the United States, noting that while private sickness insurance was widespread in the early twentieth century to provide wage replacement, private insurance to pay medical expenses was rare.[26] Up through the 1920s, insurers were reluctant to provide insurance for medical expenses because they did not consider the incurrence of medical expenses to be an insurable event.[27] They were particularly concerned about problems with adverse selection and moral hazard.[28] In addition, because of the limited range of medical treatments, medical expenses were relatively low, so there was not much of a market demand for health insurance.[29] By the 1930s, however, middle-class demand for health insurance had increased because of increased costs resulting from improvements in medical care and the rise of hospitals as treatment centers.[30]

Beginning in the 1930s, Blue Cross (BC) (hospital services) and Blue Shield (BS) (physician services) plans were developed by providers to stabilize demand during the Depression and to stave off attempts to adopt national health insurance.[31] BC and BS were organized as nonprofits and required to use community rating under state enabling laws. In the 1940s, commercial companies began offering the use of experience rating for groups (e.g., employer-provided insurance) thereby undercutting BC/BS pricing.[32]

The peculiar link between employment and private health insurance prevalent in the United States developed as a result due of several legal actions taken by the federal government. In 1942, the Stabilization Act passed by Congress at the outset of World War II imposed wage and price controls that precluded companies from raising wages, but did not prevent them from offering health insurance.[33] Because during the war, demand for employees was high, many companies began offering health insurance to attract workers.[34] In 1943, the Internal Revenue Service ruled that employer-paid contributions to health insurance plans were not taxable to employees.[35] And in 1949, the National Labor Relations Board ruled that unions and employers could enter into collective bargaining over health insurance benefits.[36] As a result of these developments, in the 1950s, negotiators for unions frequently sought more generous health insurance coverage in collective bargaining in lieu of wage increases because of the favorable tax treatment.[37]

Government Health Care Programs in the United States

Enacted in 1965 as a part of President Lyndon Johnson's Great Society legislative agenda, the Medicaid and Medicare programs were created to provide medical insurance for low income persons, the disabled, and the elderly. Coverage under the Medicaid program was available to those meeting the eligibility requirements for the "categorically needy,"[38] the "medically needy,"[39] and certain special groups.[40] Under Medicaid, many residents of nursing homes are provided coverage for their nursing home expenses if they meet certain asset and income eligibility requirements.[41] Ironically, although originally intended to provide medical insurance coverage for low-income uninsured persons, Medicaid has become the primary payor for nursing home residents from middle-class backgrounds who "spend down" in order to qualify for assistance.[42]

The Medicaid program is funded by both state and federal governments. All fifty states participate in the program, but states are not required to do so; in fact, Arizona did not participate in Medicaid until 1982.[43] While the states are responsible for administering the program, they are required to meet federal requirements in exchange for the federal financial contribution.[44]

In 1965, the Medicare program was also adopted to provide coverage for the elderly. It provides benefits to those age sixty-five and older, disabled workers under age sixty-five, and certain people with end-stage renal disease (ESRD).[45] Individuals are entitled to Medicare if they paid into the Social Security system during their working years.[46] Part A provides coverage for medically necessary hospital services; Part B provides coverage for physician services.[47] At the time of the creation of Medicare in the United States, outpatient drug costs were not covered.[48] Although prescription drug spending as a percentage of national health expenditures was about the same then (10%) as now (11%), because hospital costs were "far less predictable and potentially devastating," they were the major focus of the legislation.[49] Under Part D, beginning January 1, 2006, private companies provide insurance coverage for prescription drugs.[50] Medicare is funded by the federal government through premiums (for Parts B and D) and taxes.[51]

In 1997, the State Children's Health Insurance Program (SCHIP) was created by the federal government to provide matching funds to states to expand coverage for low-income children.[52] This program targets uninsured children under the age of nineteen in families with incomes at less than 200 percent of the federal poverty level (FPL) who are not eligible for Medicaid.[53] Under SCHIP, the federal government provides a match for state funding, subject to certain limits.[54] The states may implement the program by expanding Medicaid, setting up a separate program, or a combination of the two.[55] All fifty states participate in this program.[56]

The number of uninsured children has been reduced by a third since 1997 largely as a result of SCHIP and Medicaid expansion.[57] But some studies indicate that there are still 9 million uninsured children in the United States and many of them are eligible for SCHIP but have not been signed up with their state.[58] The continuation of SCHIP beyond 2007 required reauthorization by Congress.[59]

Problems with the United States Health Care System

Many of the problems in the United States health care system are due to the strong link between employment and health insurance coverage. Accordingly, loss of a job may mean loss of health insurance. Although continuation coverage is available for up to eighteen months after the loss of employment under COBRA, many workers do not take advantage of this because they are required to pick up the full cost of the premium.[60]

Another problem with the current system is its unfair tax treatment of funds used to purchase health insurance. Employees in group plans provided by employers don't pay taxes on their employer-paid premiums, even though they are a form of compensation.[61] Self-employed individuals are entitled to a deduction for premiums paid for health insurance covering themselves, their spouse, and their dependents.[62] And individuals who are not covered by a health plan and purchase a high-deductible policy can get a deduction for contributions to a Health Saving Account.[63] But "an individual (other than a self-employed individual) may deduct health insurance premiums only to the extent that aggregate unreimbursed medical expenses exceed 7.5% of adjusted gross income."[64] Unfortunately, small firms, and especially those with low-wage workers, generally don't offer health insurance benefits to their employees.[65] Only Hawaii requires employers to provide health insurance.[66]

Massachusetts requires all but the smallest employers to either provide insurance to their employees or pay a tax.[67] And, due to the high cost of health care and rate of growth, low-income persons who don't qualify for Medicaid may not be able to afford to purchase an individual health insurance policy.

There are also significant racial disparities in health care outcomes in the United States due in part to the lack of universal access. For example, infant mortality rates among African Americans are twice the national average.[68] "African American women are more than twice as likely to die from cervical cancer than are white women, and are more likely to die of breast cancer than are women of any other racial or ethnic group."[69] African-American adults are 29 percent more likely to die from heart disease and 40 percent more likely to die from stroke than white Americans.[70] And African-Americans, Native Americans, Alaska Natives, and Hispanic Whites are more likely to suffer from diabetes than non-Hispanic whites.[71] The life expectancy of African-Americans has always been substantially lower than that of white Americans.[72] Since the beginning of twentieth century, life expectancy of all Americans has been lower than Canadians.[73] Until the 1970s, this disparity was due to lower life expectancy of African-Americans, but since the 1970s, life expectancy of white Americans has not improved as much as that of Canadians.[74]

SCHIP Expansion: The Continuing Controversy over the Government's Role in Health Care Reform

In 2008, there was an unsuccessful attempt at the federal level to expand SCHIP. According to Sara Rosenbaum: "The conflagration over the reauthorization of the State Children's Health Insurance Program offers a compelling example of Washington's current inability to address even seemingly uncontroversial matters such as improved health care coverage for children."[75] Controversy among groups espousing various "theories of justice" erupted over SCHIP expansion.[76] There were essentially four groups: (1) conservatives (e.g., Bush administration, experts at AEI), who favor limiting governmental role to setting rules for market competition and providing subsidies to the poor; (2) libertarians (e.g., Michael Cannon at CATO), who favor substantially cutting back government regulation and rely on market forces to reduce costs, improve quality, and expand access; (3) utilitarians (e.g., Henry Aaron at Brookings), who favor an incremental approach to expanding access through state experiments, and tax and insurance reforms coupled with rationing to contain costs; and (4) egalitarians (e.g., Families USA, Progressive Democrats, Congressman

PART SIX: *Social Justice and Health Care Reform*

Rahm Emanuel (D-IL)), zealous advocates of expansion of government programs, with focus on eventually implementing a single-payer system.

In October 2007, President Bush vetoed SCHIP reauthorization legislation that would have permitted states to expand coverage of children in families at or below 200% FPL to 300% FPL. This would have provided increased funding of $35 billion to be paid for through a $0.61-per-pack increase in tobacco tax.[77] In his statement accompanying the veto, President Bush stated he was vetoing the legislation because it "would move health care in this country in the wrong direction."[78] He argued that the expansion of SCHIP would distort the original purpose of the program by allowing coverage of children in relatively high-income families rather than limiting its scope to children in families that could not afford private health insurance and were not eligible for Medicaid.[79] Moreover, he argued that the bill would move children from private health insurance on to the government program, and as a result government coverage would displace private health insurance.[80]

After the initial veto by President Bush in October 2007, there was a bipartisan attempt to develop a compromise measure. The second bill would also have given states authority to expand coverage of children in families at or below 200% of FPL to 300% FPL, but did have some additional provisions to address the "crowd out" problem — i.e., the exit from private insurance plans. This passed Congress but was vetoed by President Bush on December 12, 2007.[81] The veto message reiterated that the effect of the bill would be to move children from private health insurance to governmental programs.[82] On December 29, 2007, President Bush signed a bill extending SCHIP funding through March 31, 2009 and providing states projected to have a shortfall with funding above their FFY 2007 funding levels.[83] In response to this series of events, Sara Rosenbaum asked, "Why would the President veto bipartisan legislation that does what he insisted on — namely, aggressively enroll the poorest children?"[84] Then she answered her own question:

> The answer lies in a far larger dimension of SCHIP that is basic to any health insurance legislation — namely, the legislative architecture of the reform plan, its structure and operational approach. Viewed from this vantage point, the SCHIP battle turns out not to be about family-income assistance levels or the mechanism for financing . . . *Instead, the issue became the role of government in organizing and overseeing the health care marketplace.*"[85]

Professor Rosenbaum's point was brought home by a speech given at an American Enterprise Institute (AEI) Conference in April 2007, in which

Secretary of DHHS Michael Leavitt noted the two "divergent views as to the role that government ought to play in health care" — i.e., government as "proprietor" (setting prices and defining benefits) or government as "organizer (setting the rules for the market, remedying inequities, and subsidizing the needy).[86] Robert Helms, John Calfee, and Joseph Antos, health policy experts at AEI, a leading conservative think tank, argued that the "primary focus" of SCHIP should be on children in families with incomes less than 200% of the FPL and that its "subsidies should be restructured" to permit parents to purchase private health insurance.[87]

Michael Cannon, a health policy expert at CATO, the leading libertarian think tank, argued that rather than expanding SCHIP, Congress "should (1) make private health insurance more affordable by allowing consumers and employers to purchase less expensive policies from other states, and (2) fold Medicaid and SCHIP funding into block grants that no longer encourage states to open taxpayer-financed health care to non-needy families."[88] He believed that that this would make it possible to reduce spending on governmental programs.

On the other hand, Henry Aaron, a health policy expert at Brookings, a center-left think tank, favored the expansion of SCHIP, noting:

> It uses the conservative principle of permitting states latitude and independence to achieve the liberal goal of extending health insurance coverage.[89]

Families USA issued a statement deploring President Bush's veto noting that it would "put the health of America's children at risk."[90] And Rahm Emanuel, House Democratic Chair, clearly expressed his goals: "SCHIP should be for children what Medicare is for the elderly — a universal health care program."[91] One political commentator noted that House Democratic leaders planned to use the controversy over SCHIP expansion to put the Republicans on the defensive and set the stage for the debate over universal health insurance.[92]

The SCHIP expansion controversy shows that although all persons of good will want children to have access to health care, there is still substantial disagreement over the role of government versus the private sector in providing access to health care. The basic disagreement focuses on the role of private health insurance and markets in health care reform. At the two extremes are libertarians — who see no reason for any significant government presence in the health care sector and would focus on enhancing consumer choice and market competition in order to bring down cost, expand access, and

PART SIX: *Social Justice and Health Care Reform*

improve quality — and egalitarians, who see no need for a private sector and favor a single payer; indeed, many would prohibit private health insurance, as in Canada. Political compromises to expand access to health care may be possible between conservatives and the center-left if solutions preserve the role of the market and private insurance, focus on the role of the states, and minimize the expansion of federal government programs. With the election of Barack Obama, and a new Congress dominated by the Democratic Party, it is probable that SCHIP expansion will occur in 2009, along with other health care reforms.[93]

Chapter Seventeen

Health Care Reform Proposals

Several times in the past, the United States has seemed poised to adopt a system to provide universal access to health care. In 1993, a task force headed by Hillary Clinton issued a proposed health plan. Eventually, the Clinton Health Plan embraced universal access and managed competition within a budget. Under the Clinton health plan, most people were to receive health coverage through their employers, to be financed by payroll taxes. For those who weren't employed, the government would pay for enrollment in a health plan. Both for-profit and nonprofit health care plans were to be responsible for delivering care, and regional health care alliances were to negotiate with health plans and monitor the quality of care.[1]

Under the Clinton Health Plan, at least three plans were to be offered in each region: HMO, PPO, and fee-for-service.[2] It purposely eschewed reliance on the Canadian single-payer model and preserved a significant role for private health insurance. It was a variation on the theme of managed competition approach to health care reform, popular in the 1990s.[3] When first introduced, it seemed likely that it would be enacted in the fall of 1994.[4] The Clinton Health Plan, however, ran into serious political opposition (e.g., the "devastating Harry and Louise ads") and was never adopted.[5]

Market-Based Proposals for Health Care Reform

In the 1990s, conservative groups such as the National Center for Policy Analysis, the Heritage Foundation, and the American Legislative Exchange Council (ALEC) began promoting health or medical savings accounts (HSAs or MSAs) that would couple a high-deductible health insurance policy with a tax-preferred savings account to cover medical expenses.[6] HSAs/MSAs have become the most important and widely embraced market oriented health care reform strategy. In 1997 Congress authorized Medicare MSAs. In 2003, access to HSAs was expanded by federal legislation that permits individuals to deduct contributions to a HSA when they couple it with the purchase of a high-deductible health plan (at least $1,000 for an individual and $2,000 for a family) and no additional health insurance.[7] Funds then can build up tax-free within the account without limit, and withdrawals are not taxable if used for medical expenses.[8]

Another managed-competition health care reform proposal made in the 1990s was to open up the Federal Employees Health Benefits Program (FEHBP). It was proposed that the government would provide a subsidy for low-income taxpayers to buy into the FEHBP. At one time this approach was supported by two conservative groups: the Heritage Foundation and the American Legislative Exchange Council (ALEC).[9] In addition, opening up the FEHBP was also supported by Democrat John Kerry in his 2004 campaign for the presidency, along with federal government reinsurance for some of the risk of catastrophic care.[10]

The FEHBP is structured so that federal employees are allocated a certain amount of money to use in buying health insurance coverage from a range of companies offering policies approved by the government. There is an annual enrollment at which time federal employees are permitted to sign up with a health plan. These plans compete on the basis of price and quality. Beginning in 1994, "report cards," based on consumer satisfaction surveys on the plans, were provided to federal employees in advance of annual enrollment period so as to assist them in making a choice.[11]

Proposals for a Government-Run Health Care System

The Physicians' Working Group (PWG) has advocated the adoption of a single-payer system in the United States — i.e., "an expanded and improved version of traditional Medicare [that] would cover every American for all necessary medical care."[12] PWG estimates that a single-payer system would "save at least $200 billion annually (more than enough to cover all of the uninsured) by eliminating the high overhead and profits of the private, investor-owned insurance industry and reducing spending for marketing and other satellite services."[13] And further, that "[p]hysicians and hospitals would be freed from the concomitant burdens and expenses of paperwork created by having to deal with multiple insurers with different rules, often designed to avoid payment."[14]

In addition, PWG argues that this system would "make it possible to enforce overall spending limits for the health care system, slowing cost growth over the long run."[15] Finally, they contend that because of the saving due to reductions in administrative overhead, reductions in marketing costs, and this ability to set spending limits, single-payer is the "only affordable option for universal, comprehensive coverage."[16]

Incremental Reform Proposals

There seems to be a consensus emerging in the United States that we need to move to universal access, but disagreement over methods and particularly over the role of markets. Many have argued that incremental reform is the more likely path in the United States because of the structure of our government, weak party discipline, the role of powerful interest groups, and our concerns about the expansion of the role of the federal government, but others have noted that incremental reforms may not address many of the problems in our current system.[17]

The Baldwin-Price Bill would recognize that while there is an emerging consensus on the goal of universal access, there remains substantial disagreement over the means, and accordingly would "let a thousand flowers bloom."[18] This proposed legislation would encourage state programs to expand access by providing federal subsidies to the states, but allow the states to take different approaches in working toward universal access.[19]

Indeed, several states have adopted or considered adopting programs that would provide universal access. In 2006, Massachusetts adopted an approach to universal access that includes both an employer "pay or play" provision[20] and an individual mandate.[21] Under the Massachusetts "pay or play"[22] provision, employers with more than ten employees who don't provide health insurance to their employees are required to pay their "'fair share' of the cost of covering the uninsured, at a rate of $295 per employee per year."[23]

Massachusetts also established the Commonwealth Health Insurance Connector Program ("Connector"), which, in turn, operates the Commonwealth Care Health Insurance Program to facilitate the purchase of insurance by individuals by connecting them with insurers and providing subsidies to assist low-income persons in purchasing coverage.[24] Uninsured persons at or under 300% of the federal poverty level (FPL) are eligible for coverage under Commonwealth Care.[25] Under the individual mandate, persons were required to purchase a health insurance policy providing certain minimum benefits by July 1, 2007, or pay a penalty.[26]

Under the Massachusetts law, the "Connector" is also responsible for defining the minimum insurance package required under the individual mandate.[27] Initially, there was some difficulty in implementing the plan that arose when the minimal standards, as established by the "Connector," would have required 200,000 persons to purchase additional insurance coverage.[28] In addition, initial bids for providing the basic plans were at premium levels that the "Connector" "considered unaffordable."[29] At the end of its first year in operation, it was reported that the population of uninsured dropped from 13% to 7%, but the costs were $625 million per year up from an estimate of $472 million.[30] Other states (e.g., Vermont and Maine) have adopted, or are looking at, reforms to provide universal access. [31] And the State of Hawaii has had an employer mandate since 1975.[32]

Another proposed incremental approach was the announcement on January 18, 2006, by the Health Care Coalition for the Uninsured (HCCU), an organization composed of sixteen of the nation's largest health care and community organizations, of an agreement on a proposal that would significantly expand health coverage for the uninsured.[33] Among the groups endorsing the proposal was the Catholic Health Association.[34]

Reform under the HCCU proposal would be in two phases: Phase I focuses on children and Phase II focuses on adults.[35] Phase I calls for the expansion of SCHIP and "giving states the flexibility to deem low-income uninsured children eligible and enroll them in SCHIP or Medicaid when they qualify for other means-tested programs."[36] In addition, it calls for Congress to "make refundable, advanceable, and assignable tax credits available to families with children with incomes up to 300 percent of the federal poverty level [FPL] to facilitate the purchase of health coverage."[37] It also calls for Congress to establish a competitive grant program to enable states to experiment with new approaches to expanding health coverage.[38]

Phase II calls for Congress to give states the flexibility and funds to expand Medicaid eligibility to cover all adults with incomes below the FPL and additional funding for this purpose.[39] In addition, it calls for Congress to make available a refundable, advanceable tax credit for the purchase of health insurance for uninsured adults up to 300% FPL which could be used to purchase coverage regardless of whether or not the coverage was provided through an employer. [40]

The Obama Plan

In his 2008 campaign, President Barack Obama proposed a plan for health care reform that would rely "on an employer mandate, new public and private insurance programs, and insurance market regulation."[41] The plan would create new options for obtaining health insurance: a public plan and a national health insurance exchange (similar to the Connector in Massachusetts) where a private plan could be purchased.[42] The private plans available through the Exchange would be required to offer a comprehensive benefit package similar to plans participating in the FEHBP.[43] Premium levels would be controlled.[44] Insurance coverage would be portable and not tied to a particular job.[45]

Under the Obama plan, large employers would be required to either provide health insurance to their employees or pay a tax toward the cost of the new public plan.[46] Small employers would receive a tax credit for providing insurance to their employees.[47] Moreover, the Obama plan would not permit private insurers to "deny coverage for pre-existing conditions or charge substantially higher premiums to sick enrollees."[48] Thus, it "would end medical underwriting according to health status."[49]

Advocacy of Reform by Catholic Groups

Catholic health care organizations have joined the call for comprehensive health care reform to provide universal access. The USCCB, Catholic Health Association (CHA), and Catholic Charities supported SCHIP expansion.[50] CHA has embraced a set of principles for health care reform, discussed *infra*.[51] Ascension Health Care has made a commitment to achieving 100% access to health care through a shared public and private partnership.[52] Its plan has a strongly egalitarian streak, rejecting "a two-tiered health system that separates those who can pay for services from those who cannot pay."[53] And Providence Health System in Seattle has also been strongly committed to universal access.[54]

Catholic theologians have traditionally viewed access to basic health care as a human right and characterized the failure of government to provide universal access as a "moral failure."[55] But, of course, the devil is in the details: i.e., what would be included in the package of basic services. It is probable that in the present day, they will include contraception, sterilization, and abortion. There is reason to be wary of a wholesale government takeover of the health care system; it's likely to result in providing services considered immoral, maybe even coercing Catholic institutions into providing such services.[56] And, of course, the principle of subsidiarity would support arguments for the decentralization and localization of health care delivery.

At the time of the Clinton health care proposal, Catholic leaders generally supported health care reform, but had also lobbied against including abortion in the standard benefits package.[57] Democratic proposals included abortion coverage in the standard benefits package, but also included a conscience clause to allow Catholic hospitals to continue to refuse to provide it.[58] But this was still problematic from a Catholic perspective, because Catholics would be required to pay into health plans that covered abortion.[59]

In a 2007 document, the Catholic Health Association set forth its vision for health care reform.[60] This document envisions a more expansive role for government, criticizes the current reliance on employer-sponsored health insurance, and expresses a desire that "health care should be organized as a true system that is integrated to promote the nation's health."[61] It also eschews the notion that health care is a commodity.[62]

The 2007 document sets forth eight principles that should serve as a basis for health care reform: (1) universal access to a package of basic health benefits; (2) special protection for the poor and vulnerable, including provision of the same quality of care for everyone; (3) emphases on primary and preventive health care to create healthy communities; (4) fair financing, with the government's portion to be financed through a progressive system of taxation; (5) allocation of resources in a manner that is "transparent and participative," with a focus on cost-effective use of resources and avoidance of futile care; (6) an emphasis on patient-centered health care and the availability of "end-of-life and palliative care"; (7) an emphasis on safety and efficiency to be achieved through the increased use of information technology and evidence-based medicine; and (8) respect for religiously-affiliated health care organizations.[63]

Although the document does not otherwise mention the *ERDs*, it specifically called for the rejection of "public financing for procedures prohibited by the *Ethical and Religious Directives for Catholic Health Care Services*, including abortion and euthanasia."[64]

In an earlier document issued in 2000, the CHA offered "a framework for reform that can serve in the public forum as a catalyst for accessible and affordable health care for all in a just and compassionate health care system."[65] This document includes several specific proposals for expansion of the role of the federal government including: (1) enactment by the federal government of an individual mandate requiring everyone to be enrolled in a health insurance plan; (2) definition of a basic benefits package by the federal government that would not include coverage for abortion or euthanasia; (3) expanding Medicaid and SCHIP; (4) establishing a new plan similar to the FEHBP that would provide access to insurance coverage with appropriate premium subsidies to be provided by the federal government; (5) a federal requirement of guaranteed issuance of insurance private insurers to cover everyone regardless of pre-existing conditions during an annual enrollment period; and (6) Medicare reform.[66]

In contrast with the CHA approach, and its predominant focus on social justice concerns and a more expansive role for the federal government, is a proposal issued by the Catholic Medical Association in 2004 that views problems in the health care system as stemming from the influence of a culture of death.[67] The proposal of the Catholic Medical Association relies more on market-based solutions than on the expansion of government programs. As to a government run health care system, it notes, "Unitarian financing would carry with it universal and compulsory cooperation in abortion and other procedures that epitomize a culture of death."[68] It further notes:

> When the "right to health care" is improperly understood, when it lapses into radical autonomy, the triumph of relativism, the mere instrumentality of the healer, or a culture of entitlement for the healed, it ceases to be just and it ceases to be of Christ.[69]

At the centerpiece of this document is a concern about the demise of the Hippocratic Oath and the "erosion" of the physician-patient relationship that have "their root in the loss of a common understanding, within and without the medical profession, of the sanctity and inviolability of each human life."[70] This report decries contraceptive mandates; government support for contraception, abortion, and sterilization; government action against pharmacists with conscientious objections to coerce them to fill prescriptions for Plan B; and attacks on conscience-clause laws.[71]

The CMA's principles for health care reform are: (1) "individual ownership of insurance" to be subsidized through refundable tax credits; (2) "freedom from health insurance mandates;" (3) "choice of private insurance policies" including new options to be offered by faith-based groups; (4) expansion of health savings accounts including offering of a faith-based health savings account option in the FEHBP; (5) the enactment at the federal level of legislation to expand and strengthen conscience protections for health care providers; and (6) "experiments with diocesan self insurance" to avoid paying for contraceptive coverage and to strengthen support for natural family planning.[72] The CMA report states:

> The key to the crisis in American health care today is that it violates essential norms of justice and charity on both sides of the physician-patientrelationship. It impairs the ability of the physician to decide and act as Jesus would, and it ignores the dignity of the poor in countless ways. Government policies have denied persons of little or no income the means to direct their own families' health care; have saturated

neighborhoods with "reproductive health" facilities and philosophies that have resulted in abandoned children, extraordinarily high rates of abortion and sexually transmitted disease; and have undermined husband-and-wife and parent-child relationships.

As a subset of the mis-insurance of all Americans, the mis-insurance of the poor is a particularly scandalous affront to the requirements of genuine justice, charity, and solidarity.

"History teaches us that in the field of service to health as well, every commitment to achieve justice has been shown to be insufficient because of the fragility and selfishness of man. Without the support of charity there has not been either a sufficient or an increasing upholding of justice.... The figure of the Good Samaritan is the point of reference for a full interpretation of the relationship between justice and charity, of a justice that receives from charity the connotations of sensitivity, sharing and solidarity."[73] [footnote omitted]

Mary McDonough has criticized the CMA proposal, stating that it "lacks both substance and practicality as seen in its promotion of high-deductible health plans" because in order to benefit from such plans, consumers must have a relatively high level of disposable income.[74] She further notes that its lack of a requirement of guaranteed issuance of insurance and price controls on premiums could make insurance coverage unaffordable for the chronically ill.[75] She also criticizes the failure of the CMA proposal to call for definition of a basic benefits package by the government to avoid consumer confusion.[76]

These criticisms could be addressed in an approach to health care reform proposal that would be based on a market-based approach and provide more autonomy for religious health care providers as envisioned by the CMA proposal. For example, high-risk pools could be created by states to provide coverage for the chronically ill at affordable levels, and states could use a variety of revenue sources to finance these funds.[77] A refundable tax credit could be provided to assist low- and moderate-income participants in HSAs.[78] And insurers could be required to provide information to consumers in a readily understandable form as is presently done in the FEHBP. These approaches would be compatible with a system, as proposed by CMA, that would provide more opportunities to develop faith-based approaches to health insurance in the private sector, and avoid the obvious dangers posed by an expansion of federal power as endorsed by CHA that is likely to carry with it government mandates for the financing and even the provision of abortions and sterilizations.

CHA endorsed President Obama's appointment of former Senator Tom Daschle, a "pro-choice" Catholic, to be Secretary of Health and Human Services and head of a new White House Office of Health Reform.[79] On the other hand, pro-life groups expressed concern about his appointment in light of "his documented and indefatigable support for abortion on Capitol Hill."[80] While in the Senate, Daschle had opposed efforts to ban partial-birth abortion and supported taxpayer funding for abortions.[81] In February 2009, Daschle's name was withdrawn from consideration for these posts due to unpaid taxes.[82] Subsequently, President Obama announced the nomination of Governor Kathleen Sebelius of Kansas to be Secretary of Health and Human Services. This announcement generated concern among some Catholic bishops because Governor Sebelius has taken an avowedly "pro-choice" position and had earlier been publicly requested to refrain from receiving Communion by Archbishop Naumann of Kansas City, Kansas.[83]

Conclusion

Catholic hospitals are in difficult situation. If they are to survive as distinctively Catholic institutions, they must continue to emphasize their Catholic identity, including their adherence to the *ERD*s. Unfortunately, however, as evidenced by contraceptive coverage mandates, emergency contraception laws, and attacks on conscience-clause legislation, we are in a socio-legal environment that is hostile toward many of the traditional values underlying Catholic health care. As a legal and political matter, it is becoming increasingly difficult for Catholic institutions to claim exemption from laws of general application that may require them to act in violation of Catholic teaching.

Catholic institutions could bolster their claim to statutory, if not constitutional protection, from such laws by becoming more pervasively Catholic. And if Catholic institutions are generally perceived to be serious about their Catholic identity, it may be easier to argue for legislative exemption from such laws. On the other hand, emphasizing the distinctive mission of Catholic hospitals may strengthen claims that public funding should be denied because of the sectarian nature of these hospitals.

It is instructive to compare the state of Catholic health care systems with Catholic higher education. Since there are no specific norms in canon law governing the Catholic identity of the health care institution, and no clear policy statement on these issues from the Vatican, *Ex Corde Ecclesiae*,[1] a document focusing on Catholic institutions of higher learning, is sometimes used as basis of comparison for the analysis of Catholic identity in health care institutions.[2] *Ex Corde Ecclesiae* was directed at arresting the trend toward secularization in Catholic universities that began with the *Land O' Lakes Declaration* in the 1960s.[3]

After emphasizing the importance of maintaining Catholic identity in the universities, *Ex Corde Ecclesiae* notes:

> In particular, Catholic theologians, aware that they fulfill a mandate received from the Church, are to be faithful to the Magisterium of the Church as the authentic interpreter of Sacred Scripture and Sacred Tradition.[4]

The concept of academic freedom has, however, been used effectively to prevent any serious attempts to enforce adherence to Catholic Doctrine even in theology departments of Catholic universities. Although canon law seemingly requires those who teach Catholic theology at the university to have a *mandatum* from the local bishop, most Catholic universities have refused to publicize whether the members of their theology faculties have received the *mandatum*.[5] In addition, the tradition of faculty governance would also likely frustrate such attempts. As a result, it is likely that in the future only a relatively small number of Catholic higher education institutions, many of them newly founded, will remain distinctively Catholic.[6]

There is nothing equivalent to the *Land O'Lakes Declaration* in the world of Catholic health care. By way of contrast with Catholic higher education, there appears to have been a more concerted and serious effort to maintain a distinctively Catholic character in health care systems. The religious orders have tried to provide spiritual formation to their lay employees who ultimately will be responsible for maintaining the mission of the sponsoring order. They have foreseen the increasing importance of the laity and engaged in concerted planning to maintain their Catholic identity. In addition, the *ERDs* provide a relatively clear set of norms that continue to apply in Catholic health care systems and provide standards for maintaining their Catholic identity.

There is also a greater appreciation of the value of maintaining a Catholic identity in the health care field as opposed to higher education. Indeed, Catholicity provides a distinctive brand in the health care market place that has developed an appeal to Catholics and non-Catholics. Health care institutions deal with life, death, and suffering and so the spiritual dimension of Catholic hospitals may even enhance their position in the marketplace. Physicians and nurses also view themselves as healers, and their interests more readily align with the religious mission of Catholic institutions. Most health care providers appreciate the importance of a religious mission in providing health care and a compassionate dimension of health care, even if they are not Catholic. There isn't the sort of constant struggle within health care institutions over issues of Catholic mission that we observe within Catholic colleges and universities, so it is possible that the mission of Catholic hospitals will survive even with the transfer of ownership of these facilities to lay boards. Kevin O'Rourke has recommended several measures that could be implemented to ensure this continuation of mission, including continuing emphasis on the *ERDs*, emphasis on the preferential option for the poor, and the internalization of the mission to foster the continuing support for the mission by employees and physicians.[7]

Nonetheless, there are problems and difficulties in maintaining a Catholic mission in health care institutions. At times, some Catholic health care institutions have shown a willingness to accommodate to the prevailing culture by entering into affiliations and arrangements that effectively circumvent the *ERDs*. And unfortunately, the provision of direct sterilizations by some Catholic institutions, in violation of the *ERDs*, may further encourage attempts by those who seek legislation requiring Catholic hospitals to provide a full range of reproductive health services. On the whole, however, the prospects of maintaining a Catholic identity in the health care sector appear more hopeful than the prospects in Catholic higher education because of the presence of the normative framework provided by the *ERDs*.

It is possible that external forces that would severely limit the carrying out of that mission may ultimately prevail. The Catholic Church is the only major Western institution that continues to adhere to the belief that there is a universal moral law that provides specific, absolute moral norms concerning human reproduction, binding at all times on all persons. The sexual revolution has had a tremendous impact on the West, and the Catholic Church's position is countercultural. Elites in the West, including several justices on the U.S. Supreme Court, have embraced an ethical relativism that views individual autonomy in sexual matters as a primary means of self-discovery and self-fulfillment.[8] In effect, this right of sexual self-fulfillment and a commitment to tolerance bring with it an antinomian orientation that trumps traditional moral principles that are viewed by these same elites as primitive and even malicious. With this cultural shift among elites, it is not clear that the secular liberal Western state will continue to permit the Catholic Church to continue to practice — even in its own institutions — its beliefs on the intrinsic immorality of direct abortion, direct sterilization, and contraception.[9] Catholic hospitals may eventually be forced to choose between continued existence and adherence to the *ERDs*.

If FOCA is adopted, it could override existing conscience protection laws. Catholic institutions could be forced to close their obstetrics units to avoid having to perform sterilizations and abortions. Comprehensive health care reform could bring with it mandates requiring all hospitals to provide a full-range of reproductive services as a condition of receiving federal funding. If

Catholic health care institutions in the United States are no longer permitted to receive federal funding and follow the *ERDs*, particularly their restrictions on the provision of abortions and sterilizations, then the bishops will face a difficult dilemma. The continuing recognition of health care institutions as Catholic, even though they are providing reproductive health care services in violation of the specific norms of the *ERDs*, will undoubtedly create a substantial risk of scandal among the faithful.[10] On the other hand, closure of these institutions, or withdrawal of recognition of their Catholic nature and severing of any links with the local bishop, will substantially diminish the role of the Catholic Church in health care.

Some have argued that Catholics should continue to operate acute care hospitals, despite the obvious difficulties, because they can continue to be a positive witness to society in this role.[11] However, while Catholics should not precipitately move out of the acute care hospital sector, it is time to recognize that such a move in the future may be inevitable in light of the various forces at work in society. Apart from the problems of maintaining a religious ministry in an increasingly hostile environment, general acute care hospitals are in decline. More surgeries are being done in ambulatory surgery centers, drug therapies have the potential to reduce the need for surgical interventions, and specialty hospitals are becoming more widespread. It is an increasingly competitive and difficult economic environment for Catholic hospitals. In a 1998 article discussing the difficult economic environment, Fr. Richard McCormick indicated his pessimism over whether Catholic health care could keep "its integrity in this context."[12]

Reflecting on McCormick's observations in an article published in 2000, Daniel Sulmasy referred to McCormick's belief that Catholics should "leave hospitals and shift to hospice and care for the elderly," but further notes that they will find similar problems in those "spheres of health care."[13] So, he urges Catholics to "keep their hospitals."[14] In the views of some, such as McCormick and Sulmasy, the threats to the Catholic hospital come primarily from the "growing place of technology and a hostile economic environment."[15] But to me, the more pressing concern is the pressure on Catholic hospitals to become involved in performing immoral procedures. And, with the passage of FOCA and comprehensive health care reform, this problem may become an immediate concern.

The primary role of Catholic health care should be to provide support for the culture of life and to evangelize the secular culture.[16] As stated in *Charter for Health Care Workers*, issued by the Pontifical Council for Assistance to Health Care Workers:

Conclusion

> The work of health care persons is a very valuable service to life. It expresses a profoundly human and Christian commitment, undertaken and carried out not only as a technical activity but also as one of dedication to and love of neighbor. It is a form of "Christian witness." "Their profession calls for them to be guardians and servants of human life."
>
> Life is a primary and fundamental good of the human person. Caring for life, then, expresses, first and foremost, a truly human activity in defense of life.[17] [citations omitted]

It is increasingly difficult to perform those roles in the acute care hospital setting. In order to survive financially, Catholic hospitals are entering into complex and nuanced arrangements with non-Catholic providers who are involved in providing reproductive services that are incompatible with Catholic teaching. The cumulative effect of all this activity is to undermine Catholic teaching on abortion, contraception, and sterilization. In addition, health care is becoming less personal and more reliant on technology.[18] Perhaps it would be better to divert the resources of Catholic health care to alternative ministries. This could be a series of hospices to support the dying or those in a persistent vegetative state. It could include a system of family health centers that would provide Natural Family Planning instruction and birthing facilities as well as general health care for families; clinics in underserved areas that could focus on preventive care; rehabilitation facilities; and centers for care of the mentally ill and handicapped. And all these efforts should be permeated with spiritual support for both patients and providers.[19]

Unfortunately, however, even if Catholics remove themselves from the operation of acute care hospitals, the Catholic health care ministry will be under continuing pressure to provide immoral drugs or procedures. For example, recently, Divine Mercy Care — a Virginia pharmacy that follows Catholic teaching and refuses to provide birth control prescriptions and condoms — has been attacked by those arguing that all pharmacies and pharmacists should be required to provide such drugs.[20]

Unfortunately, national "pro-choice" Catholic politicians threaten the continued existence of Catholic health care because they provide political cover and legitimacy to efforts to impose mandates on Catholic health care institutions to provide services in violation of the *ERD*s. The beginnings of this problem may be traced to a meeting of Catholic theologians and politicians held at the Kennedy compound at Hyannisport, in the summer of 1964, to discuss the political aspects of abortion.[21] This meeting, as recounted by Al Jonsen, was precipitated by a shift toward the liberalization of abortion laws.

Attendees at the meeting included: Robert Kennedy, Edward Kennedy, Giles Milhaven, Sargent Shriver, Josef Fuchs, Al Jonsen, Robert Drinan, Charles Curran, and Richard McCormick.[22] The theologians present concurred that it was permissible for Catholic politicians to support liberalized abortion laws that would permit abortions in the hard cases of a serious physical threat to maternal health, pregnancies due to rape or incest, and severe fetal deformities.[23] The apparent basis for this position was a prudential judgment — i.e., the recognition of the difficulty of maintaining restrictive abortion policies that would conform to Catholic teaching in contemporary American society.[24]

Gradually, however, in the aftermath of *Roe v. Wade*, leading Catholic politicians discarded this more nuanced approach and began to embrace the view that abortion is a fundamental right, a politically expedient move for them that garnered the support of the emerging feminist movement. This was a significant shift: while at one time it arguably may have been morally permissible for a Catholic politician to vote for an abortion law restricting legal abortion to the hard cases, in order to maintain some sort of social peace and head off attempts to enact even more radical laws, it is a much different proposition to argue that the support of Catholic politicians for unfettered access to abortion with public financing is morally justifiable.

By the 1980s, however, much of the hierarchy and Catholic politicians had become accustomed to an approach that allowed Catholic politicians to support abortion rights without fear of condemnation by their bishops. In 1984, in an address delivered at the University of Notre Dame, the prominent Catholic politician Mario Cuomo, governor of New York, would state that his opposition to the Hatch Amendment — a constitutional amendment that would return to the states the authority to legislate on abortion — and support for Medicaid funding of abortion were consistent with Catholic teaching.[25] He also commended one New York bishop for recognizing that abortion should be treated as an internal Catholic matter rather than as a public policy issue.[26] In contrast, Archbishop Charles Chaput has exhorted Catholics "to keep fighting for the sanctity of the human person, starting with the unborn child and extending throughout life."[27]

It is my hope that the Catholic health care ministry will continue to adhere to the *ERDs* and promote a culture of life even in the face of challenges from a post-Christian society that embraces a culture of death. It is also my hope that Catholic hospitals will remain free to develop their own value-based model of health care free from state and federal legislative mandates that will require them to violate the *ERDs*. But if this is not the case, then the path of resistance to such mandates may become necessary. As the late Robert Cover noted, sometimes resistance to the state provides the defining moment for a religion.[28] It may be that Catholic health care in the United States will be called upon to resist the culture of death in the face of state attempts to force Catholic institutions to provide immoral procedures. In his last novel, *The Thanatos Syndrome,* Walker Percy articulates an alternative vision for a marginalized Catholic health care ministry through the fictional character of Fr. Rinaldo Smith, an alcoholic priest whom some regard as insane. Fr. Smith's hospice was closed down for a time by medical authorities, but at its reopening, he pleads:

> Listen to me, dear physicians, dear brothers, dear Qualitarians, abortionists, euthansiasts! Do you know why you are going to listen to me? Because Every last one of you is a better man than I and you know it! And yet you like me. Every last one of you knows me and what I am, a failed priest, an old drunk, who is only fit to do one thing and to tell you one thing. You are good, kind, hardworking doctors, but you like me nevertheless and I know that you will allow me to tell you one thing — no, ask one thing — no, beg one thing of you. Please do this one favor for me, dear doctors. If you have a patient, young or old, suffering, dying, afflicted, useless, born or unborn, whom you for the best of reasons wish to put out of his misery — I beg only one thing of you, dear doctors! Please send him to us. Don't kill them! We'll take them — all of them! Please send them to us! I promise you, and I know that you believe me, that we will take care of him, her — we will even call on you to help us take care of them! — and you will not have to make such a decision. God will bless you for it and you will offend no one except the Great Prince Satan, who rules the world, that is all.[29]

Notes

Introduction

[1] Pope John Paul II, *Evangelium Vitae* ("The Gospel of Life") (1995); http://www.vatican.va/holy_father/john_paul_ii/encyclicals/documents/hf_jp-ii_enc_25031995_evangelium-vitae_en.html.

[2] Kenneth R. White, "Hospitals Sponsored by the Roman Catholic Church: Separate, Equal and Distinct." *Milbank Quarterly* 78:2 (2000): 213, 233, notes:

> A confluence of powerful environmental forces at the beginning of the twenty-first century is threatening the future of Catholic health care. A review of the research that defines, differentiates, and describes the performance and identity measures of Catholic hospitals reveals them to be a *separate* case of private, nonprofit hospital. They have experienced environmental pressures to become isomorphic with other hospital ownership types and are *equal* on some dimensions. To keep pace with the changing demands of religious sponsorship and the social role of the hospital, Catholic hospitals continue to redefine themselves. To justify a *distinct* and legitimate social role they must begin to emphasize organizational commitments to a "Catholic" way of doing things. Without a palpable and routinely noticeable distinctiveness, the institutions fail the "identity challenge" of what makes them Catholic. (Ibid. [citations omitted]).

[3] Nat Henthoff, "New President, More Abortions? The Pro-Life Battle Begins Anew." *Washington Times*, Nov. 24, 2008, A21.

[4] John O. Mudd, "From CEO to Mission Leader: Lay Directors Must Take Responsibility for the Catholic Identity of Institutions." *America* 14 (July 18, 2005): 193.

[5] *See* "Catholic Hospitals and the Charity Myth." The Abortion Access Project; http://www.abortionaccess.org/viewpages.php?id=168 (asserting "that Catholic hospitals actually provide lower levels of charity care than most other hospitals") (on file with author).

[6] *Cf.* William Saletan, *Bearing Right: How Conservatives Won the Abortion Wars* (Berkeley: University of California Press, 2003). Saletan distinguishes between liberal pro-choice activists who advocate public funding of abortion and oppose parental consent laws from more conservative pro-choice supporters who support access to abortion but not public funding and favor parental consent laws. He concludes the position of conservative pro-choice supporters has prevailed in the political arena. *See* Ibid.

[7] The term "reproductive health services" is itself a controversial and tendentious term. In the international law context, this term has been used to promote increased access to abortion, contraception, and sterilization. *See* Fr. Robert Araujo, S.J., "Sovereignty, Human Rights, and Self-Determination: The Meaning of International Law." *Fordham International Law Journal* 24 (2001): 1477, 1508–09. Generally, those working in the Catholic natural-law tradition would not consider abortion, contraception, and sterilization to be "reproductive health services," because they are intended to prevent reproduction. In January of 2003, the Vatican announced plans to publish a "Lexicon on Ambiguous and Colloquial Terms about Family Life and Ethical Questions" that would include a glossary of terms intended to clarify

sexual and reproductive issues. In an interview concerning the glossary, Cardinal Trujillo particularly "took issue with the term 'reproductive rights,' which he said 'is used not to promote the right of reproduction, but the right of abortion.'" Jennifer Harper, "Vatican Writes 'Glossary' on Sex; Will Publish Lexicon to Clear up 'Grave Moral Confusion,'" *Washington Times*, Jan. 17, 2003, A1. The Italian version of the Lexicon was subsequently published in 2003, and an English version is planned. Pontifical Council for the Family, Publications; http://www.vatican.va/roman_curia/pontifical_councils/family/documents/rc_pc_family_doc_20031119_publications-list_en.html (last visited Dec. 8, 2008).

[8] *See* Leslie Laurence, "The Hidden Health Threat That Puts Every Woman at Risk." *Redbook*, July 1, 2000, 112, stating:

> Abortion isn't the only procedure banned by hospitals under Catholic control. Prescribing birth control (even to treat endometriosis and ovarian cysts), performing surgery to sterilize men and women who've completed their families, treating infertility with in vitro fertilization and artificial insemination—all these procedures can become off-limits. Medical schools affiliated with Catholic hospitals can't train students to perform abortions or do research on fetal tissue. Doctors treating patients who have refused "extraordinary measures" at the end of their lives can't withdraw feeding tubes.

The author of this *Redbook* article was concerned about more than the unwillingness of Catholic hospitals to provide certain services. She is also concerned about any mixing of religion with health care. To this end she quotes a psychiatrist practicing at a Minnesota clinic that was considering a merger with the prestigious St. Mary's Medical Center. This psychiatrist was offended by that hospital's customs of offering prayers over the loudspeaker and placing crucifixes in the patient rooms. This psychiatrist further stated: "Thoughtful Catholics recognize that it is not hospitable or charitable to use the vulnerability of an illness as an occasion to proselytize for a religious viewpoint." Ibid.

[9] As of 2006, nine states had adopted emergency contraception legislation. Erica S. Mellick, "Time for Plan B: Increasing Access to Emergency Contraception and Minimizing Conflicts of Conscience." *The Journal of Health Care Law & Policy* 9:2 (2006): 402, 436 (citing Cal. Penal Code § 13823.11(e), (g)(4)(A) (West 2002); 412 Ill. Comp. Stat. Ann. 70/2.2(b) (West 2005); Mass. Gen. Laws. Ann. ch. 111, § 70E(o) (West 2006); N.J. Stat. Ann. § 26:2H-12.6c (West 2005); N.M. Stat. Ann. § 24-10D-3 (A) (West 2003); N.Y. Public Health Law § 2805-p (2) (McKinney 2006); S.C. Code Ann. § 16-3-1350 (B) (Law. Co-op. 1997); Tex. Health & Safety Code Ann. § 171.012(C) (Vernon 2005); Wash. Rev. Code Ann. § 70.41.350(1) [West 2006]).

This article also lists seven states requiring emergency rooms to provide information about emergency contraception, and seven states requiring emergency rooms to dispense emergency contraception to sexual assault victims upon request. Ibid., 436. (citing Cal. Penal Code §13823.11 (e)(2) & (g)(4)(B) (2002); ass. Gen. Laws Ann. ch. 111 §70E (West 2006); N. J. Stat. Ann. §26:2H-12.6c(c) (West 2005); N.M. Stat. Ann. §24-10D-3 (A)(3) (Michie 2003); N.Y. Public Health Law §2805-p (2)(c) (McKinney 2006); S.C. Code Ann. §16-3-1350 (B) (Law. Co-op. 2006); Wash. Rev. Code Ann. §70.41.350(1)(C) (West 2006).

[10] John Burger, "Mandatory Contraceptive Coverage — Is Abortion Next?" *National Catholic Register*, Feb. 17, 2002.

[11] Ibid. (quoting Cathleen Cleaver, Director of Planning and Information for the Pro-Life Secretariat of the United States Conference of Catholic Bishops).

[12] R*eligious Refusals and Reproductive Rights,* ACLU Reproductive Freedom Project (2002); http://www.aclu.org/FilesPDFs/ACF911.pdf.

[13] In 1999, the California State Assembly defeated by a vote of 31 to 39 a bill proposed by Assemblywoman Sheila Kuhl (D-Santa Monica) that would have required Catholic hospitals to provide abortions or abortion referrals. If they failed to do so, then the hospitals would not have had access to public bond financing or Cal-Mortgage loan insurance. The bill was defeated when five Latino Democrats voted against it. Jim Holman, "GOP and Latino Dems to the Rescue, San Francisco Faith." July–Aug. 1999; http://www.sffaith.com/ed/articles/1999/0799an.htm.

[14] *See, e.g.,* Abortion Non-Discrimination Act, H.R. 4691, Hearing before the House Energy and Commerce S. Comm. on Health, 107th Cong. (2d Sess. 2002). Catherine Weiss, Director of the ACLU Reproductive Freedom Project, stated:

> When, however, religiously affiliated organizations move into secular pursuits — such as providing medical care or social services to the public or running a business — they should no longer be insulated from secular laws that apply to these secular pursuits. In the public world, they should play by public rules. The vast majority of health care institutions, including those with religious affiliations, serve the general public. They employ a diverse workforce. And they depend on government funds. A recent study found that Medicare and Medicaid accounted for 46% of total revenues to religiously affiliated hospitals in California in 1998, while unrestricted contributions, including charitable donations from church members, accounted for only .0015% (or $15 in every $10,000) of total revenues. These institutions ought to abide by the same standards of care and reproductive health mandates that apply to other health care institutions. (Ibid.)

[15] Ibid. Statement of Professor Lynn Wardle, J. Reuben Clark Law School, Brigham Young University.

[16] United States Conference of Catholic Bishops, *The Campaign to Force Hospitals to Provide Abortions* Sept. 2003); http://www.usccb.org/prolife/issues/abortion/THREAT.PD.

[17] *Valley Hospital Association, Inc. v. Mat-Su Coalition for Choice*, 948 P.2d 963 (Alaska 1997).

[18] John Kerry, a Catholic and a Democrat who supports abortion rights, has stated, "Abortions need to be moved out of the fringes of medicine and into the mainstream of medical practice." "GOP Web Site Uses Misleading Kerry Quote on Abortion." FactCheck.org, Annenberg Political Fact Check (Sept. 24, 2004) (quoting from *US Congressional Record*, Vol. 140 S10393, "Pensacola Anti-Abortion Murders and Religious Fanaticism"; Aug. 2 1994); http://www.factcheck.org/gop web site uses misleading kerry quote.html. This Web site focuses on the misuse of a quote by Republican Web site during 2004 campaign to suggest Kerry favors frequent abortions and quotes Kerry campaign spokesperson characterizing Kerry's position as being that abortion should be "safe, legal and rare." Ibid.

[19] Leslie Cannold, *The Abortion Myth: Feminism, Morality, and the Hard Choices Women Make* (Lebanon, NH: Wesleyan University Press, 2001), 43.

[20] "Finding Common Ground in a Pluralist Society," *Health Progress* (July–Aug. 1998); http://findarticles.com/p/articles/mi_qa3859/is_199807/ai_n8791394 (remarks of Rev. Brian Hehir, Professor, Harvard Divinity School).

[21] Ibid.(Remarks of Mary Healey-Sedutto, Ph.D., director of Health and Hospitals, Archdiocese of New York.)

[22] Weiss, *supra* note 14, at 1.

[23] *Religious Refusals and Reproductive Rights*, *supra* note 12, at 2.

[24] Ibid., 1.

[25] United States Conference of Catholic Bishops, *Ethical and Religious Directives for Catholic Health Care Services*, 4th ed. (2001). *See also* White, *supra* note 2, at 216, noting, "The

moral responsibility of Catholic health care is outlined in the Ethical and Religious Directives for Catholic Health Care Services."

[26] Directive 38, *Ethical and Religious Directives for Catholic Health Care Services*, supra note 25, at 25.

[27] Directive 53, Ibid., 28.

[28] Directive 45, Ibid., 26.

[29] Bonar Menninger, "Mission & Margin." *HealthLeaders* (Dec. 2003); http://www.catholicsforchoice.org/news/inthenews/2003/2003dechealthleaders_missionandmargin.asp (quoting Sr. Mary Roch Rocklage, chairwoman of the St. Louis-based Sisters of Mercy Health System and the immediate past chairwoman of the American Hospital Association).

[30] "Finding Common Ground," *supra* note 20 (remarks of Rev. Brian Hehir, Professor, Harvard Divinity School).

[31] Tony Quinn, "Democrats: A Loyal Constituency Is Restless." *Los Angeles Times*, Jan. 6, 2002, Op. pt. M, 2. This article notes:

> But the real political damage for Democrats may lie in Church leaders' accusations that the legislation smacks of officially endorsed bigotry against Catholics. They assert the pope was ridiculed and the Church compared to a witch's coven as the bill moved through the Legislature. Church leaders also worry that the bill is part of a larger effort by feminist groups and their Democratic allies to force Catholic hospitals to provide abortion on demand, a matter of growing public debate as the number of Catholic-owned hospitals increases in California.... Is there any room left in the Democratic Party for the traditionalist Catholic viewpoint?
>
> David Carlin, the former Democratic majority leader of the Rhode Island Senate, doesn't think so. In an article titled "How Can a Catholic Be a Democrat?" Carlin complains that his party is not only pro-abortion, but also in favor of same-sex marriage, physician-assisted suicide, stem-cell research and even cloning embryos. "If you're a Catholic," he writes, "how can you possibly continue to be a Democrat when the Democratic Party can be relied on to support the rejection of Christian values and their replacement by un-Christian or anti-Christian values?" (Ibid.)

[32] *Catechism of the Catholic Church* (1994), Par. 2270; http://www.vatican.va/archive/catechism/p3s2c2a5.htm#I. The *Catechism* states:

> Human life must be respected and protected absolutely from the moment of conception. From the first moment of his existence, a human being must be recognized as having the rights of a person — among which is the inviolable right of every innocent being to life. (Ibid.)

[33] *See*, e.g., "Kerry Affirms Support for Abortion Rights." CNN, Apr. 26, 2004; http://www.cnn.com/2004/ALLPOLITICS/04/23/kerry.abortion/index.html.

[34] Interview with Democratic candidate for Vice President Joe Biden, *Meet the Press*, Sept. 7, 2008; http://www.msnbc.msn.com/id/26590488/page/4/. The transcript states:

> **Tom Brokaw:** What if Senator Obama comes to you and says, "When does life begin? Help me out here, Joe." As a Roman Catholic, what would you say to him?
>
> **Mr. Biden:** I'd say, "Look, I know when it begins for me." It's a personal and private issue. For me, as a Roman Catholic, I'm prepared to accept the teachings of my church. But let me tell you, there are an awful lot of people of great confessional faiths — Protestants, Jews, Muslims and others — who have a different view. They believe in God as strongly

as I do. They're intensely as religious as I am religious. They believe in their faith and they believe in human life, and they have differing views as to when life — I'm prepared as a matter of faith to accept that life begins at the moment of conception.

But that is my judgment. For me to impose that judgment on everyone else who is equally and maybe even more devout than I am seems to me is inappropriate in a pluralistic society. And I know you get the push back, "Well, what about fascism?" Everybody, you know, you going to say fascism's all right? Fascism isn't a matter of faith. No decent religious person thinks fascism is a good idea.

Mr. Brokaw: But if you, you believe that life begins at conception, and you've also voted for abortion rights . . .

Mr. Biden: No, what I voted [was] against curtailing the right, criminalizing abortion. I voted against telling everyone else in the country that they have to accept my religiously based view that it's a moment of conception. There is a debate in our church, as Cardinal Egan would acknowledge, that's existed. Back in *Summa Theologia*, when Thomas Aquinas wrote *Summa Theologia*, he said there was no — it didn't occur until quickening, 40 days after conception. How am I going out and tell you, if you or anyone else that you must insist upon my view that is based on a matter of faith [sic]? And that's the reason I haven't. But then again, I also don't support a lot of other things. I don't support public, public funding. I don't, because that flips the burden. That's then telling me I have to accept a different view. This is a matter between a person's God, however they believe in God, their doctor, and themselves in what is always a — and what we're going to be spending our time doing is making sure that we reduce considerably the amount of abortions that take place by providing the care, the assistance and the encouragement for people to be able to carry to term and to raise their children.

[35] Ibid. *But see Declaration on Procured Abortion*, Sacred Congregation of the Doctrine of the Faith, Par. 7 (1974); http://www.vatican.va/roman_curia/congregations/cfaith/documents/rc_con_cfaith_doc_19741118_declaration-abortion_en.html. The Declaration states: "St. Thomas, the Common Doctor of the Church, teaches that abortion is a grave sin against the natural law."

[36] Ibid.

[37] Michael New, "Analyzing the Effect of State Legislation on the Incidence of Abortion Among Minors." Report of the Heritage Center for Data Analysis (Feb. 5, 2007); http://www.heritage.org/Research/Family/CDA07-01.cfm.

[38] Tim Townsend, "Do Not Forget Me in Your Prayers." *St. Louis Post-Dispatch*, Aug. 18, 2008, A1.

[39] Notification, Bishop Raymond Burke, LaCrosse Wisconsin, dated Nov. 23, 2003; http://www.ewtn.com/library/BISHOPS/BURKENOT.HTM. Bishop Burke stated:

> I hereby call upon Catholic legislators, who are members of the faithful of the Diocese of La Crosse, to uphold the natural and divine law regarding the inviolable dignity of all human life. To fail to do so is a grave public sin and gives scandal to all the faithful. Therefore, in accord with the norm of can. 915, Catholic legislators, who are members of the faithful of the Diocese of La Crosse and who continue to support procured abortion or euthanasia may not present themselves to receive Holy Communion. They are not to be admitted to Holy Communion, should they present themselves, until such time as they publicly renounce their support of these most unjust practices.

[40] David R. Obey, "My Conscience, My Vote." *America* (Aug. 16, 2004); http://www.americamagazine.org/content/article.cfm?article_id=3708.

[41] P.J. Huffstutter, "St. Louis Catholics Debate Political Directive." *L.A. Times*, Oct. 7, 2004, 14.

[42] Ibid.

[43] Robert McClory, "Irreconcilable Differences." *U.S. Catholic*, Oct. 1, 2004, 18.

[44] Jacqueline L. Salmon and Michelle Boorstein, "Wuerl Elected to Lead Panel Guarding Catholic Doctrine." *Washington Post*, Nov. 15, 2008, B7; http://www.washingtonpost.com/wp-dyn/content/article/2008/11/14/AR2008111402529.html.

[45] "Archbishop Wuerl Says Politicians' Support for Abortion Is Wrong." *Catholic News Agency*, May 5, 2008; http://www.catholicnewsagency.com/new.php?n=12551.

[46] Salmon and Boorstein, *supra* note 44.

[47] United States Conference of Catholic Bishops, *Catholics in Political Life* (June 2004). The bishops stated:

> The question has been raised as to whether the denial of Holy Communion to some Catholics in political life is necessary because of their public support for abortion on demand. Given the wide range of circumstances involved in arriving at a prudential judgment on a matter of this seriousness, we recognize that such decisions rest with the individual bishop in accord with the established canonical and pastoral principles. Bishops can legitimately make different judgments on the most prudent course of pastoral action. Nevertheless, we all share an unequivocal commitment to protect human life and dignity and to preach the Gospel in difficult times.

[48] Most Rev. Raymond L. Burke, *Canon 915: The Discipline Regarding the Denial of Holy Communion to Those Obstinately Persevering in Manifest Grave Sin*; http://www.ewtn.com/library/CANONLAW/burkcompol.HTM (last visited Dec. 8, 2008). Archbishop Burke noted:

> The matter in question was extensively discussed by the Bishops of the United States during their meeting in June of 2004. The statement of the United States Bishops, "Catholics in Political Life," adopted on June 18, 2004, which was the fruit of the discussion, failed to take account of the clear requirement to exclude from Holy Communion those who, after appropriate admonition, obstinately persist in supporting publicly legislation which is contrary to the natural moral law. (Ibid.)

[49] Ibid., stating:

> [T]he discipline [denial of access to Holy Communion to those who are publicly unworthy] must be applied in order to avoid serious scandal — for example, the erroneous acceptance of procured abortion against the constant teaching of the moral law. No matter how often a bishop or priest repeats the teaching of the Church regarding procured abortion, if he stands by and does nothing to discipline a Catholic who publicly supports legislation permitting the gravest of injustices and, at the same time, presents himself to receive Holy Communion, then his teaching rings hollow. To remain silent is to permit serious confusion regarding a fundamental truth of the moral law. Confusion, of course, is one of the most insidious fruits of scandalous behavior.
>
> I am deeply aware of the difficulty, which is involved in applying the discipline of can. 915. I am not surprised by it and do not believe that anyone should be surprised. Surely, the discipline has never been easy to apply. But what is at stake for the Church demands the wisdom and courage of shepherds who will apply it.
>
> The United States of America is a thoroughly secularized society which canonizes radical individualism and relativism, even before the natural moral law. The application, therefore, is more necessary than ever, lest the faithful, led astray by the strong cultural

trends of relativism, be deceived concerning the supreme good of the Holy Eucharist and the gravity of supporting publicly the commission of intrinsically evil acts. Catholics in public office bear an especially heavy burden of responsibility to uphold the moral law in the exercise of their office which is exercised for the common good, especially the good of the innocent and defenseless. When they fail, they lead others, Catholics and non-Catholics alike, to be deceived regarding the evils of procured abortion and other attacks on innocent and defenseless human life, on the integrity of human procreation, and on the family. (Ibid.)

[50] Interview with Nancy Pelosi, *Meet the Press,* Aug. 24, 2008; http://www.msnbc.msn.com/id/26377338/page/3/. Speaker Pelosi stated:

Mr. Brokaw: Senator Obama saying the question of when life begins is above his pay grade, whether you're looking at it scientifically or theologically. If he were to come to you and say, "Help me out here, Madame Speaker. When does life begin?" what would you tell him?

Rep. Pelosi: I would say that as an ardent, practicing Catholic, this is an issue that I have studied for a long time. And what I know is, over the centuries, the doctors of the church have not been able to make that definition. And Senator — Saint Augustine said at three months. We don't know. The point is, is that it shouldn't have an impact on the woman's right to choose. *Roe v. Wade* talks about very clear definitions of when the child — first trimester, certain considerations; second trimester; not so third trimester. There's very clear distinctions [sic]. This isn't about abortion on demand, it's about a careful, careful consideration of all factors and — to — that a woman has to make with her doctor and her god. And so I don't think anybody can tell you when life begins, human life begins. As I say, the Catholic Church for centuries has been discussing this, and there are those who've decided . . .

[51] United States Conference of Catholic Bishops, *Bishops Respond to House Speaker Pelosi's Misrepresentation of Church Teaching on Abortion,* News Release, Aug. 26, 2008; http://www.usccb.org/comm/archives/2008/08-120.shtml. The bishops' response stated:

In the course of a *Meet the Press* interview on abortion and other public issues on August 24, House Speaker Nancy Pelosi misrepresented the history and nature of the authentic teaching of the Catholic Church against abortion.

In fact, the *Catechism of the Catholic Church* teaches, "Since the first century the Church has affirmed the moral evil of every procured abortion. This teaching has not changed and remains unchangeable. Direct abortion, that is to say, abortion willed either as an end or a means, is gravely contrary to the moral law" (Par. 2271). In the Middle Ages, uninformed and inadequate theories about embryology led some theologians to speculate that specifically human life capable of receiving an immortal soul may not exist until a few weeks into pregnancy. While in canon law these theories led to a distinction in penalties between very early and later abortions, the Church's moral teaching never justified or permitted abortion at any stage of development.

These mistaken biological theories became obsolete over 150 years ago when scientists discovered that a new human individual comes into being from the union of sperm and egg at fertilization. In keeping with this modern understanding, the Church teaches that from the time of conception (fertilization), each member of the human species must be given the full respect due to a human person, beginning with respect for the fundamental right to life.

[52] Biden interview, *supra* note 34.

[53] United States Conference of Catholic Bishops, *Bishops Respond to Senator Biden's Statements Regarding Church Teaching on Abortion,* USCCB News Release, Sept. 9, 2008; http://www.usccb.org/comm/archives/2008/08-129.shtml.

[54] Steven Ertelt, "Joe Biden's Catholic Bishop Won't Deny Communion Over Pro-Abortion Views." LifeNews.com, Nov. 11, 2008; http://www.lifenews.com/state3635.html.

[55] Peter Steinfels, "Catholics and Choice in the Voter's Booth." *New York Times*, Nov. 8, 2008; http://www.nytimes.com/2008/11/08/us/politics/08beliefs.html.

[56] Ibid.

[57] United States Conference of Catholic Bishops, *Forming Consciences for Faithful Citizenship*, Par. 22, p. 8 (approved Nov. 2007); http://www.usccb.org/faithfulcitizenship/FCStatement.pdf.

[58] Ibid., Par. 34, p. 11.

[59] Ibid., Par. 28, p. 9.

[60] Ibid., Par. 35, p. 11.

[61] Ibid., Par. 34, p. 11.

[62] Steinfels, *supra* note 55.

[63] E. J. Dionne, Jr., "A Catholic Shift to Obama?" *Washington Post*, Oct. 21, 2008, A17; http://www.washingtonpost.com/wp-dyn/content/article/2008/10/20/AR2008102002290.html.

[64] Cindy Wooden, "Archbishop Burke Warns Democrats Becoming 'Party of Death,'" *National Catholic Reporter*, Sept. 29, 2008; http://ncronline3.org/drupal/?q+print/2054.

[65] David D. Kirkpatrick, "A Fight Among Catholics Over Which Party Best Reflects Catholic Teaching." *New York Times*, Oct. 5, 2008; http://www.nytimes.com/2008/10/05/us/politics/05catholic.html.

[66] Letter from Cardinal George, Sept. 2, 2008; http://www.archchicago.org/cardinal/letter/letters_2008/letter_090308.shtm.

[67] Charles J. Chaput, "Vote for Real Hope and Change." *First Things,* Aug. 19, 2008; http://www.firstthings.com/onthesquare/?p=1151.

[68] Doug Kmiec, "Convictions: Endorsing Obama." *Slate*, Mar. 23, 2008; http://www.slate.com/blogs/blogs/convictions/archive/2008/03/23/endorsing-obama.aspx.

[69] Nicholas P. Cafardi, "I'm Catholic, Staunchly Anti-Abortion, and Support Obama." *National Catholic Reporter*, Sept. 30, 2008; http://ncronline3.org/drupal/?q=node/2058.

[70] Ibid.

[71] Ibid.

[72] George Weigel, "Pro-Life Catholics for Obama: Should Abortion Be the Litmus Test for Political Support?" *Newsweek*, Oct. 14, 2008; http://www.newsweek.com/id/163896.

[73] Nicholas P. Cafardi, M. Cathleen Kaveny, and Douglas W. Kmiec, "A Catholic Brief for Obama: Why the Faithful Can in Good Conscience Back the Democrat." *Newsweek*, Oct. 17, 2008; http://www.newsweek.com/id/164445.

[74] Steinfels, *supra* note 55.

[75] Ibid.

[76] Julia Duin, "Bishops Warn Obama About Abortion Issue," *Washington Times*, Nov. 12, 2008, A 3.

[77] Ibid.

[78] Ibid.

[79] Manya Brachear, "Catholic Bishops Plan to Forcefully Confront Obama." *Chicago Tribune*, Nov. 11, 2008; http://www.chicagotribune.com/features/religion/chi-081111bishops,0,615284.story.

[80] Jacqueline L. Salmon, "Bishops Call Obama-Supported Abortion Rights Bill a Threat to the Catholic Church." *Washington Post*, Nov. 12, 2008, A10.

[81] Michael Paulson, "Catholic Bishops Warn Obama They'll Fight on Abortion." *Boston Globe,* Nov. 12, 2008, 12.

[82] United States Conference of Catholic Bishops, *Cardinal George Voices Hope for Obama Administration*, *Points to Possible Obstacles to Our Desired Unity*. News Release, Nov. 12, 2008; http://www.usccb.org/comm/archives/2008/08-174.shtml.

[83] *See*, e.g., Joe Feuerherd, "How a Bill Doesn't Become Law." *National Catholic Reporter*, Nov. 28, 2008; http://ncronline.org/news/politics/how-bill-doesnt-become-law.

[84] *See*, e.g., Melinda Henneburger, "Lose-Lose on Abortion: Obama's Threat to Catholic Hospitals and Their Very Serious Counterthreat." *Slate*, Nov. 24, 2008; http://www.slate.com/id/2205326/.

[85] The 2004 Democratic Platform provided:

> We will defend the dignity of all Americans against those who would undermine it. Because we believe in the privacy and equality of women, we stand proudly for a woman's right to choose, consistent with *Roe v. Wade*, and regardless of her ability to pay. We stand firmly against Republican efforts to undermine that right. At the same time, we strongly support family planning and adoption incentives. Abortion should be safe, legal, and rare.

2004 Democratic Party Platform, "Strong at Home, Respected in the World." 38; http://s3.amazonaws.com/apache.3cdn.net/8a738445026d1d5f0f_bcm6b5l7a.pdf (last visited Dec. 8, 2008).

The 2008 Democratic Platform states:

> The Democratic Party strongly and unequivocally supports *Roe v. Wade* and a woman's right to choose a safe and legal abortion, regardless of ability to pay, and we oppose any and all efforts to weaken or undermine that right.
>
> The Democratic Party also strongly supports access to comprehensive affordable family planning services and age-appropriate sex education which empower people to make informed choices and live healthy lives. We also recognize that such health care and education help reduce the number of unintended pregnancies and thereby also reduce the need for abortions.
>
> The Democratic Party also strongly supports a woman's decision to have a child by ensuring access to and availability of programs for pre- and post-natal health care, parenting skills, income, support, and caring adoption.
>
> 2008 Democratic Party Platform, "Renewing America's Promise." 50–51; http://s3.amazonaws.com/apache.3cdn.net/8a738445026d1d5f0f_bcm6b5l7a.pdf (last visited Dec. 8, 2008).

[86] 2008 Democratic Platform, *supra* note 85, at 10, stating: "Families and individuals should have the option of keeping the coverage they have or choosing from a wide array of health insurance plans, including many private health insurance options and a public plan. Coverage should be made affordable for all Americans with subsidies provided through tax credits and other means."

[87] *See*, e.g., *Continuing the Commitment: A Pathway to Health Care Reform* 8 (The Catholic Health Association, 2000). Principle One of the Guiding Principles for Health Care Reform states:

> A reformed system should provide health care for all. Health care services necessary for the development and maintenance of a healthful life are a basic human right, not to

be limited by the lack of health care coverage. The availability and affordability of health coverage should not be a function of employment, health status, income, or other factors. Access to appropriate health care services should be assured irrespective of the nature of health coverage.

[88] *Cf.* H. Tristram Engelhardt, Jr., "Roman Catholic Social Teaching and Religious Hospital Identity in a Post-Christian Age." *Christian Bioethics* 6 (3) (2000): 295.

PART ONE: *Moral Foundations*

[1] George P. Graham, "Bioethics: An Orphan Discipline." *Homiletic & Pastoral Review* (May 2001); http://www.catholicculture.org/culture/library/view.cfm?id=4126&CFID=905296&CFTOKEN=1569326.

[2] Pope Paul VI, *Humanae Vitae* (1968); http://www.vatican.va/holy_father/paul_vi/encyclicals/documents/hf_p-vi_enc_25071968_humanae-vitae_en.html.

[3] David F. Kelly, *Contemporary Catholic Health Care Ethics* (Washington, DC: Georgetown University Press, 2004), 96.

[4] Ibid., 94.

[5] Ibid.

[6] Ibid., 95.

[7] Ibid.

[8] Ibid., 96.

[9] Ibid.

[10] John Paul II, *Veritatis Splendor* (1993); http://www.vatican.va/holy_father/john_paul_ii/encyclicals/documents/hf_jp-ii_enc_06081993_veritatis-splendor_en.html.

[11] John Paul II, *Evangelium Vitae* (1995); http://www.vatican.va/holy_father/john_paul_ii/encyclicals/documents/hf_jp-ii_enc_25031995_evangelium-vitae_en.html.

Chapter One: *The Catholic Natural-Law Tradition*

[1] *Catechism of the Catholic Church* (1994), states: "The task of interpreting the Word of God authentically has been entrusted solely to the Magisterium of the Church, that is, to the Pope and to the bishops in communion with him" (Par. 100); http://www.vatican.va/archive/ENG0015/__PN.HTM.

[2] William E. May, *An Introduction to Moral Theology* (Huntington, IN: Our Sunday Visitor, 1991), 100.

[3] Ibid., 44.

[4] May, *supra* note 4, at 210–11.

[5] Ibid., 213.

[6] There is an ongoing debate over whether the teaching of *Humanae Vitae* is infallible. Most theologians consider it to be authoritative, but not infallible. Others have argued that the document itself was infallibly proclaimed *ex cathedra* by Pope Paul VI, or that even if it wasn't proclaimed *ex cathedra*, the teaching is infallible because it has been continuously proclaimed by the universal ordinary Magisterium. Janet Smith, Humanae Vitae: *A Generation Later* (Washington, DC: Catholic University of America Press, 1991), 155–60.

[7] May, *supra* note 4, at 215–23.

[8] Benedict M. Ashley, O.P., and Kevin D. O'Rourke, O.P., *Ethics of Health Care*, 3rd ed. (Washington, DC: Georgetown University Press, 2002), 9.

[9] Ibid.

[10] Ibid., 9–10.

[11] Ibid., 10.

[12] Ibid.

[13] Ibid., 11.

[14] Gerald Kelly, S.J., *Medico-Moral Problems* (St. Louis: The Catholic Hospital Association, 1958), 13–14; *see also* Charles J. McFadden, *Medical Ethics*, 3rd ed. (Philadelphia: F.A. Davis, Co., 1953), 33.

[15] Kelly, *supra* note 14, at 108.

[16] Ibid., 111.
[17] Albert R. Jonsen, *The Birth of Bioethics* (New York: Oxford University Press, 1998), 36.
[18] Ibid., 36–37.
[19] McFadden, *supra* note 14, at xiii.
[20] Ibid., xii.
[21] Ibid., 18.
[22] Ibid.
[23] Ibid., 20–21.
[24] Ibid., 18.
[25] McFadden, *supra* note 14, at 18.
[26] McFadden, *supra* note 14, at 77–80.
[27] Ibid., 93.
[28] Ibid., 99.
[29] Ibid., 282.
[30] Ibid., 294–95.
[31] Ibid., 162.
[32] Ibid., 162.
[33] Ibid.

Chapter Two: *Challenges to the Catholic Natural-Law Tradition*

[1] The term "revisionist theologians" is taken from William E. May, *An Introduction to Moral Theology*, 2d ed. (Huntington, IN: Our Sunday Visitor, 2003), 142. Professor May notes:

> First of all revisionist theologians—among them Franz Böckle, Charles E. Curran, Josef Fuchs, Bernard Häring, Louis Janssens, Richard McCormick, Timothy E. O'Connell, Richard Gula, Franz Scholz, and Bruno Schuller., while denying the existence of moral absolutes (such as the specific prohibitions in Catholic teaching on contraception, direct abortion, and direct sterilization) . . . acknowledge that there are other kinds of moral absolutes. . . . Thus, they acknowledge the absoluteness of such principles as "one must always act in conformity with love of God and Neighbor" and "One must always act in accordance with right reason. Ibid, 145 [endnotes omitted].

[2] *See, e.g.,* Charles E. Curran, *Medicine and Morals* (Corpus Books, 1970), 29, stating:

> Since the experience of Christian people and all men of good will is a source of moral knowledge, an ethician cannot simply spell out in advance everything that must be done by the doctor. And generally speaking, in other complicated areas of human life, the theologian cannot say that this or that action must always be performed. In many matters of medicine the ethician can merely tell the doctor to exercise his own prudent moral judgment. The patient and the doctor together must decide the feasibility of performing an operation by weighing the advantages against the risk.

[3] May, *supra* note 1, at 146.
[4] Ibid.
[5] Ibid., 105.
[6] Ibid.
[7] Ibid., 106.
[8] Ibid., 107.
[9] May, *supra* note 1, at 108.

[10] Ibid., 108.
[11] Ibid., 109.
[12] Christopher Kaczor, *Proportionalism and the Natural Law Tradition* (Washington, DC: Catholic University of America Press, 2002), 10–11.
[13] Ibid., 13–14.
[14] Ibid., 14–15.
[15] Ibid., 12.
[16] Benedict M. Ashley, O.P., and Kevin D. O'Rourke, O.P., *Ethics of Health Care*, 3rd ed. (Washington, DC: Georgetown University Press, 2002), 9.
[17] John Paul II, *Veritatis Splendor* (1993), Par. 74; http://www.vatican.va/holy_father/john_paul_ii/encyclicals/documents/hf_jp-ii_enc_06081993_veritatis-splendor_en.html.
[18] Ibid., Par. 75.
[19] May, *supra* note 1, at 215.
[20] Pope Paul VI, *Humanae Vitae* (1968); http://www.vatican.va/holy_father/paul_vi/encyclicals/documents/hf_p-vi_enc_25071968_humanae-vitae_en.html.
[21] May, *supra* note 1, at 101.
[22] David F. Kelly, *Contemporary Catholic Health Care Ethics* (Washington, DC: Georgetown University Press, 2004), 103.
[23] Ibid., 104
[24] *Humanae Vitae*, *supra* note 20, Pars. 14–17.
[25] Kaczor, *supra* note 12, at 4–5.
[26] Curran, *supra* note 2, at 29.
[27] Albert R. Jonsen, *The Birth of Bioethics* (New York: Oxford University Press, 2003), 36, 54 (discussing the work of Richard McCormick).
[28] James F. Keenan, S.J., "The Moral Agent: Actions and Normative Decision Making." in James J. Walter, Timothy E. O'Connell, and Thomas A. Shannon, eds., *A Call to Fidelity: On the Moral Theology of Charles E. Curran* (Washington, DC: Georgetown University Press, 2002), 44.
[29] Curran, *supra* note 2, at 2–8.
[30] Ibid., 43.
[31] Ibid., 1.
[32] Ibid., 2.
[33] Ibid., 16.
[34] Ibid., 17.
[35] Curran, *supra* note 2, at 19–20.
[36] Ibid., 20–21.
[37] Ibid., 22–24.
[38] Ibid., 31.
[39] Ibid., 31–32.
[40] Ibid., 3.
[41] Curran, *supra* note 2, at 3.
[42] Ibid., 5.
[43] Ibid., 7.
[44] Ibid., 29, stating:

> Perhaps in other matters now spelled out in the hospital code, more room should be left for conscientious decision by the doctor. The problem seems to reside in a system of theory that attaches exclusive moral importance to the physical structure of an act. At the very least, theologians must listen when doctors of good will are listening to them. In fact, theologians must ask doctors to reveal their moral experience. The doctor must at least be

listened to with respect when he honestly says that he thinks a raped 15-year-old girl who is a patient in a mental hospital should be aborted.

[45] Ibid., 7.
[46] Ibid., 7.
[47] Ibid., 6.
[48] Ibid., 6. The 1971 *ERD*s appear to require removal of the tube itself rather than permitting removal of the fetus alone. Directive 16, "Ethical and Religious Directives for Catholic Health Facilities." Reprinted in Thomas J. O'Donnell, S.J., *Medicine and Christian Morality* (Staten Island, NY: Alba House, 1976), 311, 315.
[49] *Cf.* Philip Jenkins, *The New Anti-Catholicism: The Last Acceptable Prejudice* (New York: Oxford University Press, 2003), 60.

> The dispute over *Humanae Vitae* also dissolved traditional constraints about openly challenging Church authorities. Very shortly after the encyclical was issued, prominent Catholic theologian Charles Curran announced to a press conference that Catholics were not bound to obey the papal pronouncement, and his doubts were publicly echoed by hundreds of other priests and Catholic educators. This was an early manifestation of what would be a continuing theme over the next thirty years; the repeated clashes between Church authorities and liberal theologians, especially on the issues of sexuality. In 1977, the once dependably orthodox Catholic Theological Society of America (CTSA) published the study *Human Sexuality*, which stated that no definitive grounds existed to condemn practices such as contraception, sterilization, and masturbation. (Ibid. [footnotes omitted]).

[50] Ibid., 59. According to Professor Jenkins:

> [F]rom the late 1960s, the contraception debate made the issue of obedience crucially important. For most Catholic families, to accept the official Church position meant pursuing a course that would profoundly affect one's everyday life and prosperity. Many families chose to disregard Church teaching on this vital issue, though without feeling the need to abandon the Church. By 1992, a Gallup poll found that 80 percent of U.S. Catholics disagreed with the statement "Using artificial means of birth control is wrong." (Ibid. 58–59 [footnotes omitted]).

[51] Christopher J. Kauffman, *Ministry and Meaning: A Religious History of Catholic Health Care in the United States* (Chestnut Ridge, NY: The Crossroads Publishing Company, 1995), 290–91.
[52] Ibid., 291 quoting Richard A. McCormick, S.J., "Not What Catholic Hospitals Ordered." *Linacre Quarterly* 39 (May 1972), 21.
[53] Jenkins, *supra* note 49, at 60.
[54] Ari L. Goldman, "Catholicism, Democracy, and the Case of Father Curran." *New York Times*, Aug. 24, 1986, § 4.
[55] Ibid.
[56] Ibid. (citing *New York Times*/CBS Poll: "What American Catholics Think").
[57] Peter Steinfels, "Vatican Watershed — A Special Report; Papal Birth-Control Letter Retains Its Grip." *New York Times,* Aug. 1, 1993; http://query.nytimes.com/gst/fullpage.htm l?sec=health&res=9F0CE7D9133CF932A3575BC0A965958260.
[58] William Lobdell and Teresa Watanabe, "Church May Penalize Politicians; Bishops Are Exploring Requiring Officeholders Who Are Catholic to Back Official Doctrine," *Los Angeles Times*, Nov. 29, 2003, at Main News. The prominent pro-choice Catholic politicians mentioned in this article are Senator Edward Kennedy (D-MA), Republican Governor George Pataki of New York, Governor Arnold Schwarzenegger of California, and Rep. Nancy Pelosi

(D-CA). Ibid. The article also refers to statistics from the American Life League, a pro-life group, indicating that voters have elected 412 politicians to state and federal offices who are both Catholic and pro-choice. Ibid.

Chapter Three: *The Reassertion of Absolute Norms*

[1] Aline H. Kaliban, "Where Have All the Proportionalists Gone?" *Religious Ethics* 3 (2002): 30.

[2] William E. May, "Moral Theologians and *Veritatis Splendor*." *Homiletic & Pastoral Review* 7 (Dec. 1994): 30; http://ewtn.com/library/THEOLOGY/MORALVS.HTM.

[3] Ibid.

[4] *Catechism of the Catholic Church* (1994); http://www.vatican.va/archive/ENG0015/_INDEX.HTM.

[5] Pope John Paul II, *Veritatis Splendor* (1993); http://www.vatican.va/edocs/ENG0222/__P1.HTM.

[6] Pope John Paul II, *Evangelium Vitae* (1995); http://www.vatican.va/holy_father/john_paul_ii/encyclicals/documents/hf_jp-ii_enc_25031995_evangelium-vitae_en.html.

[7] *Catechism*, *supra* note 4, at Par. 1761.

[8] Ibid., Par. 2270.

[9] Ibid., Par. 2271.

[10] Ibid., Par. 2272.

[11] Ibid., Par. 2366 (quoting Pope Paul VI, *Humanae Vitae* (1968); http://www.vatican.va/holy_father/paul_vi/encyclicals/documents/hf_p-vi_enc_25071968_humanae-vitae_en.html).

[12] Ibid.

[13] *Catechism*, *supra* note 4, at Par. 2277.

[14] Ibid.

[15] Ibid., Par. 2278.

[16] Ibid., Par. 2279.

[17] Ibid.

[18] *Veritatis Splendor*, *supra* note 5, at Par. 5.

[19] Ibid., Par. 4.

[20] Ibid.

[21] *See*, e.g., Richard A. McCormick, S.J., "Some Early Reactions to *Veritatis Splendor*." *Theological Studies* 55 (1994): 481.

[22] *Veritatis Splendor*, *supra* note 5, at Par. 6.

[23] Ibid., Par. 25. That paragraph states:

> The moral prescriptions which God imparted in the Old Covenant, and which attained their perfection in the New and Eternal Covenant in the very person of the Son of God made man, must be *faithfully and continually put into practice* in the various different cultures throughout the course of history. The task of interpreting these prescriptions was entrusted by Jesus to the Apostles and their successors, with the special assistance of the Spirit of truth. . . .

The next paragraph continues:

> In the moral catechesis of the Apostles, besides exhortations and directions connected to specific historical and cultural situations, we find an ethical teaching with precise rules of behaviour. (Ibid., Par. 26.)

[24] Ibid., Par. 29 (emphasis in original).
[25] Ibid., Pars. 31–32.
[26] Ibid., Par. 34.
[27] *Veritatis Splendor*, *supra* note 5, at Pars. 35–37.
[28] Ibid., Par. 37.
[29] Ibid., Par. 43.
[30] Ibid., Par. 47.
[31] Ibid., Par. 49.
[32] Ibid., Par. 52.
[33] *Veritatis Splendor*, *supra* note 5, at Par. 53.
[34] Ibid., Par. 56.
[35] Ibid., Par. 64.
[36] Ibid., Par. 65.
[37] Ibid., Par. 73. *See also* May, *supra* note 2.
[38] *Veritatis Splendor*, *supra* note 5, at Par. 75.
[39] Ibid., Par. 75.
[40] Ibid., Par. 78.
[41] Ibid., Par. 80.
[42] Ibid., Par. 110.
[43] Richard A. McCormick, S.J., "Document Begs Many Legitimate Moral Questions — Papal Encyclical, '*Veritatis Splendor*,'" *National Catholic Reporter*, Oct. 15, 1993.
[44] Janet Smith, "*Veritatis Splendor,* Proportionalism, and Contraception." *Irish Theological Quarterly* 63 (1998): 307–26; http://www.aodonline.org/aodonline-sqlimages/SHMS/Faculty/SmithJanet/Publications/MoralPhilosophy/VeritatisSplendor.pdf.
[45] Janet Smith, "Moral Methodologies: Proportionalism." *Ethics and Medicine* 19 (June 1994): 1–2; http://www.aodonline.org/aodonline-sqlimages/shms/faculty/SmithJanet/Publications/MoralPhilosophy/MoralMethods.pdf.
[46] McCormick, "Some Early Reactions to *Veritatis Splendor*." *supra* note 21, at 502–03.
[47] Ibid., 503.
[48] John Conley, "Narrative, Act, Structure: John Paul II's Method of Moral Analysis." In *Choosing Life: A Dialogue on* Evangelium Vitae, eds., Kevin Wm. Wildes and Alan C. Mitchell (Washington, DC: Georgetown University Press, 1997), 3.
[49] *Evangelium Vitae*, *supra* note 6, at Par. 12.
[50] Conley, *supra* note 48, at 3.
[51] Conley, *supra* note 48, at 4–8.
[52] Ibid., 8–12.
[53] *Evangelium Vitae*, *supra* note 6, at Par. 12; Conley, *supra* note 48 at 13.
[54] *Evangelium Vitae*, *supra* note 6, at Par. 12.
[55] Ibid., Par. 70; Conley, *supra* note 48 at 14–15.
[56] Ibid.
[57] Ibid., Par. 13.
[58] Ibid., Par. 17.
[59] *Evangelium Vitae*, *supra* note 6, at Par. 14 (emphasis added).
[60] Ibid. (emphasis added).
[61] Ibid.
[62] Ibid., Par. 15.
[63] Ibid.
[64] Ibid.
[65] *Evangelium Vitae*, *supra* note 6, at Pars. 19–20.

[66] Ibid., Par. 21.
[67] Ibid., Par. 58.
[68] Ibid., Par. 60.
[69] Ibid., Par. 62 (emphasis added).
[70] Ibid., Par. 65.
[71] *Evangelium Vitae*, *supra* note 6, at Par. 65.
[72] Ibid. (quoting from Second Vatican Ecumenical Council, *Lumen Gentium* [*Dogmatic Constitution on the Church*], Par. 25).
[73] Ibid.
[74] William E. May, *Catholic Bioethics and the Gift of Human Life* (Huntington, IN: Our Sunday Visitor, 2000), 27.
[75] Ibid.
[76] Ibid., 28.
[77] Francis A. Sullivan, S.J., "The Doctrinal Weight of *Evangelium Vitae*." *Theological Studies* 56 (1995): 560, 564. In this regard, Fr. Sullivan quotes the following language from *Lumen Gentium*:

> Although the individual bishops do not enjoy the prerogative of infallibility, they nevertheless proclaim Christ's doctrine infallibly whenever, even though dispersed through the world, but still maintaining the bond of communion among themselves and with the successor of Peter, and authentically teaching matters of faith and morals, they are in agreement on one position as definitively to be held. This is even more clearly verified when, gathered together in an ecumenical council, they are teachers and judges of faith and morals for the universal Church, whose definitions must be adhered to with the submission of faith.

Ibid., 561 (quoting Pope Paul VI, *Lumen Gentium*, Par. 25 (Nov. 21, 1964); http://www.vatican.va/archive/hist_councils/ii_vatican_council/documents/vat-ii_const_19641121_lumen-gentium_en.html).
[78] Ibid., 562 (quoting "On File." *Origins* 24 [Apr. 13, 1995]: 734).
[79] Sullivan, *supra* note 77, at 564.
[80] Ibid.
[81] Ibid., 563.
[82] Ibid., 565.
[83] *Evangelium Vitae*, *supra* note 6, at Par. 73.
[84] Ibid., Par. 89.
[85] Ibid., Par. 88.

Chapter Four: *Secular Bioethics versus Catholic Bioethics*

[1] George Hunston Williams, the late Harvard Divinity School professor and church historian, has traced the origins of the term to 1971: the year Professor Van Rensselaer Potter, a cancer scholar at the University of Wisconsin, published his *Bioethics: Bridge to the Future* (Englewood Cliffs, NJ: Prentice Hall, 1971), 131–133, and Andre Hellegers was named to head the newly created Kennedy Institute for Human Reproduction and Bioethics. George Hunston Williams, "'Safer Footing Than Blind Reason Stumbling Without Fear': Reflections on Bioethics in Our Civic, Religious, Historical, Professional Context." *The Death Decision*, ed., Leonard J. Nelson (Ann Arbor, MI: Servant Books, 1984), 127, 132. Williams notes that bioethics developed from the merging of two streams:

> Thus "bioethics" appeared in 1971 and in quite different contexts.... The essential difference between Potter's use of the word, the first in print, and Hellegers's is that in the first instance there is an optimism about the possibilities of auto-evolution and human progress, while in the second instance there is a stress not so much on doing good as on not doing harm. Progress and restraint are the two contrasting dispositions. Moreover, the originator of the term in Madison emphatically places bioethics in the context of environmental ethics. The restraint in Georgetown is there because of a long tradition in Catholic ethics. (Ibid., 132–33 [footnotes omitted]).

[2] H. Tristram Englehardt, Jr., "The Ordination of Bioethicists as Secular Moral Experts." *Social Philosophy & Policy* 19 (2002): 59, 60.

[3] Leigh Turner, "Zones of Consensus and Zones of Conflict: Questioning the 'Common Morality' Presumption in Bioethics." *Kennedy Institute of Ethics Journal* 13 (2003): 193. Professor Turner notes:

> Three recurring, questionable presumptions persist in many different branches of contemporary bioethics theory. The assumptions are particularly evident in the principlist, common morality approach of Tom Beauchamp and James Childress (1979–2001), although similar claims are found in casuistic models of moral deliberation (Jonsen and Toulmin 1988) and the common morality approach of Bernard Gerr, Charles Culver, and Danny Clouser (1997). The first presumption is that a trans-historical, universal "common morality" exists and can serve as a normative baseline for judging various actions and practices. The second presumption is that the common morality is in a state of relatively stable, ordered "wide reflective equilibrium." The third presumption is that reflective equilibrium at the level of moral intuitions, maxims, or principles is important, because a shared understanding of general norms provides the necessary prelude to engaging in the articulation of more specific action guides and policies. (Ibid., 193–94.)

[4] Christopher McDonald, "Will the 'Secular Priests' of Bioethics Work Among the Sinners?" *American Journal of Bioethics* 3 (2003): 36.

[5] Albert R. Jonsen, *The Birth of Bioethics* (New York: Oxford University Press, 2003), 211–214.

[6] Ibid., 212.

[7] Ibid. *See also* George P. Graham, "Bioethics: An Orphan Discipline." *Homiletic & Pastoral Review* (May 2001); http://www.catholic.net/rcc/Periodicals/Homiletic/2001-05/graham.html.

[8] Jonsen, *supra* note 5, at 214–17.

[9] Ibid., 13–26.

[10] Edmund D. Pellegrino, "Bioethics at Century's Turn: Can Normative Ethics Be Retrieved?" *Journal of Medicine & Philosophy* 25 (2000): 655, 659, discussing Warren T. Reich, "The Wider View: Andre Hellegers's Passionate, Integrating Intellect and the Creation of Bioethics." *Kennedy Institute of Ethics Journals* 9 (1999): 25.

[11] Pellegrino, *supra* note 10, at 659.

[12] Ibid.

[13] Jonsen, *supra* note 5, at 301.

[14] Ibid.

[15] Ibid.

[16] Ibid., 296, 303.

[17] Ibid., 103, discussing "The Belmont Report: Ethical Principles and Guidelines for the Protection of Human Subjects of Research." The National Commission for the Protection of Human Subjects of Biomedical Behavioral Research, U.S. Department of Health, Educa-

tion and Welfare (Washington, DC: Government Printing Office, 1979); *see also* Dianne N. Irving, "The Impact of International Bioethics on the 'Sanctity of Life Ethics' and the Ability of Ob-Gyn's to Practice According to Conscience." Lifeissues.net, June 18, 2001; http://www.lifeissues.net/writers/irv/irv_40bioandconscience01.html (paper presented at International Conference: The Future of Obstetrics and Gynaecology, International Federation of Catholic Medical Associations and MaterCare International, Rome, Italy, June 18, 2001).

[18] Jonsen, *supra* note 5, at 104 (footnote omitted).

[19] Irving, *supra* note 17.

[20] Matter of Quinlan, 355 A.2d 647, 671 (N.J. 1976).

[21] Glenn McGee, Arthur L. Caplan, Joshua P. Spanogle and David A. Asch, "A National Study of Ethics Committees." *American Journal of Bioethics* 1 (2001): 60.

[22] Ibid., 62.

[23] Ibid., 62–63.

[24] Ibid.

[25] Ibid., 61.

[26] Ruth Shalit, "When We Were Philosopher Kings." *The New Republic*, Apr. 18, 1997; http://catholiceducation.org/articles/medical_ethics/me0008.html.

[27] *Cf.* Kayhan Parsi, "Bioethics Consultation in the Private Sector: What Is an Appropriate Model." *HEC Forum* 17 (2005): 355 (discussing bioethics consultation in the private sector).

[28] Loretta M. Kopelman, "Bioethics and Humanities: What Makes Us One Field?" *Journal of Medicine & Philosophy* 23 (1998): 356 (address by the founding president of the newly formed American Society of Bioethics and Humanities).

[29] Larry R. Churchill, "Are We Professionals? A Critical Look at the Social Role of Bioethicists." *Daedalus* 128 (Fall 1999): 253 (discussing ASBH core competencies and questioning whether there is or should be a profession of bioethicists).

[30] Carla M. Messikomer, Renee C. Fox, and Judith P. Swazey, "The Presence and Influence of Religion in American Bioethics." *Perspectives in Biology and Medicine* 44 (2001): 485, 506.

[31] David J. Smolin, "Does Bioethics Provide Answers? Secular and Religious Bioethics and Our Procreative Future." *Cumberland Law Review* 35 (2005): 473, 474–75.

[32] Ibid., 475.

[33] Ibid., 476.

[34] Ibid., 477.

[35] Ibid.

[36] Peter Singer, "Sanctity of Life or Quality of Life?" *Pediatrics* 72 (1983): 128.

[37] Ibid.

[38] Ibid.

[39] Peter Singer, *Practical Ethics*, 2d ed. (New York: Cambridge University Press, 1993), 14.

[40] Ibid., 88–89.

[41] Ibid., 137.

[42] Ibid., 138.

[43] Ibid., 138–43.

[44] Ibid., 137.

[45] Ibid., 138–41.

[46] Ibid., 143–46.

[47] Ibid., 146–49.

[48] Ibid., 150.

[49] Ibid., 151.

[50] Ibid., 151.
[51] Ibid., 211.
[52] Ibid., 182.
[53] Ibid., 183.
[54] Ibid., 182.
[55] Ibid., 191.
[56] Ibid., 191–92.
[57] Ibid., 196.
[58] Ibid.
[59] Ibid.
[60] 521 U.S. 701 (1997) (upholding Washington state's ban on assisted suicide).
[61] Ibid., 734.
[62] Singer 1983, *supra* note 36, at 129. See also Ronald Dworkin, Thomas Nagel, Robert Nozick, John Rawls, T.M. Scanlon, and Judith Jarvis Thompson, "Assisted Suicide: The Philosopher's Brief." *The New York Review of Books* (no. 5), Mar. 27, 1997, 44 (amicus curiae brief submitted in Glucksberg critiquing slippery slope argument); http://www.nybooks.com/articles/1237.
[63] Ibid.
[64] Singer 1993, *supra* note 39, at 215.
[65] Ibid.
[66] Robert J. Lifton, *The Nazi Doctors: Medical Killing and the Psychology of Genocide* (New York: Basic Books, 1986); http://www.holocaust-history.org/lifton/contents.shtml. Lifton notes:

> The crucial work—"The Permission to Destroy Life Unworthy of Life" (*Die Freigabe der Vernichtung lebensunwerten Lebens*)—was published in 1920 and written jointly by two distinguished German professors: the jurist Karl Binding, retired after forty years at the University of Leipzig, and Alfred Hoche, professor of psychiatry at the University of Freiburg. Carefully argued in the numbered-paragraph form of the traditional philosophical treatise, the book included as "unworthy life" not only the incurably ill, but large segments of the mentally ill, the feebleminded, and retarded and deformed children. More than that, the authors professionalized and medicalized the entire concept. And they stressed the therapeutic goal of that concept: destroying life unworthy of life is "purely a healing treatment" and a "healing work." . . .
>
> Hoche, in his section, insisted that such a policy of killing was compassionate and consistent with medical ethics; he pointed to situations in which doctors were obliged to destroy life (such as killing a live baby at the moment of birth, or interrupting a pregnancy to save the mother). He went on to invoke a concept of "mental death" in various forms of psychiatric disturbance, brain damage, and retardation. He characterized these people as "human ballast" (*Ballastexistenzen*) and "empty shells of human beings"—terms that were to reverberate in Nazi Germany. Putting such people to death, Hoche wrote, "is not to be equated with other types of killing . . . but [is] an *allowable, useful act.*" He was saying that these people are *already* dead. (Ibid., 46–47 [footnotes omitted]).

[67] Ibid., 21. And, of course, eugenics was in fashion in the United States as it was in Germany in the 1920s and 1930s. Edward J. Larson and Leonard J. Nelson, III, "Involuntary Sexual Sterilization of Incompetents in Alabama." *Alabama Law Review* 43 (1992): 405.
[68] Pellegrino, *supra* note 10, at 656.
[69] Kevin Wm. Wildes, *Moral Acquaintances: Methodology in Bioethics* (South Bend, IN: University of Notre Dame, 2000), 142.

[70] Pellegrino, *supra* note 10, at 656.
[71] H. Tristram Engelhardt, Jr., *The Foundations of Bioethics*, 2d ed. (New York: Oxford University Press, 1996), 8.
[72] Ibid.
[73] Ibid.
[74] Wildes, *supra* note 69, at 21.
[75] Ibid., 23–24.
[76] Ibid., 23–54.
[77] Ibid., 52.
[78] Ibid., 54–66 discussing Tom L. Beauchamp and James Childress, *The Principles of Biomedical Ethics,* 4th ed. (New York: Oxford University Press, 1994).
[79] Wildes, *supra* note 69, at 84–85.
[80] Wildes, *supra* note 69, at 90–107.
[81] Ibid., 113.
[82] *See, e.g.,* Churchill, *supra* note 29.
[83] Ibid.
[84] Shalit, *supra* note 26.
[85] Charles L. Bosk, "Professional Ethicist Available: Logical, Secular, Friendly." *Daedalus* 128 (Fall 1999): 47.
[86] Ruth Shalit notes:

> Consider the personal journey of John Fletcher, chief ethics consultant for the University of Virginia Medical Center. Ordained as an Episcopal minister in his hometown of Birmingham, Alabama, Fletcher quickly came to realize he was not cut out for the ministry, and resigned his ordination. "I am not the enemy of religion," he explains. "But I must maintain my distance in order to maintain my sanity."
>
> Several colleagues say that Fletcher's strong secular emphasis colors his consulting. A physician at the UVA Medical Center recalls the case of a 15-year-old girl in the late stages of metastatic cancer who was refusing to endure yet another round of toxic and painful chemotherapy. Her parents wanted her to undergo the treatment. Did the girl have the right to refuse? A meeting was called between the patient, her family, the treatment team and Fletcher, the ethics consultant on duty. "The family clearly had religious beliefs," recalls the physician, who was in the room at the time, "and John proceeded to ridicule those beliefs . . . . At one point, the mother turned to him and said, 'Don't you think there's a chance that God will cure her?' And John looked her straight in the eye and barked out, 'No!'" The girl, who at this point already decided to go through with the treatment, ran out of the room in tears. Fletcher said he did the right thing: "I felt I had to confront the mother," he says. "Sometimes people need a little jolt."

Shalit, *supra* note 26.
[87] Albert R. Jonsen, Mark Siegler, and William J. Winslade, *Clinical Ethics*, 5th ed. (New York: McGraw-Hill, 2002).
[88] Ibid., 1.
[89] Ibid., 4.
[90] Ibid., 5.
[91] Ibid., 60–61. The authors suggest that religious beliefs could play a negative role in treatment decision-making: "Certain religious groups hold beliefs about health, sickness, and medical care that may be unfamiliar to providers. Sometimes such beliefs will influence the patient's preferences about care in ways that providers might consider imprudent or dangerous." Ibid., 61.

[92] Ibid., 180.

[93] Ibid.

[94] Ibid. They state: "Religious counselors and chaplains have an important role to play in health care. However, Western medicine has long maintained a distance from religion because of scientific skepticism and the professional duty to avoid favoritism toward any religious position." Ibid.

[95] Ibid., 180–81. The first example concerns a patient who has just had the Whipple procedure performed for the treatment of pancreatic cancer. He has had a difficult recovery and his family members are devout Christians. They ask the physician, who has no religious affiliation, to pray with them for the patient's recovery. One of the patient's children shows the physician an article from a medical journal on the role the positive role that prayer can play in healing. The authors suggest that the physician should show respect for the patient's belief, but decline to pray with them. The authors conclude: "[T]he primary issue is to avoid depreciation of spiritual beliefs that cannot harm and may help." Ibid., 181.

The second case example involves a board certified obstetrician-gynecologist who is asked by a delegation of female African immigrants to perform ritual genital surgery on young women in their community. Unlicensed persons are currently performing the surgery. The physician was raised a Black Muslim, was familiar with the Koran and believes the surgery is not required by Islamic law. The authors suggest that the physician should refuse to perform the surgery and try to educate the women "both about the religious law of their own faith and the medical consequences of the practice." Ibid.

[96] The Magisterium is defined by the *Catechism of the Catholic Church*, 2d ed. (1997), Pars. 888–92 (English translation), as follows:

> The teaching office
>
> **888** Bishops, with priests as co-workers, have as their first task "to preach the Gospel of God to all men," in keeping with the Lord's command. They are "heralds of faith, who draw new disciples to Christ; they are authentic teachers" of the apostolic faith "endowed with the authority of Christ."
>
> **889** In order to preserve the Church in the purity of the faith handed on by the apostles, Christ who is the Truth willed to confer on her a share in his own infallibility. By a "supernatural sense of faith" the People of God, under the guidance of the Church's living Magisterium, "unfailingly adheres to this faith."
>
> **890** The mission of the Magisterium is linked to the definitive nature of the covenant established by God with his people in Christ. It is this Magisterium's task to preserve God's people from deviations and defections and to guarantee them the objective possibility of professing the true faith without error. Thus, the pastoral duty of the Magisterium is aimed at seeing to it that the People of God abides in the truth that liberates. To fulfill this service, Christ endowed the Church's shepherds with the charism of infallibility in matters of faith and morals. The exercise of this charism takes several forms:
>
> **891** "The Roman Pontiff, head of the college of bishops, enjoys this infallibility in virtue of his office, when, as supreme pastor and teacher of all the faithful — who confirms his brethren in the faith — he proclaims by a definitive act a doctrine pertaining to faith or morals.... The infallibility promised to the Church is also present in the body of bishops when, together with Peter's successor, they exercise the supreme Magisterium," above all in an Ecumenical Council. When the Church through its supreme Magisterium proposes a doctrine "for belief as being divinely revealed," and as the teaching of Christ, the definitions "must be adhered to with the obedience of faith." This infallibility extends as far as the deposit of divine Revelation itself.

892 Divine assistance is also given to the successors of the apostles, teaching in communion with the successor of Peter, and, in a particular way, to the bishop of Rome, pastor of the whole Church, when, without arriving at an infallible definition and without pronouncing in a "definitive manner," they propose in the exercise of the ordinary Magisterium a teaching that leads to better understanding of Revelation in matters of faith and morals. To this ordinary teaching the faithful "are to adhere to it with religious assent" which, though distinct from the assent of faith, is nonetheless an extension of it.

[97] Edmund D. Pellegrino, "Secular Bioethics and Catholic Medical Ethics: Moral Philosophy at the 'Margins,'" in *The Bishop and the Future of Catholic Health Care* (National Catholic Bioethics Center, 1997), 30.

[98] Ibid., 31.

[99] Ibid., 31.

[100] Ibid., 34.

[101] Committee for Pro-Life Activities, National Conference of Catholic Bishops (NCCB), "Nutrition and Hydration: Moral and Pastoral Reflections." (1992), 7; http://www.priestsforlife.org/magisterium/bishops/92-04nutritionandhydrationnccbprolifecommittee.htm (hereinafter 1992 NCCB Statement).

[102] A Statement of the Catholic Bishops of Pennsylvania, *Nutrition and Hydration: Moral Considerations,* rev. ed. (1999; first issued Dec. 12, 1991). http://www.pacatholic.org/statements/nutritionhydration.html (accessed Aug. 2, 2007).

[103] Irving, *supra* note 17.

[104] David Solomon, "Christian Bioethics, Secular Bioethics, and the Claim to Cultural Authority." *Christian Bioethics* 11 (2005): 349, 350.

[105] Michael Panicola, "Rethinking Catholic Bioethics." *Hastings Center Report* 46 (Sept.–Oct. 2004), reviewing with approbation James F. Drane, *More Humane Medicine: A Liberal Catholic Bioethics* (Edinboro University, 2003).

[106] Michael Rie, "What Is Christian about Christian Bioethics?" *Christian Bioethics* 5 (1999): 263.

[107] H. Tristram Engelhardt, Jr., "Physician-Assisted Suicide Reconsidered: Dying as a Christian in a Post-Christian Age." *Christian Bioethics* 4 (1998): 143, 151.

[108] *Compare* H. Tristram Engelhardt, Jr., "Roman Catholic Social Teaching and Religious Hospital Identity in a Post-Christian Age." *Christian Bioethics* 4 (2000): 295 (advocacy by the Catholic Church of social justice in health care may backfire because in a post-Christian society it will be translated in secular terms as a plea for universal access to abortion) *with* Edmund D. Pellegrino, John Collins Harvey, and Kevin T. Fitzgerald, S.J., "Must the Church Be Mute Lest Its Truths Be Distorted?" *Christian Bioethics* 8 (2002): 43 (risk of distortion of its teaching should not dissuade the Church from clearly articulating its social teaching).

[109] United States Conference of Catholic Bishops, *Ethical and Religious Directives for Catholic Health Care Services,* 4th ed. (2001); http://www.usccb.org/bishops/directives.shtml.

Chapter Five: *Ethical and Religious Directives*

[1] United States Conference of Catholic Bishops, *Ethical and Religious Directives for Catholic Health Care Services,* 4th ed. (2001); http://www.usccb.org/bishops/directives.shtml. See also Kenneth R. White, "Hospitals Sponsored by the Roman Catholic Church" (2000), 213, 216 (noting that "[t]he moral responsibility of Catholic health care is outlined in the Ethical and Religious Directives for Catholic Health Care Services").

[2] White, *supra* note 1, at 216. In 2002, the National Conference of Catholic Bishops and the United States Catholic Conference merged to become the United States Conference of Catholic Bishops (USCCB).

[3] 2001 *ERDs*, *supra* note 1, at Directive 52.

[4] Ibid., Directive 53.

[5] Ibid., Directive 45.

[6] Ibid., Directive 60. Catholic teaching condemns direct euthanasia, an act or omission that is intended to cause death for the purpose of eliminating suffering. On the other hand, it may be permissible to discontinue medical procedures that are extraordinary or disproportionate. *The Catechism of the Catholic Church* (1994), Pars. 2277–78, states:

> **2277** Whatever its motives and means, direct euthanasia consists in putting an end to the lives of handicapped, sick, or dying persons. It is morally unacceptable.
>
> Thus an act or omission which, of itself or by intention, causes death in order to eliminate suffering constitutes a murder gravely contrary to the dignity of the human person and to the respect due to the living God, his Creator. The error of judgment into which one can fall in good faith does not change the nature of this murderous act, which must always be forbidden and excluded.
>
> **2278** Discontinuing medical procedures that are burdensome, dangerous, extraordinary, or disproportionate to the expected outcome can be legitimate; it is the refusal of "overzealous" treatment. Here one does not will to cause death; one's inability to impede it is merely accepted. The decisions should be made by the patient if he is competent and able or, if not, by those legally entitled to act for the patient, whose reasonable will and legitimate interests must always be respected.

[7] White, *supra* note 1, at 220–21.

[8] The results of a 1975 survey conducted by anonymous mail questionnaires on the sterilization and contraceptive practices in United States Catholic hospitals revealed that even at that time 20% of the facilities permitted medically indicated sterilizations, 32% provided oral contraceptives, 25% diaphragms, and 9% IUDs. John M. O'Lane, "Sterilization and Contraception Services in Catholic Hospitals." *American Journal of Obstetrics & Gynecology* (Feb. 15, 1979): 355–57.

[9] The Daughters of Charity, with the approval of the local bishop, agreed to continue to provide abortion referrals, at least on a temporary basis, at Niagara Falls Memorial Hospital, a community hospital that was merged with St. Mary's, a hospital owned by the Daughters. Lucette Lagnado, "Religious Practice: Their Role Growing, Catholic Hospitals Juggle Doctrine and Medicine." *Wall Street Journal*, Feb. 4, 1999, A1. In addition, Brackenridge Hospital, a city-owned hospital that is managed by Ascension Health, provided abortion referrals in a city-operated clinic set aside within the hospital to provide contraceptives and sterilizations. Kim Sue Lia Perkes, "Bishops to Weigh Tighter Controls at Catholic Hospitals." *Austin-American Statesman*, Oct. 26, 2000, A1.

[10] In 2007, the Diocesan Administrator and former Bishop of Birmingham, Alabama, published a notice in the *Birmingham News* in response to concerns about the takeover of a secular system by St. Vincent's Hospital, a part of the Ascension system. This notice stated: "St. Vincent's does not and cannot control what goes on in these [professional] buildings.... Although it is not possible to police the contraceptive conversations or practices in a physician's offices, the Catholic people need to know explicitly that I ask physicians leasing offices in these buildings adjacent to our hospitals to follow the Ethical and Religious Directives." Statement by Most Revered David E. Foley, D.D., Diocesan Administrator, Diocese of Birmingham in Alabama, *Birmingham News*, May 7, 2007.

[11] *See* Christopher Zehnder, "What's Ailing Catholic Hospitals?" *Crisis*, Nov. 2001; http://www.crisismagazine.com/november2001/feature8.htm.

[12] "An Ob-Gyn Blames Excessive Focus on the Bottom Line." *Our Sunday Visitor*, July 13, 2008, 11 (interview by Ann Carey of Dr. Cvetokovich, an obstetrician/gynecologist who practices medicine in the Tepeyac Family Center in Fairfax, Virginia, and regional director of the Catholic Medical Association).

[13] "Shocking Lack of Understanding." *Our Sunday Visitor*, July 13, 2008, 12 (interview of John Haas, president, National Catholic Bioethics Center).

[14] Ann Carey, Texas Bishops Examine Reports of Ethical Lapses at Catholic Hospitals, *Our Sunday Visitor*, July 12, 2008, 3.

[15] John-Henry Weston, "Texas Bishop Repents Publicly for Catholic Hospital That Was Doing Sterilizations." LifeSiteNews.com, Nov. 12, 2008; http://www.lifesitenews.com/ldn/2008/nov/08112110.html. The statement provides:

> PUBLIC STATEMENT
>
> I wish to address the matter of direct sterilizations in Catholic Hospitals in the Diocese of Tyler. Last June it was reported by anonymous researchers that a large number of tubal ligations are performed in Catholic Hospitals in the state of Texas. Both Catholic hospitals in the Diocese of Tyler responded that they were in compliance with the Ethical and Religious Directives [*ERD*s] for Catholic Health Services. Sadly, subsequent investigation reveals that there had been a serious misinterpretation of the *ERD*s and that in fact many direct sterilizations had been done and continue to be done at the time of the article. As a Bishop, I am deeply saddened and upset by this news. As Bishop of the Diocese of Tyler, I have to admit my failure to provide adequate oversight of the Catholic hospitals as regards their protection of the sacred dignity of each human person.
>
> Many causes and complications that have resulted in this unacceptable situation [sic]. I continue to work directly with the Catholic Hospitals in the Diocese of Tyler, and with my brother Bishops in the state of Texas, to bring an end to immoral procedures and to put in place some method of ongoing accountability and transparency of monitoring both protocols and actual practices. As Catholics, we must insure all people seeking health care in our Catholic Hospitals will be treated with respect and dignity as Jesus teaches us. The Church has approved the Ethical and Religious Directives for Catholic Health Services as binding upon our Catholic Hospitals to insure the sacred dignity of each patient is protected and defended. The Directives are for the protection of every woman's human dignity.
>
> Thankfully, in response to their own investigation of the matter, CHRISTUS St. Michael's in Texarkana has discontinued all tubal ligations. They report a favorable response from their local medical community.
>
> Prior to release of the report, Trinity Mother Frances had experienced a 50% reduction in the number of tubal ligations. Trinity Mother Frances is a large health care system and is developing plans to protect the sacred dignity of each human person through compliance with an authentic interpretation of the *ERD*s, particularly *ERD* 53, which prohibits direct sterilization.
>
> Bishop Alvaro Corrada, S.J.
> Bishop of Tyler

Statement of Bishop Alvaro Corrada, S.J., Bishop Diocese of Tyler. Published in *Catholic East Texas*, Nov. 21, 2008; http://www.lifesitenews.com/ldn/2008_docs/tylerbishopstatement.pdf.

[16] Ibid.

[17] Bishop Alvaro Corrada, S.J., *Statement on Human Dignity, Conscience and Health Care to Catholics and People of East Texas*. Diocese of Tyler, Texas, Dec.1, 2008; http://www.dioceseoftyler.org/documents/HumanDignityBpCorrada.pdf. The bishop stated in part:

> Medical procedures that treat an existing pathology (for example, cancer of part of the reproductive system) may be administered in a Catholic hospital, even if they result in sterilization. These procedures are not viewed as sterilizations either by the Catholic Church or the medical community. They are simply procedures for existing pathologies that result in sterilization. Tubal ligation and other forms of direct sterilization, on the other hand, treat no illness and serve only to destroy the reproductive capacity of a patient. They are elective procedures, not medically indicated or necessary for healing the patient. No one, especially a Catholic or a Catholic hospital, can be rightly compelled in the name of medicine to provide such procedures. (Ibid.)

[18] Ann Carey, "Texas Hospital Challenges Bishop on Sterilizations." *Our Sunday Visitor*, Dec. 28, 2008; http://www.osv.com/OSVNav/OSVNewsweeklyDecember282008/Texashospitalchallengesbishoponsterilizations/tabid/7313/Default.aspx.

[19] Ann Carey, "Moral Sterility." *Our Sunday Visitor*, July 13, 2008, 9.

[20] Congregation for the Doctrine of the Faith, "Reply of the Sacred Congregation for the Doctrine of the Faith on Sterilization in Catholic Hospitals" (*Quaecumque Sterilizatio*), Mar. 13, 1975, reprinted in Kevin D. O'Rourke and Philip Boyle, *Medical Ethics: Sources of Catholic Teaching*, 3rd ed. (Washington, DC: Georgetown University Press, 1989), 398–99, discussed in Carey, *supra* note 18.

[21] Congregation for the Doctrine of the Faith, *Responses to Questions Concerning 'Uterine Isolation' and Related Matters*. July 31, 1993; http://www.vatican.va/roman_curia/congregations/cfaith/documents/rc_con_cfaith_doc_31071994_uterine-isolation_en.html, discussed in Carey, *supra* note 18.

[22] David F. Kelly, *Contemporary Catholic Health Care Ethics* (Washington, DC: Georgetown University Press, 2004), 117.

[23] Haas interview, *supra* note 13.

[24] Directive 53, *Ethical and Religious Directives for Catholic Health Care Services*, 4th ed. (2001), *supra* note 1.

[25] Haas interview, *supra* note 13.

[26] Jean deBlois, C.S.J., and Kevin D. O'Rourke, O.P., J.C.D., "Introducing the Revised Directives: What Do They Mean for Catholic Healthcare?" *Health Progress* 76 (Apr. 1995).

[27] Francis Morrisey, "Toward Juridic Personality." *Health Progress* 82 (July–Aug. 2001); http://www.chausa.org/Pub/MainNav/News/HP/Archive/2001/07JulAug/Articles/SpecialSection/0107j.htm

[28] *See* Adam J. Maida and Nicholas P. Cafardi, *Church Property, Church Finances, and Church-Related Corporations* (Catholic Health Association of the United States, 1984), 57.

> In the field of health care, the U.S. Bishops, exercising this faith authority, have approved the "Ethical and Religious Directives for Catholic Health Facilities." These directives . . . are applied to specific situations under the guidance of each diocesan bishop within that bishop's diocese. It is a person's acceptance of the Catholic faith that makes these directives binding. A health care facility could not call itself Catholic and ignore these directives. They have been defined by the bishops as being the essence of "Catholic" health care. (Ibid. [footnotes omitted]).

[29] Ibid.

[30] deBlois and O'Rourke, *supra* note 26.

[31] Ibid.

[32] Ibid.
[33] Christopher J. Kauffman, *Ministry and Meaning: A Religious History of Catholic Health Care in the United States* (Chestnut Ridge, NY: The Crossroads Publishing Company, 1995), 252.
[34] Ibid., 169.
[35] Ibid., 171.
[36] Sharon Pentland, "What's Past Is Prologue." *Health Progress* (Jan.–Feb. 1995): 76; http://www.chausa.org/Pub/MainNav/News/HP/Archive/1995/01JanFeb/articles/Foundation/hp9501o.htm.
[37] Ibid.
[38] Kauffman, *supra* note 33, at 252.
[39] Ibid., 185.
[40] Kevin D. O'Rourke, Thomas Kopfensteiner, and Ron Hamel, "A Brief History." *Health Progress* 82 (Nov.–Dec. 2001); http://www.chausa.org/Pub/MainNav/News/HP/Archive/2001/11NovDec/Articles/Features/hp0111G.htm (citing Michael P. Bourke, "Surgical Code for Catholic Hospitals." Archdiocese of Detroit [1921]).
[41] Ibid.
[42] Kauffman, *supra* note 33, at 185.
[43] Ibid.
[44] Ibid., 169.
[45] O'Rourke et al., *supra* note 40.
[46] *Code of Ethical and Religious Directives for Catholic Hospitals* (1949).
[47] Pentland, *supra* note 36.
[48] Kauffman, *supra* note 33, at 252.
[49] Ibid.
[50] Ibid.
[51] Pentland, *supra* note 36.
[52] Kauffman, *supra* note 33, at 289.
[53] Gerald Kelly, S.J., *Medico-Moral Problems* (St. Louis: The Catholic Hospital Association, 1958), vii–viii.
[54] deBlois and O'Rourke, *supra* note 26.
[55] O'Rourke et al., *supra* note 40.
[56] Ibid. (Citing *Code of Ethical and Religious Directives for Catholic Hospitals*, 2d ed., [1956]).
[57] 1949 *ERD*s, *supra* note 46, at 1.
[58] Gerald Kelly, *supra* note 53, at 1–15.
[59] Ibid., 4–5.
[60] Ibid., 1–3.
[61] Ibid., 5.
[62] Ibid., 12. According to Gerald Kelly, under the principle of double effect, an action is deemed morally licit if the following requirements are met:

> 1. *The action, considered by itself and independently of its effect, must not be morally evil.* There are some actions, as we know, that are intrinsically evil: e.g., blasphemy, perjury, masturbation, and murder. Such actions are always forbidden, no matter what beneficial consequences they might have. Consequently, if we can determine that a given action falls into this category, we know that no principle can justify it . . . .
> 2. *The evil effect must not be the means of producing the good effect.* The principle underlying this condition is that a good end cannot justify the use of an evil means . . . .

When a dangerously affected tube is removed, the mother is saved precisely by this operation and not by killing the fetus. And, when the oophorectomy is performed, the growth of the cancer is impeded by the suppression of hormone activity and not by the sterilization. In both these cases, therefore, the evil effects (loss of fetal life and sterilization) are simply unavoidable by-products of operations designed to produce the good effects.

3. *The evil effect is sincerely not intended, but merely tolerated* . . . . In the cases we are considering, therefore, neither the patient nor the physician may intend the loss of fetal life or the sterilization. The attitude toward these effects must be one of mere tolerance.

4. *There must be a proportionate reason for performing the action, in spite of its evil consequences.* In practice, this means that there must be a sort of balance between the total good and the total evil produced by an action. Or, to put it another way, it means that, according to a sound prudential estimate, the good to be obtained is of sufficient value to compensate for the evil that must be tolerated. (Ibid., 13–14.)

[63] 1949 *ERDs, supra* note 46, at 1.
[64] Ibid.
[65] Ibid.
[66] Ibid., 2.
[67] Ibid., 4–5.
[68] Ibid., 4.
[69] 1949 *ERDs, supra* note 46, at 4–5.
[70] Ibid., 4.
[71] Ibid.
[72] Ibid., 5.
[73] Ibid.
[74] Gerald Kelly, *supra* note 53, at 69.
[75] Ibid., 68.
[76] 1949 *ERDs, supra* note 46, at 5.
[77] David Kelly, *supra* note 22, at 113 (2004).
[78] Ibid.
[79] Ibid.
[80] Ibid.
[81] 1949 *ERDs, supra* note 46, at 4.
[82] Ibid.
[83] Ibid., 5.
[84] Ibid.
[85] Ibid., 4.
[86] 1949 *ERDs, supra* note 46, at 5.
[87] Ibid.
[88] Ibid.
[89] Ibid.
[90] Ibid.
[91] Ibid., 6.
[92] Gerald Kelly, *supra* note 53, at 184.
[93] 1949 *ERDs, supra* note 46, at 5–6.
[94] Ibid.
[95] Ibid., 6.
[96] Ibid., 6–7.

[97] Ibid.
[98] Gerald Kelly, *supra* note 53, at 179.
[99] Ibid.
[100] Ibid.
[101] Ibid.
[102] Ibid.
[103] Ibid., 7.
[104] deBlois and O'Rourke, *supra* note 26.
[105] Ibid.
[106] Ibid.
[107] O'Rourke et al., *supra* note 40.
[108] Ibid.
[109] Kauffman, *supra* note 33, at 290.
[110] Ibid.
[111] Ibid.
[112] O'Rourke et al., *supra* note 40.
[113] Richard A. McCormick, S.J., "Not What Catholic Hospitals Ordered." *Linacre Quarterly* 39 (May 1972), 16, discussed in Kauffman, *supra* note 33, at 290.
[114] McCormick, *supra* note 113, at 17.
[115] Kauffman, *supra* note 33, at 291.
[116] Ibid., 290–91.
[117] McCormick, *supra* note 113.
[118] Ibid., 18.
[119] Ibid.
[120] Ibid., 19.
[121] Ibid.
[122] Ibid.
[123] McCormick, *supra* note 113, at 19.
[124] Ibid., 20.
[125] Ibid.
[126] Ibid.
[127] Ibid.
[128] Ibid.
[129] Warren T. Reich, "Policy vs. Ethics." *Linacre Quarterly* 39 (Nov. 1972): 21.
[130] Ibid., 21.
[131] Ibid.
[132] Ibid. at 22.
[133] Ibid.
[134] Ibid., 23.
[135] Reich, *supra* note 129, at 23.
[136] Ibid.
[137] Ibid., 24.
[138] Ibid.
[139] Ibid.
[140] Ibid., 25 (citing *Medico-Moral Guide* [Ottawa: The Catholic Hospital Association of Canada, 1970]) 4–5, 9 (par. 19).
[141] Reich, *supra* note 129, at 26.
[142] Ibid., 26.
[143] Ibid.

[144] Ibid., 27 (footnote omitted).
[145] Ibid.
[146] O'Rourke et al., *supra* note 40.
[147] Ibid., n. 14, citing Letter of John Cardinal Krol, president of NCCB (Mar. 7, 1973) (on file with Kevin O'Rourke, O.P.).
[148] Ibid. (citing *Taylor v. St. Vincent's Hospital, Billings, MT,* c-1090, U.S. District Court, Montana, Oct. 27, 1972). Subsequently, however, the court ruled that it did not have jurisdiction to hear the claim on the merits in light of changes in federal law in reaction to its earlier injunction (*Taylor v. St. Vincent's Hospital,* 369 F. Supp. 948 [Mont. 1973]). In a footnote, the court quotes from the legislative history to the Health Programs Extension Act of 1973 § 401(b), Pub. L. No. 93-45, 87 Stat. 91, the statute that prohibited a court from finding that a hospital receiving Hill-Burton money is acting under color of state law, as follows:

> The background for subsection (b) of section 401 of the bill is an injunction issued in November 1972 by the United States District Court for the district of Montana in *Taylor v. St. Vincent's Hospital.* The court enjoined St. Vincent's Hospital, located in Billings, Montana, from prohibiting Mrs. Taylor's physician from performing a sterilization procedure on her during the delivery of her baby by Caesarean section.
> The suit to enjoin the hospital was brought under 42 U.S.C. § 1983 (which authorizes civil actions for redress of deprivation of civil rights by a person acting under color of state law) and 28 U.S.C. § 1343 (which grants United States district courts jurisdiction of actions (authorized by another law) to redress deprivation, under color of any State law, of a Constitutional right) . . . .
> Section (b) of 401 would prohibit a court or a public official, such as the Secretary of Health, Education, and Welfare, from using receipt of assistance under the three laws amended by the bill . . . as a basis for requiring an individual or an institution to perform or assist in the performance of a sterilization procedures or abortions, if such action would be contrary to religious beliefs or moral conviction.
> In recommending the enactment of this provision, the Committee expresses no opinion as to the validity of the *Taylor* decision.

Taylor, 369 F. Supp. at 950, n. 1 (*quoting* 1973 U.S. C.C.A.N. (P.L. 93-45) 1473).
[149] *Ethical and Religious Directives for Catholic Health Facilities* (1971), reprinted in Thomas J. O'Donnell, S.J., *Medicine and Christian Morality* (Staten Island, NY: Alba House, 1976), 311–12.
[150] Thomas J. O'Donnell, S.J., "The Directives: A Crisis of Faith." *Linacre Quarterly* 39 (Aug. 1972): 139.
[151] Ibid., 142–43.
[152] Ibid., 144.
[153] Ibid.
[154] Ibid., 144–45.
[155] 1971 *ERDs*, reprinted in O'Donnell, *Medicine and Christian Morality, supra* note 149.
[156] O'Donnell, *supra* note 150, at 145.
[157] Ibid.
[158] Ibid.
[159] Ibid., 146.
[160] Ibid.
[161] 1971 *ERDs*, reprinted in O'Donnell, *Medicine and Christian Morality, supra* note 149, at 312.
[162] O'Donnell, *supra* note 149, at 37–38.

[163] Ibid., 38.
[164] Ibid.
[165] Ibid.
[166] Ibid.
[167] 1971 *ERD*s, at Directive 12, reprinted in O'Donnell, *Medicine and Christian Morality*, *supra* note 149, at 314.
[168] Ibid. The Directive further states: "Catholic hospitals are not to provide abortion services based on the principle of material cooperation." Ibid.
[169] 1971 *ERD*s, at Directive 24, reprinted in O'Donnell, *Medicine and Christian Morality*, *supra* note 149, at 316–17.
[170] 1971 *ERD*s at Directive 11, reprinted in O'Donnell, *Medicine and Christian Morality*, *supra* note 149, at 314 (emphasis in original).
[171] O'Donnell, *supra* note 149, at 135.
[172] 1971 *ERD*s, at Directive 13, reprinted in O'Donnell, *Medicine and Christian Morality*, *supra* note 149, at 314.
[173] 1971 *ERD*s, at Directive 16, reprinted in O'Donnell, *Medicine and Christian Morality*, *supra* note 149, at 315. The conditions set out are:

a. the affected part is presumed already to be so damaged and dangerously affected as to warrant its removal, and that
b. the operation is not just a separation of the embryo or fetus from its site within the part (which would be a direct abortion from a uterine appendage), and that
c. the operation cannot be postponed without notably increasing the danger to the mother. (Ibid.)

[174] Ibid. *See also* Charles E. Curran, *Medicine and Morals* (Washington, DC: Corpus Books, 1970), 6.
[175] David Kelly, *supra* note 22, at 114.
[176] 1971 *ERD*s, at Directive 15, reprinted in O'Donnell, *Medicine and Christian Morality*, *supra* note 149, at 315.
[177] 1971 *ERD*s, at Directive 18, reprinted in O'Donnell, *Medicine and Christian Morality*, *supra* note 149, at 315.
[178] 1971 *ERD*s, at Directive 19, reprinted in O'Donnell, *Medicine and Christian Morality*, *supra* note 149, at 315.
[179] O'Donnell, *supra* note 149, at 38–39.
[180] Ibid., 115.
[181] 1971 *ERD*s, at Directive 18, reprinted in O'Donnell, *Medicine and Christian Morality*, *supra* note 149, at 315.
[182] 1971 *ERD*s, at Directive 20, reprinted in O'Donnell, *Medicine and Christian Morality*, *supra* note 149, at 316.
[183] 1971 *ERD*s, at Directive 19, reprinted in O'Donnell, *Medicine and Christian Morality*, *supra* note 149, at 315. The full text of this directive states: "Similarly excluded is every action which, either in anticipation of the conjugal act, or in its accomplishment, or in the development of its natural consequences, purposes, whether as an end or as a means, to render procreation impossible." Ibid.
[184] 1971 *ERD*s, at Directive 20, reprinted in O'Donnell, *Medicine and Christian Morality*, *supra* note 149, at 316.
[185] 1971 *ERD*s, at Directive 6, reprinted in O'Donnell, *Medicine and Christian Morality*, *supra* note 149, at 313.
[186] O'Donnell, *supra* note 149, at 115.

[187] Ibid., 117.
[188] Ibid.
[189] Ibid.
[190] deBlois and O'Rourke, *supra* note 26 (citing Congregation for the Doctrine of the Faith, *Sterilizations in Catholic Hospitals*, NCCB, Sept. 15, 1977). Fr. O'Donnell quotes from this document as follows:

> Any sterilization which of itself, that is, of its own nature and condition, has the sole immediate effect of rendering the generative faculty incapable of procreation, is to be considered direct sterilization, as the term is understood in the declarations of the Pontifical Magisterium, especially of Pius XII. Therefore, notwithstanding any subjectively right intention of those whose actions are prompted by the care or prevention of physical or mental illness which is foreseen or feared as a result of pregnancy, such sterilization remains absolutely forbidden according to the Doctrine of the Church. . . . The Congregation, while it confirms this traditional doctrine of the Church, is not unaware of the dissent against this teaching from many theologians. The Congregation, however, denies that doctrinal significance can be attributed to this fact as such, so as to constitute a "theological source" which the faithful might invoke and thereby abandon the authentic Magisterium, and follow the opinions of private theologians which dissent from it.

O'Donnell, *supra* note 149, at 117–18 (quoting "Responses to Questions of the Episcopal Conference of North American": Prot. 2027/69, Mar. 13, 1975).

[191] 1971 *ERD*s, at Directive 28, reprinted in O'Donnell, *Medicine and Christian Morality*, *supra* note 149, at 317.
[192] Ibid.
[193] 1971 *ERD*s, at Directive 29, reprinted in O'Donnell, *Medicine and Christian Morality*, *supra* note 149, at 317.
[194] 1971 *ERD*s, at Directives 30 and 31, reprinted in O'Donnell, *Medicine and Christian Morality*, *supra* note 149, at 317.
[195] Prefatory Note, Revised Uniform Anatomical Gift Act, National Conference of Commissioners on Uniform State Laws; http://www.anatomicalgiftact.org/DesktopDefault.aspx?tabindex=1&tabid=63.
[196] Amir Halevy and Baruch Brody, "Brain Death: Reconciling Definitions, Criteria and Tests." *Annals of Internal Medicine* 119 (1993): 519, 519–20.
[197] Ibid., 520 (*citing* Uniform Determination of Death Acts, National Conference of Commissioners on State Laws; http://www.law.upenn.edu/bll/archives/ulc/fnact99/1980s/udda80.htm).
[198] 1971 *ERD*s, at Directive 30, reprinted in O'Donnell, *Medicine and Christian Morality*, *supra* note 149, at 317.
[199] Ibid.
[200] 1971 *ERD*s, at Directive 31, reprinted in O'Donnell, *Medicine and Christian Morality*, *supra* note 149, at 317.
[201] Ibid.
[202] *Ethical and Religious Directives for Catholic Health Care Services* (1995).
[203] deBlois and O'Rourke, *supra* note 26.
[204] Ibid.
[205] Ibid., 12.
[206] Ibid. The preamble to the 1994 *ERD*s states:

The Directives have been refined through an extensive process of consultation with bishops, theologians, sponsors, administrators, physicians, and other health care providers. While providing standards and guidance, the Directives do not cover in detail all the complex issues that confront Catholic health care today. Moreover, the Directives will be reviewed periodically by the National Conference of Catholic Bishops, in light of authoritative church teaching, in order to address new insights from theological and medical research or new requirements of public policy.

1994 *ERD*s, *supra* note 202, at 1.
[207] Ibid.
[208] Ibid.
[209] Ibid.
[210] Ibid., 2.
[211] Ibid.
[212] deBlois and O'Rourke, *supra* note 26.
[213] Ibid.
[214] Ibid.
[215] 1994 *ERD*s, *supra* note 202, at "Contents."
[216] 1994 *ERD*s, *supra* note 202, at "General Introduction."
[217] 1994 *ERD*s, *supra* note 202, at "Principles Governing Cooperation."
[218] 1994 *ERD*s, *supra* note 202, at "General Introduction."
[219] Ibid.
[220] Ibid.
[221] 1994 *ERD*s, *supra* note 202, at Directive 5.
[222] 1994 *ERD*s, *supra* note 202, at Directive 9.
[223] 1994 *ERD*s, *supra* note 202, Pt. 1, "The Social Responsibility of Catholic Health Care Services."
[224] 1994 *ERD*s, *supra* note 202, at Directive 3.
[225] 1994 *ERD*s, *supra* note 202, at Directive 7.
[226] 1994 *ERD*s, *supra* note 202, Pt. 2, "Pastoral and Spiritual Responsibility of Catholic Health Care."
[227] 1994 *ERD*s, *supra* note 202, at Directive 10.
[228] 1994 *ERD*s, *supra* note 202, at Directive 22.
[229] 1971 *ERD*s, at Directive 24, reprinted in O'Donnell, *Medicine and Christian Morality*, *supra* note 149, at 317.
[230] 1994 *ERD*s, *supra* note 202, at Directive 36.
[231] Ibid. (Footnote omitted).
[232] 1994 *ERD*s, *supra* note 202, at Directive 36, n. 19.
[233] Ibid., citing Pennsylvania Catholic Conference, *Guidelines for Catholic Hospitals Treating Victims of Sexual Assault*, in *Origins* 22 (1993): 810.
[234] 1994 *ERD*s, *supra* note 202, at Pt. 4, "Issues in Care for the Beginning of Life."
[235] 1994 *ERD*s, *supra* note 202, at Directive 45.
[236] Ibid.
[237] 1994 *ERD*s, *supra* note 202, at Directive 47.
[238] Jean deBlois, C.S.J., and Kevin D. O'Rourke, O.P., J.C.D., "Care for the Beginning of Life: The Revised Ethical and Religious Directives Discuss Abortion, Contraception, and Assisted Reproduction." *Health Progress* 76 (Sept.–Oct. 1995); http://www.chausa.org/Pub/MainNav/News/HP/Archive/1995/09SeptOct/Articles/Features/hp9509e.htm.
[239] *Compare* 1994 *ERD*s, *supra* note 202, at Directive 45, *with* 1971 *ERD*s, at Directive 12, reprinted in O'Donnell, *Medicine and Christian Morality*, *supra* note 149, at 314.

[240] 1994 ERDs, *supra* note 202, at Directive 45.
[241] 1994 *ERDs*, *supra* note 202, at Directive 46.
[242] 1994 *ERDs*, *supra* note 202, at Directive 49.
[243] 1994 *ERDs*, *supra* note 202, at Directive 48.
[244] 1971 *ERDs*, at Directive 16, reprinted in O'Donnell, *Medicine and Christian Morality*, *supra* note 149, at 315.
[245] Curran, *supra* note 174, at 6.
[246] deBlois and O'Rourke, *supra* note 238, at 39. *See also* Ashley M. Benedict, O.P., and Kevin D. O'Rourke, O.P., *Ethics of Health Care*, 3rd ed. (Washington, DC: Georgetown University Press, 2002), 131, stating:

> Although it would be wrong to detach a child from its normal site of implantation, to detach it from an abnormal site that constitutes a pathology in the woman's body would seem to be licit. In this case, removing the fertilized ovum from the fallopian tube by means of salpingostomy or methotrexate does not have as its direct intrinsic intention (moral object) the death of the fetus; rather its intention is to treat the pathological condition. For this reason, it is our opinion that salpingostomy and the use of methotrexate do not result in direct abortion. (Ibid.)

[247] David Kelly, *supra* note 22, at 114.
[248] Ibid., discussing John F. Tuohey, "The Implication of the Ethical and Religious Directives for Catholic Health Care Services on the Clinical Practice of Resolving Ectopic Pregnancies." *Louvain Studies* 20 (1995): 41.
[249] Ibid.
[250] 1994 *ERDs*, *supra* note 202, at Directive 52.
[251] *Cf.* 1971 *ERDs*, at Directive 19, reprinted in O'Donnell, *Medicine and Christian Morality*, *supra* note 149, at 315.
[252] The Catechism defines scandal as "an attitude or behavior which leads another to do evil. The person who gives scandal becomes his neighbor's tempter. He damages virtue and integrity; he may even draw his brother into spiritual death. Scandal is a grave offense if by deed or omission another is deliberately led into a grave offense." *Catechism of the Catholic Church* (1994), Par. 2284; http://www.vatican.va/archive/catechism/p3s2c2a5.htm#II.
[253] deBlois and O'Rourke, *supra* note 238, at 38.
[254] 1994 *ERDs*, *supra* note 202, at Directive 53.
[255] Ibid.
[256] 1994 *ERDs*, *supra* note 202, Pt. 5, "Issues in Care for the Dying."
[257] Ibid., 21 (citation omitted).
[258] Ibid.
[259] Ibid.
[260] Ibid.
[261] Ibid.
[262] Ibid.
[263] Ibid.
[264] Ibid.
[265] *See discussion,* Chapter 13, *infra*.
[266] 1994 *ERDs*, *supra* note 202, at Directive 56 (emphasis added).
[267] 1994 *ERDs*, *supra* note 202, at Directive 57 (emphasis added; citation omitted).
[268] 1994 *ERDs*, *supra* note 202, at Directive 59.
[269] 1994 *ERDs*, *supra* note 202, at Directive 60.
[270] 1994 *ERDs*, *supra* note 202, at Directive 61.

[271] Ibid.
[272] 1994 *ERD*s, *supra* note 202, Pt. 6, "Forming New Partnerships with Health Care Organizations and Providers."
[273] Ibid., 25–26.
[274] Ibid., 26.
[275] 1994 *ERD*s, *supra* note 202, at Directive 67.
[276] 1994 *ERD*s, *supra* note 202, at Directive 68.
[277] Ibid.
[278] 1994 *ERD*s, *supra* note 202, at Directive 69.
[279] 1994 *ERD*s, *supra* note 202, at Directive 70.
[280] 1994 *ERD*s, *supra* note 202, at Appendix, "Principles Governing Cooperation."
[281] Ibid., 29.
[282] Ibid.
[283] Ibid.
[284] Ibid.
[285] Ibid.
[286] Ibid.
[287] Ibid.
[288] Ibid.
[289] Ibid.
[290] Ron Hamel, "Part Six of the Directives: Preserving Integrity in Partnerships Directives Requires an Objective Moral Analysis of Cooperative Arrangements." *Health Progress* 83 (Nov.–Dec. 2002); http://www.chausa.org/Pub/MainNav/News/HP/Archive/2002/11NovDec/Articles/SpecialSection/HP0211i.htm.
[291] Ibid.
[292] Ibid.
[293] 2001 *ERD*s, *supra* note 1.
[294] Peter J. Cataldo and John M. Haas, "Institutional Cooperation: The *ERD*s." *Health Progress* 83 (Nov.–Dec. 2002); http://www.chausa.org/Pub/MainNav/News/HP/Archive/2002/11NovDec/Articles/SpecialSection/HP0211l.htm.
[295] Ibid.
[296] *Compare* 1994 *ERD*s, *supra* note 202, at Directives 45–49, *with* 2001 *ERD*, *supra* note 1, at Directives 45–49.
[297] *Compare* 1994 *ERD*s, *supra* note 202, at Directive 52, *with* 2001 *ERD*s, *supra* note 1, at Directive 52.
[298] *Compare* 1994 *ERD*s, *supra* note 202, at Directive 53, *with* 2001 *ERD*s, *supra* note 1, at Directive 53.
[299] Thomas A. Szyszkiewicz, "Induction Procedures Raise Moral Dilemma." *National Catholic Register*, Oct. 19–25, 2003, 1.
[300] According to a statement issued by the National Catholic Bioethics Center, under Directive 49, "early induction of an anencephalic child when there is no serious pathology of the mother which is being directly treated is not morally licit, emotional distress notwithstanding." NCBC Statement on Early Induction of Labor, Mar. 11, 2004; http://www.ncbcenter.org/04-03-11-EarlyInduction.asp. In addition, a 1996 statement issued by the United States bishops indicates that early induction of labor would not be permissible in the case of an anencephalic infant. "Moral Principles Concerning Infants with Anencephaly" by the Committee on Doctrine, United States Conference of Catholic Bishops, Sept. 19, 1996; http://www.usccb.org/dpp/anencephaly.htm.

[301] 2001 *ERDs, supra* note 1, at Pt. 6, "Forming New Partnerships with Health Care Organizers and Providers."
[302] Ibid., Directive 70.
[303] Ibid., n. 44.
[304] Ibid., quoting "Reply of the Sacred Congregation for the Doctrine of the Faith on Sterilization in Catholic Hospitals" (*Quaecumque Sterilizatio*), *Origins* 10 (Mar. 13, 1975): 33–35.
[305] 2001 *ERDs, supra* note 1, at 44 (referring to *Commentary on the Reply of the Sacred Congregation for the Doctrine of the Faith on Sterilization in Catholic Hospitals*, National Conference of Catholic Bishops, *Origins* 11 [Sept. 15, 1977]: 399).

PART TWO: *Catholic Identity*

[1] "Sponsorship" has been defined as:

> ... a reservation of canonical control by the juridic person that founded and/or sustains an incorporated apostolate that remains canonically a part of the Church entity. This retention of control need not be such as to create civil law liability on the part of the sponsor for corporate acts or omissions, but should be enough for the canonical stewards of the sponsoring organization to meet their canonical obligations of faith and administration regarding the activities of the incorporated apostolate.

Jordan Hite, *A Primer on Public and Private Juridic Persons: Applications to the Catholic Health Care Ministry* (Catholic Health Association, 2000), 37, quoted in Daniel C. Conlin, "Sponsorship at the Crossroads: Religious Institutes Must Consider the Direction in Which They Will Go." *Health Progress* 82 (July–Aug. 2001); http://www.chausa.org/Pub/MainNav/News/HP/Archive/2001/07JulAug/Articles/SpecialSection/HP0107i.htm.

[2] Francis G. Morrisey, "Trustees and Canon Law." *Health Progress* 83 (Nov.–Dec. 2002); http://www.chausa.org/Pub/MainNav/News/HP/Archive/2002/11NovDec/Articles/Features/HP0211g.htm.

[3] Francis G. Morrisey, "Catholic Identity in a Challenging Environment." *Health Progress* 80 (Nov.–Dec. 1999); http://www.chausa.org/Pub/MainNav/News/HP/Archive/1999/11NovDec/Articles/SpecialSection/hp9911d.htm.

[4] Hite, *supra* note 1, at 13.

[5] Ibid., 13, citing Canon 300, James A. Coriden, ed., *The Code of Canon Law: A Text and Commentary* (Mahwah, NJ: Paulist Press, 1985), 245.

[6] Kenneth R. White and James W. Begun, "How Does Catholic Hospital Sponsorship Affect Services Provided?" *Inquiry* 35 (Winter 1998/1999): 398.

[7] William W. Bassett, "Private Religious Hospitals: Limitations Upon Autonomous Moral Choices in Reproductive Medicine." *Journal of Contemporary Health Law & Policy* 17 (2001): 455, 494.

[8] Ibid., 496.

[9] Sharon Holland, "Sponsorship and the Vatican." *Health Progress* 82 (July–Aug. 2001); http://www.chausa.org/Pub/MainNav/News/HP/Archive/2001/07JulAug/Articles/SpecialSection/HP0107k.htm.

[10] Hite, *supra* note 1, at 13.

[11] Michael Dennis McGowan, *The Canonical Status of Catholic Health Care Facilities in the Province of New Brunswick in Light of Recent Provincial Government Legislation* (Ceredigion, UK: Edwin Mellen Press, 2000), 183.

[12] Ibid.

[13] Ibid., 184.

[14] In a 1975 publication, Rev. Adam Maida, now Cardinal Archbishop of Detroit, recommended that the corporate bylaws of a Catholic health care facility "should specifically incorporate language which binds the facility and its personnel to following the medico-moral directives published from time to time by the National Conference of Catholic Bishops." A. J. Maida, *Ownership, Control, and Sponsorship of Catholic Institutions* (Pennsylvania Catholic Conference, 1975), 62.

[15] Francis G. Morrisey, "Catholic Identity in a Challenging Environment." *Health Progress* 80 (Nov.–Dec. 1999); http://www.chausa.org/Pub/MainNav/News/HP/Archive/1999/11NovDec/Articles/ SpecialSection/hp9911d.htm.

[16] Ibid.

[17] Ibid.

[18] Ibid.

[19] Ibid.

[20] Ibid.

[21] Morrisey, *supra* note 15.

[22] Ibid.

[23] Ibid.

[24] Sharon Holland, "Sponsorship and the Vatican." *Health Progress* 82 (July–Aug. 2001); http://www.chausa.org/Pub/MainNav/News/HP/Archive/2001/07JulAug/Articles/SpecialSection/HP0107k.htm.

[25] Ibid.

[26] Morrisey, *supra* note 15.

[27] Ibid.

[28] Catholic Health Association of the United States, "Catholic Health Care in the United States" (Jan. 2008); http://www.chausa.org/NR/rdonlyres/68B7C0E5-F9AA-4106-B182-7DF0FC30A1CA/0/FACTSHEET.pdf.

[29] Ibid.

[30] Kenneth R. White, "Hospitals Sponsored by the Roman Catholic Church: Separate, Equal and Distinct." *Milbank Quarterly* 78:2 (2000): 213. Professor White states:

> Catholic health care organizations have responded to environmental factors by changing their scope of services, organizational arrangements, and financing mechanisms. Nonetheless, they have remained faithful to their religious values with a strategy to retain their core identity, which is defined by the provision of comprehensive health care to vulnerable and underserved populations. (Ibid., 213–214.)

[31] Arthur Jones, "Catholic Health Care Aims to Make 'Catholic' a Brand Name." *National Catholic Reporter*, July 18, 2003, 8.

[32] Ibid.

[33] John O. Mudd, "From CEO to Mission Leader." *Health Progress* 86 (Sept.–Oct. 2005); http://www.chausa.org/Pub/MainNav/News/HP/Archive/2005/09SepOct/articles/SpecialSection/HP0509J.htm. Dean Mudd states:

> We have done well in handling the transition of our organizations as businesses; but the picture is quite different when one looks at non-business areas like the expression of mission, spirit, and Catholic identity. We are far from sure how successful we will be in passing on the heart and soul of these organizations as specifically Catholic ministries. Sponsoring congregations and lay leaders must ask ourselves whether we can be confident that a gen-

eration from now our Catholic ministries will still know where they came from and why they exist. Succeeding in mission and identity remains a challenge in Catholic health care as the sisters, who previously embodied Catholic identity by their very presence, become less and less visible. Today it is common that barely a handful of sisters work in ministries with several thousand employees. Despite their many gifts, we cannot expect these women to maintain our institutions as Catholic. (Ibid.)

[34] One reason given by an official of the Archdiocese of Sacramento as a justification for the institution of a policy permitting the provision of "medically indicated sterilizations" at a Catholic Hospital in Gilroy, California, was that "if a Catholic hospital isn't able to address . . . certain individual cases, it will lose gynecological services, then begin to lose contracts, then viability, and could ultimately go out of business." Ron Shrinkman, "Survival v. Directives," *Modern Health Care* (Nov. 20, 2000): 12 (quoting Rev. Charles McDermott, Vicar Episcopal for Theological and Canonical Affairs at the Archdiocese of Sacramento).

[35] Ann Carey, "Texas Bishops Examine Reports of Ethical Lapses at Catholic Hospitals." *Our Sunday Visitor*, July 13, 2008, 3. The following information is from the Texas Price Point Web site and was brought to my attention by Ann Carey; http://www.txpricepoint.org (select basic query: childbirth and newborn-mother's hospital stay-vaginal delivery-with surgical procedure with sterilization). Texas PricePoint is sponsored by the Texas Hospital Association and the data for the Web site was collected by the Texas State Department of Health. The hospitals listed below are sponsored by religious orders with the abbreviations noted: The Sisters of Charity of the Incarnate Word in Houston and San Antonio (Christus); The Sisters of the Holy Family of Nazareth (C.S.F.N.); the Daughters of Charity (D.C.) (see discussion "Ascension Health System," Chapter 10, *infra*.); and the Sisters of Saint Francis (S.S.F.).

Texas Catholic Hospitals — Vaginal Deliveries with Sterilizations in 2005

HOSPITAL	COMMUNITY	DIOCESE	SPONSOR	# of STERILIZATIONS
Brackenridge	Austin	Austin	D.C.	9
Christus St. Catherine	Katy	Galveston-Houston	Christus	NR*
Christus St. Elizabeth	Beaumont	Beaumont	Christus	NR
Christus Jasper	Jasper	Beaumont	Christus	NR
Christus St. John	Nassau Bay	Galveston-Houston	Christus	0
Christus St. Joseph (sold 2006)	Houston	Galveston-Houston	Christus	14
Christus St. Mary	Port Arthur	Beaumont	Christus	0
Christus St.Michael Health System	Texarkana	Tyler	Christus	5
Christus Santa Rosa-City Center	San Antonio	San Antonio	Christus	0
Christus Santa Rosa	San Antonio	San Antonio	Christus	0
Christus Spohn Alice	Alice	Corpus Christi	Christus	0
Christus Spohn Beeville	Beeville	Corpus Christi	Christus	48
Christus Spohn Corpus Christi Memorial	Corpus Christi	Corpus Christi	Christus	n/a
Christus Spohn Corpus Christi Shoreline	Corpus Christi	Corpus Christi	Christus	0
Christus Spohn Corpus Christi South	Corpus Christi	Corpus Christi	Christus	n/a
Christus Spohn Kleberg	Kingsville	Corpus Christi	Christus	8
Mother Frances Jacksonville	Jacksonville	Tyler	C.S.F.N.	0

Mother Frances Tyler	Tyler	Tyler	C.S.F.N.	174
Providence Health Care Network	Waco	Austin	D.C.	NR
St. Joseph Regional	Bryan	Austin	S.S.F.	108
Seton Edgar B. Davis	Luling	Austin	D.C.	0
Seton Highland Lakes	Burnet	Burnet	D.C.	0
Seton Medical Center	Austin	Austin	D.C.	25
Seton Northwest	Austin	Austin	D.C.	8
Seton Shoal Creek	Austin	Austin	D.C.	0
Seton Southwest	Austin	Austin	D.C.	NR
United Regional	Wichita Falls	Forth Worth	C.S.F.N.	53

*NR (Not Reported) is not the same as zero. Instead, it indicates that 1–4 procedures were performed, which apparently is less than the number needed for reporting.

Brackenridge in Austin is discussed in Chapter 10, *infra*. This facility was a city-owned hospital that was leased to Ascension Health (the Daughters of Charity) for thirty years beginning in 1995. At the same location on the fifth floor, there is a city owned clinic that provides sterilizations. See Chapter 10 *infra*. It is not clear whether the numbers of sterilizations reported above are for the city-owned clinic (which does not appear at the Texas Point Web site) or for the hospital. It is possible, however, that sterilizations are being performed not only at the city-owned clinic, but also at Seton Brackenridge itself.

[36] "[T]he official approbation of direct sterilization and, *a fortiori*, its management and execution in accord with hospital regulations, is a matter which is by its very nature (or intrinsically) evil." *Ethical and Religious Directives for Catholic Health Care*, 4th ed. (2001), quoting from "Reply of the Sacred Congregation for the Doctrine of the Faith on Sterilization in Catholic Hospitals" (*Quaecumque Sterilizatio*), Mar. 13, 1975, *Origins* 10 (1976): 33–35.

[37] Directive 71, "Ethical and Religious Directives for Catholic Health Care," 4th ed. (2001), 37. Directive 71 provides:

> The possibility of scandal must be considered when applying the principles governing cooperation. Cooperation, which in all other respects is morally licit, may need to be refused because of the scandal that might be caused. Scandal can sometimes be avoided by an appropriate explanation of what is in fact being done at the health care facility under Catholic auspices. The diocesan bishop has final responsibility for assessing and addressing issues of scandal, considering not only the circumstances in his local diocese but also the regional and national implications of his decision. (Ibid. [endnotes omitted]).

Chapter Six: *Transformation of the Catholic Hospital from Religious Ministry to Business Enterprise*

[1] Kenneth R. White and James W. Begun, "How Does Catholic Hospital Sponsorship Affect Services Provided?" *Inquiry* 35 (Winter 1998/1999): 398.

[2] *The Search for Identity: Canonical Sponsorship of Catholic Health Care* (1993), 20–21. In the United States, however, the Alexian Brothers founded several hospitals in Chicago; St. Louis; Elizabeth, New Jersey; and Oshkosh, Wisconsin. Christopher J. Kauffman, *Min-

istry and Meaning: A Religious History of Catholic Health Care in the United States (Chestnut Ridge, NY: The Crossroads Publishing Company, 1995), 138.

[3] Kenneth R. White, "Hospitals Sponsored by the Roman Catholic Church: Separate, Equal and Distinct." *Milbank Quarterly* 78:2 (2000): 213.

[4] Kauffman, *supra* note 1, at 64.

[5] Ibid., 64–65.

[6] Ibid., 69.

[7] Ibid.

[8] White, *supra* note 3, at 217.

[9] Kauffman, *supra* note 1, at 100. Professor Kauffman notes:

> The frontier hospital experience originated in the premodern period with an emphasis on custodial care, cleanliness, order, and a refined moral climate. The eastern voluntary hospital serving the immigrant population according to the model of Protestant benevolence did not take root on the frontier where local idiosyncrasies determined the hospital: Catholic sisters staffed mining and railroad facilities with particular insurance schemes, but the ethos was formed by women religious who symbolized the sacred and secular. In many towns, the sister's hospital was the only facility available. Without priests these sisters were as "priests-chaplains" invoking the presence of God in their prayer and ministry. The sister's pastoral ministry blended with the nineteenth-century women's sphere of domestic life to impose a touch of refinement on the rough edges of frontier existence. This experience, which requires an extensive narrative, added a new dimension to the missionary model of health care. (Ibid., 97.)

[10] Ibid., 83. The Daughters of Charity was the largest order in the country at that time and the most active in providing these services. George C. Stewart, Jr., *Marvels of Charity: History of American Sisters and Nuns* (Huntington, IN: Our Sunday Visitor, 1994), 195. Frequently, these nursing nuns had to confront the anti-Catholic prejudices of their patients, most of whom were either unchurched or Protestant. Ibid., 214.

[11] Kauffman, *supra* note 1, at 94.

[12] Stewart, *supra* note 10, at 329.

[13] Ibid.

[14] Ibid.

[15] Kauffman, *supra* note 1, at 69, 76.

[16] Stewart, *supra* note 10, at 331.

[17] Ibid., 331. Stewart notes:

> For example, Providence Hospital in Washington, DC, operated by the Daughters of Charity was the only hospital in the city serving civilians during the Civil War. A special relationship developed from this experience, and Congress routinely appropriated monies to support the institution's care of indigent patients. When Congress appropriated $30,000 in 1897 to build an isolation ward at Providence Hospital, the bill was challenged on the grounds of separation of church and state. (Ibid.)

[18] *Bradfield v. Roberts*, 175 U.S. 291, 296 (1899) (citing Act to Incorporate Providence Hospital of the City of Washington, ch. 50, 13 Stat.43 [1864]). *See also* John Witte, Jr., *Religion and the American Constitutional Experiment*, 2d ed. (Boulder, CO: Westview Press, 2005), 131.

[19] Justice Peckham stated in the opinion for the court:

> Whether the individuals who compose the corporation under its charter happen to be all Roman Catholics, or all Methodists, or Presbyterians, or Unitarians, or members of any other religious organization, or of no organization at all, is of not the slightest consequence with reference to the law of its incorporation, nor can the individual beliefs upon religious matters of the various incorporators be inquired into. Nor is it material that the hospital may be conducted under the auspices of the Roman Catholic Church. To be conducted under the auspices is to be conducted under the influence or patronage of that church. The meaning of the allegation is that the Church exercises great and perhaps controlling influence over the management of the hospital. It must, however, be managed pursuant to the law of its being. That the influence of any particular church may be powerful over the members of a nonsectarian and secular corporation, incorporated for a certain defined purpose and with clearly stated powers, is surely not sufficient to convert such a corporation into a religious or sectarian body. That fact does not alter the legal character of the corporation, which is incorporated under an act of Congress, and its powers, duties, and character are to be solely measured by the charter under which it alone has any legal existence. There is no allegation that its hospital work is confined to members of that church or that in its management the hospital has been conducted so as to violate its charter in the smallest degree. It is simply the case of a secular corporation being managed by people who hold to the doctrines of the Roman Catholic Church, but who nevertheless are managing the corporation according to the law under which it exists. The charter itself does not limit the exercise of its corporate powers to the members of any particular religious denomination, but, on the contrary, those powers are to be exercised in favor of anyone seeking the ministrations of that kind of an institution. (Ibid., 298–99.)

[20] William W. Bassett, "Private Religious Hospitals: Limitations Upon Autonomous Moral Choices in Reproductive Medicine." *Journal of Contemporary Health Law & Policy* 17 (2001): 455, 494.

[21] Stewart, *supra* note 10, at 385.

[22] Ibid.

[23] Stewart, *supra* note 10, at 430.

[24] Ibid.

[25] Stewart, *supra* note 10, at 430.

[26] Ibid., 449.

[27] Philip Jenkins, *The New Anti-Catholicism: The Last Acceptable Prejudice* (New York: Oxford University Press, 2003), 58. Professor Jenkins notes:

> Today, in contrast, priests are much scarcer. Five hundred fifty-two priests were ordained in 1995, compared to 994 in 1965. And, of course, the number of Catholics requiring their ministry has soared during the same period, to the extent that over a quarter of U.S. parishes either have no pastor or share one with another parish. By the end of the century, the average age of America's diocesan priests had reached fifty-seven, and sixty-three for priests in religious orders: today, more priests are over ninety than are under thirty. A decline in older ideologies is also suggested by the collapsing number of nuns, as many Catholic women rejected the ideals of celibacy and the cloister. There were 180,000 nuns in 1965, compared with 80,000 by the end of the century. Between 1966 and 1976 also, some 50,000 nuns left their religious vows. Today, half the nuns in the United States are sixty-eight or older. (Ibid., 57–58.)

[28] Beverly K. Dunn, S.P., J.C.D., "The Evolving Nature of Sponsorship: Recent Decades Have Brought Changes Both in Theory and Practice." *Health Progress* 79 (Mar.–Apr.

1998); http://www.chausa.org/Pub/MainNav/News/HP/Archive/1998/03MarApr/Articles/Features/hp9803i.htm.

[29] Stewart, *supra* note 10, at 463.

[30] Beverly Catherine Dunn, S.P., *Sponsorship of Catholic Institutions, Particularly Health Care Institutions, By the Sisters of Providence in the Western United States* (1995; unpublished dissertation submitted to the Faculty of Canon Law, Saint Paul University, Ottawa, Canada, in partial fulfillment of the requirements for the degree of Doctor of Canon Law), 186–90. Dunn notes: "Neither canon law nor civil law contains the concept of sponsorship. Rather, it has developed as a practical means for adapting to changing conditions." Ibid., 186.

[31] Ibid., 186–90.

[32] Dunn, *supra* note 65.

[33] White, *supra* note 3, at 218; see also John O. Mudd, "From CEO to Mission Leader." *Health Progress* 86 (Sept.–Oct. 2005);http://www.chausa.org/Pub/MainNav/News/HP/Archive/2005/09SepOct/articles/SpecialSection/HP0509J.htm., noting:

> Lay leaders are increasingly aware that we cannot think of ourselves solely as leading businesses, while leaving to sisters and priests the mission dimensions of our work. We too must become effective mission leaders. That requires thinking of ourselves differently and preparing for a role that may not have been part of the job description when we signed up. This change is required, not just because there are fewer priests and sisters, but fundamentally because, as the Second Vatican Council made clear, laypersons have both the right and the responsibility to continue the healing and teaching ministry of Jesus. With this new era in Catholic health care and higher education comes a new set of responsibilities for lay leaders. (Ibid.)

[34] Dunn, *supra* note 30. The landmark case abrogating charitable immunity is P*resident & Dirs. of Georgetown Coll. v. Hughes,* 130 F.2d 810 (D.C. Cir. 1942). "Since that case, a clear majority of jurisdictions have abrogated charitable immunity, while the remainder retain immunity to the extent of statutory ceilings on recoverable damages, or only up to available insurance coverage, or as to charity care." Barry R. Furrow, Thomas L. Greaney, Sandra H. Johnson, Timothy S. Jost, and Robert L. Schwartz, *Liability and Quality Issues in Health Care*, 4th ed. (West, 2001), 392.

[35] Bassett, *supra* note 20, at 545.

[36] Ibid.

[37] Douglas Laycock, "Why the Supreme Court Changed Its Mind About Government Aid to Religious Institutions: It's a Lot More Than Just Republican Appointment." *Brigham Young University Law Review* (2008): 275, 279–286 (discussing the influence of anti-Catholicism on Supreme Court Justices who viewed state funding of religious schools as unconstitutional).

[38] Adam J. Maida and Nicholas P. Cafardi, *Church Property, Church Finances, and Church-Related Corporations* (Catholic Health Association of the United States, 1984), 149.

[39] Francis Morrisey, "Toward Juridic Personality." *Health Progress* 82 (July–Aug. 2001); http://www.chausa.org/Pub/MainNav/News/HP/Archive/2001/07JulAug/Articles/SpecialSection/HP0107j.htm.

[40] Ibid.

[41] Dunn, *supra* note 30.

[42] 26 U.S.C. § 501(c) (3) (West 2008).

[43] John D. Colombo, "The Role of Access in Charitable Tax Exemption." *Illinois Public Law and Legal Theory Research Papers Series*, Research Paper No. 03-13 (Sept. 26, 2003), 3;

http://papers.ssrn.com/sol3/papers.cfm?abstract_id=451360 (citing Rev. Rul. 69-545,1969-2 C.B. 117).

[44] Ibid., 4. In June 2006, the Catholic Health Association released "Guide for Planning and Reporting Community Benefit," http://www.chausa.org/Pub/MainNav/ourcommitments/CommunityBenefits/Resources/TheGuide /.

[45] Monica Langley, "No Margin, No Mission." *Wall Street Journal*, Jan. 7, 1998, A1.

[46] White and Begun, *supra* note 6.

[47] *Cf.* Richard A. McCormick, "The End of Catholic Hospitals." *America* 5 (July 4–11, 1998): 179 (discussing the effect of managed care and competitive pressures on the mission of Catholic hospitals).

[48] *Cf.* Bassett, *supra* note 20 (citation omitted; stating: "To remain financially viable, non-profit hospitals must bid successfully to patient bases to pay for delivery of service packages.").

[49] *Cf.* White, *supra* note 3 (stating: "Whereas hospitals once were charitable organizations for the sick and injured, they have gradually adopted characteristics of businesses.").

[50] *Cf.* *"Consumer Directed" Health Plans: Implications for Cost and Quality* (California Health Care Foundation, 2005), 4; http://www.chcf.org/documents/insurance/ConsumerDirHealthPlansQualityCost.pdf.

[51] 51 Ron Shrinkman, "Survival v. Directives," *Modern Health Care* (Nov. 20, 2000) (discussing the Daughters of Charity focus on maintaining good bond ratings).

[52] White, *supra* note 3, at 228. Professor White notes:

> In May 1995, two Catholic-sponsored health care systems (Catholic Health Care West and Daughters of Charity National Health System-West) consolidated. Still called Catholic Health Care West, this new system comprises hospitals sponsored by five religious congregations. . . . Also in 1995, a multisystem collaboration was strengthened by a legal commitment to merge three Roman Catholic health care systems: Sisters of Charity Health Care Systems of Cincinnati, Ohio; Franciscan Health Care Systems of Aston, Pennsylvania; and Catholic Health Corporation of Omaha, Nebraska—to become Catholic Health Initiative (CHI), the largest U.S. Catholic provider at the time. . . . In 1997, the Sisters of Mercy (Eastern System), the Franciscans, and the Daughters of Charity merged to form Catholic Health Care East.

[53] White, supra note 3, at 227. Professor White notes:

> Measuring the effectiveness of health care delivery solely in terms of profitability has necessitated the corporate restructuring of Catholic hospitals, thereby threatening the mission of providing services to the poor and medically indigent. (Ibid., 218.)

[54] Carol S. Weisman, Amal J. Khoury, Christopher Cassirer, Virginia A. Sharpe, and Laura L. Morlock, "The Implications of Affiliations between Catholic and Non-Catholic Health Care Organizations for Availability of Reproductive Health Services." *Women's Health Issues* 9 (May–June 1999): 121, 123. The authors of this study note:

> Financial distress is thought to be a major factor motivating affiliations involving Catholic hospitals. A recent study documented that the average Catholic community hospital in 1992 was less profitable than the average matched not-for-profit community hospital. Although more than 80% of Catholic hospitals were part of church-related health care systems, many were not realizing the benefits of system membership because the systems were geographically dispersed across regions, with no significant concentrations in local service areas. Affiliations with other local providers may be a strategy for financial survival for such hospitals. (Ibid., 123 [citations omitted]).

[55] Jason M. Kellhofer, "The Misperception and Misapplication of the First Amendment in the American Pluralistic System: Mergers Between Catholic and Non-Catholic Health Care Systems." *Journal of Law and Health* 16 (2001): 103, 104.

[56] *See* Christopher Zehnder, "What's Ailing Catholic Hospitals?," *Crisis,* Nov. 2001, 42–46; http://www.catholicculture.org/library/view.cfm?recnum=4155 (discussing arrangements to continue provision of sterilizations after acquisition of non-Catholic facility by Catholic facility).

[57] Lawrence E. Singer and Elizabeth Johnson Lantz, "The Coming Millennium: Enduring Issues Confronting Catholic Health Care." *Annals of Health Law* 8 (1999): 299, 311.

[58] Heather Carlson, "Freedom at Risk: The Implications of *City of Boerne v. Flores* on the Merger of Catholic and Non-Catholic Hospitals." *St. Louis University Public Law Review* 17 (1997): 157, 163–64.

[59] Zehnder, *supra* note 56 (discussing sale of St. Louis University Hospital to Tenet).

[60] Weisman, et al., *supra* note 54, looked at four case studies of affiliations between Catholic and non-Catholic health care providers. The case studies included: an acquisition of a Catholic hospital by a non-Catholic hospital, a merger between a Catholic hospital and an academic medical center, a consolidation between a Catholic and a Protestant hospital, and a 50/50 joint venture involving a Catholic health system and a public hospital. Ibid. On the basis of their four case studies, Weisman, et al. concluded:

> The impact of affiliations on availability of reproductive health services varied by service. Due to infusions of capital and the ability to realize economies of scale, obstetric services were most likely to be expanded as a consequence of affiliations. In addition, strategies for providing more comprehensive women's health care were evident in three of the four case studies. Hospital-based surgical abortion (for purposes other than to save the woman's life) was the only service for which there was evidence of a negative effect on availability. This was an interesting finding, given that none of the case studies involved an instance of a non-Catholic organization assuming Catholic identity as a result of affiliation. Availability of contraceptive services, female and male sterilization, and fertility services generally was unchanged as a result of affiliations. This is not to say that these services were widely promoted or used, but rather that the affiliations themselves did not substantially affect policies or practices with regard to their provision. (Ibid., 132–133.)

[61] Deanna Bellendi, "Oversight on Catholic Deals Sought by Group." *Modern Healthcare* (Nov. 20, 2000): 12.

[62] Ca. Corp. Code § 5917.5 (West 2008). This bill was signed by the Governor on July 14, 2003. 2003 *Cal. Legis. Serv.* ch. 65 (S.B. 932) (West). In response, Fr. Michael Place characterized the legislation as "an unprecedented interference in the sale of property" and further stated: "It is part of a larger coordinated effort to restrict Catholic health care [facilities] from carrying on their mission: to protect innocent human life and the dignity of human sexuality." Joyce Carr, "California Says Catholic Hospitals Can't Stipulate How They're Sold." *National Catholic Register*, Aug. 17–23, 2003, 1. The California law may violate the Hyde-Weldon Amendment if it used to discriminate against hospitals that refuse to provide abortions. *Cf.* Judith C. Gallagher, "Protecting the Other Right to Choose: The Hyde-Weldon Amendment." *Ave Maria Law Review* 5 (2007): 527, 529–30. Ms. Gallagher states:

> Other examples of such coercion abounded under the pre-Hyde-Weldon understanding of "health care entities." In New Jersey, there was an attempt to require a Catholic hospital to build an abortion clinic and pay for abortions. In New York, a state comptroller and gubernatorial candidate threatened a Catholic-operated health maintenance organiza-

tion (HMO) with the loss of state contracts because it chose not to pay for abortions. In addition, California recently enacted legislation that prohibits even nonprofit hospitals from ensuring that the property they sell is not used for particular types or levels of "medical services."

The narrowly defined meaning of "health care entities" enabled federally funded government entities to continue forcing institutional health care providers to participate in abortions. With the enactment of the Hyde-Weldon Amendment, the gap between individuals and institutions has been filled. The Hyde-Weldon Amendment provides that:

> None of the funds made available in this Act may be made available to a Federal agency or program, or to a State or local government, if such agency, program, or government subjects any institutional or individual health care entity to discrimination on the basis that the health care entity does not provide, pay for, provide coverage of, or refer for abortions.
>
> ... [T]he term "health care entity" includes an individual physician or other health care professional, a hospital, a provider-sponsored organization, a health maintenance organization, a health insurance plan, or any other kind of health care facility, organization, or plan (citing Consolidated Appropriations Act, 2005, Pub. L. No. 108-447, § 508(d)(1)-(2), 118 Stat. 2809, 3163 [2004]).

The Amendment effectively eliminates the uncertainty in the definition of "health care entity" by explicitly including any kind of health care facility, organization, or plan within the term. As a result, the Amendment forbids federally funded entities from coercing a broad range of health care providers. (Ibid. [footnotes omitted]).

Chapter Seven: *Catholic Hospitals and Canon Law*

[1] Michael Dennis McGowan, *The Canonical Status of Catholic Health Care Facilities in the Province of New Brunswick in Light of Recent Provincial Government Legislation* (Ceredigion, U.K.: Edwin Mellen Press, 2000), 184.

[2] Jordan Hite, *A Primer on Public and Private Juridic Persons: Applications to the Catholic Health Care Ministry* (Catholic Health Association, 2000), 5.

[3] Ibid.

[4] Ibid.

[5] Ibid.

[6] Ibid.

[7] Francis Morrisey, "Toward Juridic Personality." *Health Progress* 82 (July–Aug. 2001); http://www.chausa.org/Pub/MainNav/News/HP/Archive/2001/07JulAug/Articles/SpecialSection/0107j.htm. Canon 116, § 1 provides:

> Public juridic persons are aggregates of persons or things which are so constituted by the competent ecclesiastical authority that, within the limits set for them in the name of the Church, they fulfill a proper function entrusted to them in view of the common good, in accord with the prescripts of law; other juridic persons are private. James A. Coriden, ed., *The Code of Canon Law: A Text and Commentary* (Mahwah, NJ: Paulist Press, 1985), 82.

[8] John R. Amos, Melanie DiPietro, Jordan Hite, and Francis Morrissey, *The Search for Identity: Canonical Sponsorship of Catholic Health Care* (St. Louis, MO: Catholic Health Association of the United States, 1993), 20–24.

[9] McGowan, *supra* note 1, at 95 (Edwin Mellen Press, 2000).

[10] Amos, et al., *The Search for Identity*, *supra* note 8, at 20.

[11] Hite, *supra* note 2, at 13.

[12] Adam J. Maida and Nicholas P. Cafardi, *Church Property, Church Finances, and Church-Related Corporations* (Catholic Health Association of the United States, 1984), 149.

[13] Ibid. *See also* Canons 312–29, Coriden, *Code of Canon Law* (1985), 249–57.

[14] Hite, *Primer*, *supra* note 2, at 11.

[15] Ibid.

[16] Ibid.

[17] Ibid.

[18] Hite, *Primer*, *supra* note 2, at 13.

[19] Jordan Hite, "Structures in Health Care Ministry in the Church." *Health Progress* (Nov.–Dec. 1999); http://www.chausa.org/Pub/MainNav/News/HP/Archive/1999/11NovDec/Articles/SpecialSection/hp9911e.htm.

[20] Ibid.

[21] Beverly K. Dunn, S.P., "The Evolving Nature of Sponsorship: Recent Decades Have Brought Changes Both in Theory and Practice." *Health Progress* 79 (Mar.–Apr. 1998); http://www.chausa.org/Pub/MainNav/News/HP/Archive/1998/03MarApr/Articles/Features/hp9803i.htm..

[22] Morrisey, "Toward Juridic Personality." *supra* note 7. Morrisey mentions PeaceHealth based in Bellevue, Washington, as an example of a private juridic person involved in the health care ministry. Ibid., PeaceHealth operates six hospitals and other health care ventures in Washington, Alaska, and Oregon. It is sponsored by the Sisters of St. Joseph of Peace. *See* http://www.peacehealth.org/AboutPH/ (last visited Apr. 14, 2008). PeaceHealth traces its origins to Margaret Anna Cusack, the foundress of the Sisters of St. Joseph of Peace. She was born in Ireland into an aristocratic English family. She joined an Anglican order then later converted to the Roman Catholic faith. She came to Bellingham, Washington, from New Jersey in 1890. *See* "Mother Frances Clare, Foundress of the Sisters of St. Joseph of Peace." http://www.peacehealth.org/AboutPH/cusack.htm (last visited Apr. 14, 2008).

[23] Morrisey, "Toward Juridic Personality." *supra* note 7. Morrisey notes: "In the United States, juridic personality has been granted to Covenant Health Systems, Waltham, MA; Catholic Health Initiatives, Denver; Hope Ministries, Newtown Square, PA; and Catholic Health Ministries, Novi, MI" (footnotes omitted).

[24] Ibid. *See also* Canons 116–17, Coriden, *Code of Canon Law* (1985), 82. According to Morrisey:

> One practical difficulty concerns the Vatican authority having the competence to grant pontifical approval. If the property were that of a religious congregation, then the Congregation of Institutes of Consecrated Life and Societies of Apostolic Life (CICLSAL) would be competent to grant recognition. In fact, CICLSAL has done so recently. If the property were diocesan, on the other hand, questions involving it would be referred to the Congregation for the Clergy.

Morrisey, "Toward Juridic Personality," *supra* note 7.

[25] Sharon Holland, "Sponsorship and the Vatican." *Health Progress* 82 (July–Aug. 2001); http://www.chausa.org/Pub/MainNav/News/HP/Archive/2001/07JulAug/Articles/SpecialSection/HP0107k.htm.

[26] Ibid.

[27] Morrisey, *supra* note 7.

[28] Ibid.

[29] Ibid.

[30] Holland, *supra* note 25.

[31] Ibid.
[32] Ibid.
[33] Maida and Cafardi, *supra* note 12, at 56.
[34] Ibid. (emphasis in original). Maida and Cafardi state:

> The natural persons who oversee the affairs of the public juridic persons that sponsor health care institutions are obliged by canon law to see that these teachings are followed in the activity of the sponsored institution (an affirmative responsibility) and that the sponsored institution does not *act* contrary to the teachings of the Church in the sphere of its corporate activity (a negative responsibility).
>
> It should also be understood that this duty to follow the Church's teachings in the governance of a public juridic person's assets, although a personal duty of the appropriate canonical administrator, does not have its source in these administrators. The duty attaches to the assets, as the canon law perceives them, of the public juridic person in much the same way that the *res* or *corpus* of a civil law trust (and not the civil law trustee) carries with it the obligation of the civil law trust. These assets are so marked, so dedicated by the public juridic person to whom they pertain because of the public juridic person's prior acceptance of the Church's teaching authority. These obligations of canonical administrators to govern their public juridic person and all assets that canonically pertain to them thusly are referred to as their *faith obligations*.

Ibid. (internal citations omitted).

[35] Ibid., 57.
[36] Beverly Catherine Dunn, S.P., *Sponsorship of Catholic Institutions, Particularly Health Care Institutions, by the Sisters of Providence in the Western United States* (1995; unpublished dissertation submitted to the Faculty of Canon Law, Saint Paul University, Ottawa, Canada, in partial fulfillment of the requirements for the degree of Doctor of Canon Law), 81.
[37] Ibid.
[38] Ibid.
[39] Christopher J. Kauffman, *Ministry and Meaning: A Religious History of Catholic Health Care in the United States* (Chestnut Ridge, NY: Crossroads Publishing Company, 1995), 293.
[40] Ibid.
[41] Ibid., referring to J.J. McGrath, *Catholic Institutions in the United States: Canonical and Civil Law Status* (Washington, DC: Catholic University of America Press, 1968), 24. McGrath states:

> The property, real and personal, of Catholic hospitals and educational institutions which have been incorporated as American law corporations is the property of the corporate entity and not the property of the sponsoring body or individuals who conduct the institution. All property must be used in accordance with the corporate purposes as defined in the charter, and any property acquired from the donor who has stipulated a specific use must be used for that purpose.
>
> There is no question of dealing with ecclesiastical property when speaking of the property of Catholic hospitals and higher educational institutions in the United States. The canon law is clear that property is ecclesiastical only when it belongs to some ecclesiastical moral person. Since the institutions under consideration have not themselves been established as moral persons and, since no other moral person in fact holds title to the property of the institution, their assets are not ecclesiastical property. (Ibid.)

[42] Robert T. Kennedy, "McGrath, Maida, Michiels: Introduction to a Study of the Canonical and Civil-Law Status of Church-Related Institutions in the United States." *Jurist* 50 (1990): 351, 353, discussed in Kauffman, *supra* note 39.

[43] McGrath, *supra* note 41, at 33.

[44] Ibid.

[45] Ibid., 34.

[46] Ibid.

[47] Kennedy, *supra* note 42, at 354.

[48] McGrath, *supra* note 41, at 36.

[49] Ibid., 37.

[50] Kauffman, *supra* note 39, at 294, discussing Kennedy, *supra* note 42.

[51] Daniel C. Conlin, *Canonical and Civil Legal Issues Surrounding the Alienation of Catholic Health Care Facilities in the United States* (2000; unpublished dissertation Pontificia Studiorum Universitas St. Thoma in Urbe), 105–06 (on file with author).

[52] Ibid., 104.

[53] A. J. Maida, *Ownership, Control, and Sponsorship of Catholic Institutions* (Pennsylvania Catholic Conference, 1975), 35–36, discussed in Dunn, *supra* note 21.

[54] Maida, *supra* note 53, at 40. Maida states:

> Perhaps the most vital and clear sign of what belongs to whom can be obtained from the average person who has daily contact with these institutions, has supported them, benefited from them, and calls upon them for services as needed. Could anyone convince a sister who has given her life in the service of a Catholic hospital or college that such an institution did not pertain to the Church? Could anyone rationalize the teaching of atheistic doctrine or the practice of immoral medicine in these institutions? Does not the public, regardless of religious persuasion, consider these institutions as Catholic and expect them to exist as such and do their work of charity pursuant to Catholic religious belief?
>
> To develop a legal theory which leads to a contrary conclusion is to create a monstrosity in the law and perpetuate an injustice and fraud on the public, especially the people who have given their lives, money, and resources to promote the work of charity in the name of religion. (Ibid.)

[55] Dunn, *supra* note 21. Maida recommends: "The corporate membership of the charitable institutions should be limited to those persons charged with the administration of Church properties of the sponsoring Church body." Maida, *supra* note 53, at 60. He further recommends the following:

> It is essential that members of the charitable corporation reserve to themselves in the charter of the corporation, certain rights and functions in the charitable corporation. The extent of the rights and functions reserved will depend upon the type of legal relationship adopted by the Diocese or Religious Order and its charitable institutions and the charitable corporation law of the state of incorporation. Where possible, the following minimal powers shall be reserved to the members:
>
>   a. The right to amend the charter or bylaws of the charitable corporation.
>   b. The right to approve any sale, lease, or encumbrance on any real estate pertaining to the charitable corporation.
>   c. The right to approve any merger or dissolution of the charitable corporation.
>   d. The right to appoint the Board of Trustees and to remove any trustee with cause.
>   e. The right to appoint the administrator of the charitable corporation.
>   f. The right to approve capital and operation budgets. (Ibid., 60–61.)

[56] Kennedy, *supra* note 42, at 352.
[57] Ibid., 400–01.
[58] Dunn, *supra* note 36, at 82.
[59] *Search for Identity* (1993), *supra* note 8 at 43 n.70, citing "Sacred Congregations for Catholic Education and for Secular Institutes." Private letter, Oct. 7, 1974, Protocol NN, SCI 427/70/23 and SCRIS 300/74, original English text cited in *Canon Law Digest* IX (1978–1981): 910.
[60] Mary Kathryn Grant, "'Reframing' Sponsorship." *Health Progress* 82 (July–Aug. 2001); http://www.chausa.org/Pub/MainNav/News/HP/Archive/2001/07JulAug/Articles/SpecialSection/HP0107l.htm.
[61] Holland, *supra* note 25.
[62] Dunn, *supra* note 36, at 187.
[63] Ibid., 188.
[64] Ibid., 189.
[65] Ibid., 183.
[66] *Search for Identity*, *supra* note 8, at 43, n. 70.
[67] *Search for Identity*, *supra* note 8.
[68] Holland, *supra* note 25. Maida and Cafardi note:

> To use an example from the health care field, when public juridic persons sponsor health care institutions, they are obliged to see that the institution is operated in conformity with the teachings of the Church. This is the case whether the health care facility is an unincorporated program of the religious sponsor, as are many old age or long term care homes, or whether it is separately incorporated, as most hospitals are. . . . The natural persons who oversee the affairs of the public juridic persons that sponsor health care institutions are obliged by the canon law to see that the teachings are followed in the activity of the sponsored institution (an affirmative responsibility) and that the sponsored institution does not *act* contrary to the teachings of the Church in its corporate activities.

Maida and Cafardi, *Church Property*, *supra* note 12, at 56.
[69] Holland, *supra* note 25.
[70] Hite, *supra* note 19.
[71] Mary Kathryn Grant and Margaret Mary Kopish, "Sponsor Leadership Formation: Qualifications for the Next Generation of Sponsors." *Health Progress* 82 (July–Aug. 2001); http://www.chausa.org/Pub/MainNav/News/HP/Archive/2001/07JulAug/Articles/SpecialSection/HP0107t.htm.
[72] Francis G. Morrisey, "Trustees and Canon Law." *Health Progress* 83 (Nov.–Dec. 2002); http://www.chausa.org/Pub/MainNav/News/HP/Archive/2002/11NovDec/Articles/Features/HP0211g.htm. Morrisey states:

> From a canonical perspective, the primary duty of trustees is to ensure that the institutions under their supervision operate in accordance with the teaching, discipline, and laws of the Roman Catholic Church. This is to be done, however, taking into account the mission, vision, and values of the system they represent. These values are usually spelled out in the corporate documents or statutes governing the institution and its sponsors. (Ibid. [internal citations omitted]).

[73] One commentator has noted:

> Health care systems of the size and scale constructed over the last five years make sponsorship influence difficult to achieve. In cosponsored ministries and in the new PJP [pub-

lic juridic person] structures, leadership must be concerned about the evolution of Catholic culture and values. Sponsors at the local level still serve a powerful role in a practical and symbolic sense. In many ways they *are* the Church in the local community. In many contexts, what is known of Catholicism is known by virtue of the deep and abiding presence of the individual religious women. The danger exists of negating the roots of inspiration in individual religious in favor of only a programmatic approach to mission and ministry at the system level. Systematic approaches are required in our complex health systems, but some things can be learned from the living incarnations before us. For instance, we see that public trust is earned over decades; our employees still tend to go to the trusted sister advisor despite the fact that she may have no formal role, and if the sisters are not aligned with leadership, the leader will likely fail before the sisters do. The deeper issue is about forming and sustaining a culture without eradicating its foundation.

David J. Nygren, "Effective Governance in Complex Systems." *Health Progress* 82 (July–Aug. 2001); http://www.chausa.org/Pub/MainNav/News/HP/Archive/2001/07JulAug/Articles/SpecialSection/HP0107u.htm.

[74] "Catholic Hospital Aloha." *National Catholic Reporter,* Feb. 23, 2007, 3.

[75] Patricia Rice, "Vatican Was Able to Veto the Merger of a Catholic Hospital in New Jersey Case." *St. Louis Post-Dispatch*, Feb.1, 1998, B5.

[76] Pamela Schaeffer, "St. Louis Showdown Could Draw in Vatican." *National Catholic Reporter*, Aug. 31, 1997.

[77] Ibid.

[78] Ibid.

[79] Ibid.

[80] For a full discussion of the sale, see Stanley Towne Hatch, *A Study of Values Influencing Leadership in the Sale of Saint Louis University Hospital* (Mar. 2000; unpublished Ph.D. dissertation, Gonzaga University). St. Louis University received approximately $300 million for the hospital. Judith VandeWater, "Hospital Deal Is One of Tenet Corp.'s Most Costly Ever." *St. Louis Post-Dispatch*, Feb. 25, 1998, A6.

[81] Pamela Schaeffer, "Cardinals Claim Rights in Hospital Dispute: University President Contends It's His to Sell." *National Catholic Reporter*, Oct. 24, 1997. The offer by Tenet (approximately $300 million) was $100 million higher than the offer from the Catholic systems. Patricia Rice, "Leaders at SLU Aren't Buckling: They Stand by Hospital Sale Despite Vatican." *St. Louis Post-Dispatch*, Dec. 2, 1997, D1.

[82] Schaeffer, *supra* note 81.

[83] Ibid.

[84] Judith VandeWater, "Biondi Defends Taking Tenet's Offer: Says SLU Medical School Wouldn't Have Survived." *St. Louis Post-Dispatch*, Oct. 29, 1997, 1C.

[85] Ibid.

[86] Ibid.

[87] Justin Rigali, "Catholic Character of Hospital Would Be Lost." *St. Louis Post-Dispatch*, Oct. 24, 1997, 11C.

[88] Patricia Rice, "Rigali Gets Backing on Hospital Sale: Prelates from New York, Boston, Washington Concur." *St. Louis Post-Dispatch*, Oct. 20, 1997, B1.

[89] Ibid.

[90] Schaeffer, *supra* note 81.

[91] Tenet, "St. Louis University Sign Definitive Agreement for Hospital Sale." press release issued by St. Louis University, Feb. 24, 2008; http://www.slu.edu/publications/gc/v4-7/news_1.shtml. The press release states in relevant part:

Assurances Provided for the Church
Rev. Lawrence Biondi, S.J., President of Saint Louis University, also issued the following statement:

Since there was significant interest in the transaction, the Board of Trustees reaffirmed to the Catholic Community that the above four critical requirements would be met. Although the Board of Trustees did not seek approval or permission from the Holy See (Vatican), the Board did, however, cooperate with the Superior General of the Jesuit Order, the Very Rev. Peter-Hans Kolvenbach, S.J., who presented the University's position to the Holy See.

Cardinal Eduardo Martinez-Somalo, Prefect of the Congregation for Institutes of Consecrated Life and Societies of Apostolic Life and Cardinal Pio Laghi, Prefect for the Congregation for Catholic Education, in consultation with Father Kolvenbach, sought assurances from the University that the above four terms and conditions would be included in the final asset purchase agreement. Since the agreement between the University and Tenet had already contained legally binding language to assure Tenet's adherence to these terms, the Board of Trustees willingly provided these commitments. On February 18, 1998, Cardinals Martinez-Somalo and Laghi communicated to Father Kolvenbach that they, as the appropriate representatives and spokespersons for the Holy See (Vatican), had accepted the assurances of the University and that they had no objections to the sale of Saint Louis University Hospital to Tenet.

[92] Ibid. The press release states in relevant part:

The Saint Louis University Board of Trustees selected Tenet through a competitive and rigorous selection process that began more than a year ago.

In selecting Tenet, the Board required legally binding guarantees that the Hospital would continue to be operated and managed in a manner consistent with the Catholic, Jesuit values of the University.

Among other things, Tenet has agreed to:

1. Adhere to the Ethical and Religious Directives for Catholic Health Care Services of the National Conference of Catholic Bishops.
2. Continue the University's pastoral care services for patients and their families, offered seven days a week, 24 hours a day and managed by the University's Vice President for Mission and Ministry.
3. Adopt the Hospital's current charity care policy in perpetuity, ensuring that its role in serving the city's poor and indigent will continue.
4. Assure that the existing graduate medical education programs in pediatrics, obstetrics, and gynecology can be maintained in partnerships with other Catholic hospitals.

[93] Mary Jo Feldstein, "Hospitals Share the Details on Charity, Other Care." *St. Louis Post-Dispatch*, May 19, 2006, B1. St. Louis University reported that it provided $39,542,491 (12% of net revenue) in total community benefit (including charity care, bad debts, education services, and taxes paid) in 2004. This placed it among the top five hospitals in Missouri. The level of charity care was reported at $619,068 (1.5% of net revenues), also placing it in the top five. Ibid.

[94] Conlin, *supra* note 51, at 201.

[95] Patricia Rice, "In Wake of SLU Dispute, Vatican Tightens Control over Institutions." *St. Louis Post-Dispatch*, Nov. 1, 1998, B4.

[96] *Saint Louis University v. Masonic Temple Association of St. Louis,* 220 S.W.3rd 721 (Mo. 2007).

[97] *Saint Louis University v. Masonic Temple Association of St. Louis* (Appellate Brief filed by St. Louis University) at 10–11, 2007 WL 173604 9 (citing to affidavit of Lawrence Biondi, S.J., president of St. Louis University). *See also* Tim Townsend, Deirdre Shesgreen, Tom Timmermann, and Kavita Kumar, "Majerus Runs Afoul of Burke." *St. Louis Post-Dispatch,* Jan. 23, 2008, A1 (pointing out statements in the brief).

[98] Ibid., 38.

PART THREE: *The Struggle to Maintain Catholic Identity as Reflected in Two Health Care Systems*

Chapter Eight: *Providence Health System*

[1] Providence Health and Services Fact Sheet (2007); http://www.providence.org/resources/phs/reports/2007_Fact_Sheet.pdf.

[2] Ibid.

[3] Ibid.

[4] Ibid.

[5] "The Providence Commitment: Mission." http://www.providence.org/phs/about_Providence/mission.htm (last visited Aug. 4, 2007).

[6] George C. Stewart, Jr., *Marvels of Charity: History of American Sisters and Nuns* (Huntington, IN: Our Sunday Visitor, 1994), 149; *see also* JoDee Black, "Religious Order Moves to Save Nonprofit Empire in Northwest." *Great Falls Tribune,* Jan. 13, 2002.

[7] "Providence in the West: A Timeline, 1856–1902: Pioneering Health Care and Education." http://www.providence.org/phs/archives/History_Online/chrono1.htm.

[8] "The Architect of the Capitol, The National Statuary Hall Collection." http://www.aoc.gov/cc/art/nsh/index.cfm.

[9] "Mother Joseph of the Sacred Heart: Pioneer, Leader, Woman of Faith." http://www.providence.org/PHS/Archives/History_Online/mjoseph/mjbio.htm; *see also* Stewart, *Marvels of Charity, supra* note 6, at 149.

[10] Stewart, *supra* note 6, at 149; *see also* "Mother Joseph of the Sacred Heart." *Supra* note 9.

[11] "Mother Joseph of the Sacred Heart," *supra* note 9.

[12] Ibid. See also Stewart, *Marvels of Charity, supra* note 6, at 222–23.

[13] "Providence in the West: A Timeline, 1856–1902," *supra* note 7.

[14] Ibid.

[15] Ibid.

[16] Sisters of Providence, Pariseau Association, Chronological Events, June 13, 1977 (rev. Mar. 1979); Sisters of Providence, Sacred Heart Province, History 1859–2000 (Box 2). Providence Archives, Seattle, Washington.

[17] Ibid.

[18] Ibid.

[19] Corporations in Sacred Heart Province, Dec. 31, 1992, Sisters of Providence, Sacred Heart Province, History 1859–2000 (Box 2). Providence Archives, Seattle.

[20] "Providence in the West: A Timeline, 1856–1902," *supra* note 7.

[21] "Providence in the West: A Timeline, 1903–1960: Growth and Diversity." http://www.providence.org/phs/archives/History_OnLine/chrono2.htm (last visited June 3, 2008).

[22] Ibid.

Notes

[23] "Providence in the West: A Timeline, 1975–2006: New Life Through Collaboration." http://www.providence.org/phs/archives/History_Online/chrono4.htm (last visited June 3, 2008).

[24] Beverly Katherine Dunn, S.P., *Sponsorship of Catholic Institutions, Particularly Health Care Institutions by the Sisters of Providence in the Western United States* (dissertation submitted to the Faculty of Canon Law, Saint Paul University, Ottawa, Canada, in partial fulfillment of the requirements for the degree of Doctor of Canon Law), 38–39, SP Dissertations. Providence Archives, Seattle.

[25] Ibid., 52–53.

[26] Ibid., 53

[27] Ibid., 52–53.

[28] Ibid., 53.

[29] Ibid., 54.

[30] Ibid., 81–82.

[31] "Providence in the West: A Timeline, 1975–2006," *supra* note 23.

[32] Memorandum from Peter Bigelow to Department Management Staff and Medical Staff Executive Committee, Providence Hospital, Apr. 19, 1991, Sisters of Providence, Sacred Heart Province Corporation (1990–1991). Providence Archives, Seattle.

[33] Ibid.

[34] Position Description, Chairperson of the Board, Approved by Sr. Barbara Schamber, S.P., Provincial Superior, Mar. 1, 1991, Sisters of Providence, Sacred Heart Corporation, Board of Directors, 1990–1991. Providence Archives, Seattle.

[35] Dunn, *supra* note 24, at 106.

[36] Sisters of Providence Overview of the Governance Model, Discussion Daft, Apr. 29, 1991, Sisters of Providence, Sacred Heart Corporation, Governance, Board of Directors, 1990–1991. Providence Archives, Seattle.

[37] Ibid.

[38] Dunn, *supra* note 24, at 111–12.

[39] Ibid., 107.

[40] Ibid.

[41] Ibid.

[42] Ibid.

[43] Ibid., 110.

[44] Ibid., 110.

[45] Ibid.

[46] Ibid., 111.

[47] Ibid.

[48] Black, *supra* note 6.

[49] "Providence in the West: A Timeline, 1975–2006," *supra* note 23.

[50] Robert Struckman, "Parent Group to Integrate with Larger System." *Missoulian*, Dec. 8, 2005.

[51] Ibid.

[52] "Providence in the West: A Timeline, 1856–1902," *supra* note 7.

[53] "Providence in the West: A Timeline, 1903–1960," *supra* note 21.

[54] Dunn, *supra* note 24, at 37.

[55] Ibid.

[56] Ibid.

[57] Ibid.

[58] Ibid., 38.

[59] "Providence in the West: A Timeline, 1975–2006," *supra* note 23.
[60] Ibid.
[61] Ibid.
[62] Ibid.
[63] Ibid.
[64] Ibid.
[65] "Providence Health System to Sell Yakima and Toppenish Hospitals and Homecare to Health Management Associates: New Organization to Invest Millions In Yakima Valley." Press Release, Mar. 19, 2003, (80) Providence Yakima Medical Center Sale to Health Management Association, Inc., 2003. Providence Archives, Seattle.
[66] Struckman, *supra* note 50.
[67] "Living the Mission Day by Day: Report to the Community." Providence Health and Services (2006), 24; http://www.providence.org/resources/phs/reports/2006_Annual_Report.pdf (last visited June 3, 2008).
[68] Ibid., 24.
[69] Ibid., 23.
[70] Ibid., 23.
[71] Ibid., 24.
[72] Ibid., 24.
[73] "Providence in the West: A Timeline, 1961–1974: Transition Years." http://www.providence.org/phs/archives/History_Online/chrono3.htm (last visited June 3, 2008).
[74] "The Good Work" (Spring 1984), 12. Providence Archives, Seattle.
[75] Ibid.
[76] "Living the Mission Day by Day." Providence Health and Services Fact Sheet 3 (2007); http://www.providence.org/resources/phs/reports/2007_Fact_Sheet.pdf (last visited June 3, 2008).
[77] Ibid.
[78] Ibid., 6–11.
[79] Dunn, *supra* note 24, at 84.
[80] Ibid.
[81] Ibid.
[82] Ibid.
[83] Ibid., 87.
[84] Ibid., 88.
[85] Ibid., 89.
[86] Ibid., 89.
[87] Ibid., 90.
[88] Ibid., 92.
[89] "Mission Effectiveness Principles and Guidelines" (June 1986, rev. Aug. 1990), Sacred Heart Sisters of Providence Corporations, Office of Mission Effectiveness (1990–1991), Sisters of Providence. Providence Archives, Seattle.
[90] Ibid., Table of Contents.
[91] Ibid., 3.
[92] Ibid., 4–5.
[93] Ibid.
[94] Ibid., 6.
[95] Ibid.
[96] Ibid.
[97] Ibid., 7.

[98] Ibid., 8.
[99] Ibid., 10.
[100] Ibid., 11.
[101] Ibid., 12.
[102] Ibid., 14.
[103] Ibid., 15.
[104] Tyrone Beason, "Economics of Hospital Merger: Little Choice in 'Severe Marketplace,'" *Seattle Times,* Wednesday, Mar. 1, 2000. Beason notes:

> More than 140 years ago, five Catholic nuns had a simple mission: Care for the elderly, ill, and orphaned, and let God's will be the guide.
>
> In Vancouver, Wash., in 1856, health care, as it was, depended on the kindness of strangers.
>
> But 144 years later, Providence Health System-Washington is one of the largest health care providers in the state, and things aren't that simple. It is still driven by compassion, but also by competition and money. Slim profit margins, shrinking insurance reimbursements and expensive technology make it tough to stay competitive.

[105] Washington State Catholic Hospital & Health Care Association, Press Release, Feb. 6, 1973, Providence Health System Ethical Issues. Providence Archives, Seattle.
[106] Ibid.
[107] "The Providence Commitment." http://www.providence.org/phs/About_Providence/mission.htm.
[108] Providence Health Plans, Individual and Family Plans; http://www.providence.org/healthplans/getcoverage/individualplans/planoverview/limitations.aspx.
[109] Providence Health and Services Disclaimer; http://www.providence.org/glob/gbl_disclaimer.htm.
[110] "Healthwise Medical Reference Library: Birth Control." Providence Health Plans; http://www.providence.org/healthlibrary/contentViewer.aspx?hwid=hw237864&serviceArea=health_plans (last visited June 3, 2008).
[111] "Healthwise Medical Reference Library: Tubal Ligation and Tubal Implants." Providence Health Plans; http://www.providence.org/healthlibrary/contentViewer.aspx?hwid=hw7305&serviceArea=health_plans (last visited June 3, 2008).
[112] Healthwise Medical Reference Library, Providence Health Plans; http://www.providence.org/healthlibrary/contentViewer.aspx?hwid=tw1040&serviceArea=health_plans.
[113] "The Good Work." 2002 Report to the Community, Providence Health System 20.
[114] "Living the Mission Day by Day," *supra* note 67.
[115] "Healthwise Medical Reference Library: Emergency Contraception." Providence Health Plans; http://www.providence.org/healthlibrary/contentViewer.aspx?hwid=tb1838&serviceArea=health_plans (last visited June 3, 2008).
[116] Sharon Sayler, "Hospitals Following Rape Victim Law." *Everett Herald,* Apr. 1, 2002.
[117] Carla K. Johnson, "Catholic Hospitals Violate State Law, Pro-Choice Group Claims." *The Spokesman-Review,* Jan. 3, 2003.
[118] Ibid.
[119] Ibid.
[120] Ibid.
[121] Ibid.
[122] Richard Roesler, "Contraceptive Coverage Goes for Hospital Too." *The Spokesman-Review,* Aug. 12, 2002, A1.

[123] Gary Crooks, "Medical Center Can Find Right Balance." *The Spokesman-Review*, Aug. 18, 2002, B6.

[124] Thomas A. Szyszkiewicz, "Induction Procedures Raise Moral Dilemma." *National Catholic Register*, Oct. 19–25, 2003, 1. The Providence policy provides:

> The pre-term induction of the delivery of a fetus is allowable only under the following conditions:
> - If there is a serious risk to the health of the mother (Ethical and Religious Directives, Nos. 47, 49).
> - If the fetus has a lethal condition. "Lethal condition" is defined as a disease or a combination of abnormalities that, even with medical treatment, will not allow the fetus to live.
> - If the fetus has reached 24 weeks of gestation (currently accepted as the stage of viability) or later (Ethical and Religious Directives, No. 49).

"Anatomy of a Thorny Issue." *National Catholic Register*, Oct. 19–25, 2003, 7. Subsequently, this policy was modified after review by the National Catholic Bioethics Center and the archbishop. Ibid.

[125] Szyszkiewicz, *supra* note 124, at 7.
[126] Ibid., 1.
[127] Ibid.
[128] Ibid.
[129] Ibid., 7.
[130] Ibid.
[131] Ibid.
[132] Ibid.
[133] "Anatomy of a Thorny Issue," *supra* note 124, at 7.
[134] Ibid.
[135] Ibid.
[136] Ibid.
[137] Norman M. Ford, "Early Delivery of a Fetus with Anencephaly." *Ethics & Medics* 28 (7), (July 2003), excerpted from Norman M. Ford, *The Prenatal Person: Ethics from Conception to Birth*, 86–88, 95–99 (2002).
[138] Ibid. (footnote omitted).
[139] Ibid.
[140] NCBC *Statement on Early Induction of Labor*, Mar. 11, 2004; http://www.ncbcenter.org/04-03-11-EarlyInduction.asp. It states:

> The application of Catholic moral teaching and tradition to this issue is directed toward two specific ends: (1) complete avoidance of direct abortion, and (2) preservation of the lives of both mother and child to the extent possible under the circumstances. Based upon these ends, the Ethical and Religious Directives for Catholic Health Care Services provides directives which set the parameters for the treatment of mother and unborn child in cases of high-risk pregnancies:
>
> 47. Operations, treatments, and medications that have as their direct purpose the cure of a proportionately serious pathological condition of a pregnant woman are permitted when they cannot be safely postponed until the unborn child is viable, even if they will result in the death of the unborn child.
>
> 49. For a proportionate reason, labor may be induced after the fetus is viable.

The principle of the double effect is at work in each of these two directives. Actions that might result in the death of a child are morally permitted only if all of the following conditions are met: (1) treatment is directly therapeutic in response to a serious pathology of the mother or child; (2) the good effect of curing the disease is intended and the bad effect foreseen but unintended; (3) the death of the child is not the means by which the good effect is achieved; and (4) the good of curing the disease is proportionate to the risk of the bad effect. Fulfillment of all four conditions precludes any act that directly hastens the death of a child.

Early induction of labor for chorioamnionitis, preeclampsia, and H.E.L.L.P. syndrome, for example, can be morally licit under the conditions just described because it directly cures a pathology by evacuating the infected membranes in the case of chorioamnionitis, or the diseased placenta in the other cases, and cannot be safely postponed. However, early induction of an anencephalic child when there is no serious pathology of the mother which is being directly treated is not morally licit, emotional distress notwithstanding. Early induction of labor before term (37 weeks) to relieve emotional distress hastens the death of the child as a means of achieving this presumed good effect and unjustifiably deprives the child of the good of gestation. Moreover, this distress is amenable to psychological support such as is offered in perinatal hospice. Lastly, induction of labor before term performed simply for the reason that the child has a lethal anomaly is direct abortion.

Ibid.

[141] Benedict M. Ashley, O.P. and Kevin D. O'Rourke, O.P., *Ethics of Health Care*, 3rd ed. (Washington, DC: Georgetown University Press, 2002), 132.

[142] Kim Barker and Tyrone Beason, "Swedish Medical Center, Providence to Join Forces." *Seattle Times,* Feb. 29, 2000.

[143] Memorandum from Sr. Barbara Schamber, S.P., team leader/presiding member and Sr. Karin Dufault, S.P., Chair of the Board, to Sisters of Providence, Mother Joseph Province, Strategic Alliance with Swedish Health Services, Feb. 29, 2002, (56) Providence Seattle Medical Center, Alliance with Swedish Med. Ctr., 2000. Providence Archives, Seattle.

[144] Tom Paulson, "Swedish Hospital Buying Rival Providence; Catholics Bet Wrong on Health Care Reform, Lost Millions." *Seattle Post Intelligencer*, Mar. 1, 2000.

[145] Barker and Beason, *supra* note 142.

[146] Telephone interview with Jan Heller, Ph.D., staff ethicist for Providence Health System, and Sr. Karin Dufault, S.P., Ph.D., R.N, Chair of the Board, Providence Health System, Sept. 23, 2003.

[147] Paulson, *supra* note 144.

[148] Ibid.

[149] Interview with Loretta Green, archivist for the Sisters of Providence, Mother Joseph Province, Seattle, Washington, July 24, 2003.

[150] Barker and Beason, *supra* note 142.

[151] Ibid.

[152] Kim Barker, "Swedish Will Drop Elective Abortions to Seal Deal." *Seattle Times,* Mar. 1, 2000.

[153] Ibid.

[154] Frances Kissling, "Abortion: Swedish Selling Out Women in Seattle Deal." Letters to the Editor, *Seattle Times,* Mar. 12, 2000.

[155] J. Martin, McOmber, "Seattle Hospital to Become Research Center." *Seattle Times*, Aug. 8, 2002.

[156] Telephone interview with Jan C. Heller, Ph.D., staff ethicist, Providence Health System, and Sr. Karin Dufault, Ph.D., R.N., S.P., Chair of the Board, Providence Health System, Sept. 23, 2003.

[157] "Swedish Medical Center, Sabey Corporation Complete Terms to Redevelop Part of Swedish/Providence Campus — $37 Million Purchase to Add Biotech/Medical Research Center to Hospital Campus." Press release, Aug. 7, 2002, (56) Providence Seattle Medical Center; History. Providence Archives, Seattle.

[158] Ibid.

[159] Memorandum from Sr. Barbara Schamber, *supra* note 143.

[160] Kyung M. Song, "Providence Hospital's New Name Inspires Ire: Meet the Cherry Hill Campus Central Area Residents Feeling Snubbed by Swedish Decision." *Seattle Times*, Local News, Jan. 12, 2007.

[161] Paul J. Lim, "The Sisters of Providence Are Running a Successful Business While Tending to the Health Care Needs of the Region." *Seattle Times*, Jan. 15, 1995.

[162] Ibid.

[163] Sandy Lutz Dallas, "Mergers: Two-Hospital Towns Try Togetherness, Health Care Reform Has Competitors Turning to Collaboration, Consolidation." *Modern Health Care* (Dec. 6, 1993), at 1993 WL 6204003.

[164] Ibid.

[165] Jolayne Houtz, "Everett General Plans Gift; Reproductive Services to Be Lost in Merger," *Seattle Times*, Nov. 15, 1993, at 1993 WL 6027284.

[166] Ibid.

[167] Jolayne Houtz, "Merger to End Abortions," *Seattle Times,* Aug. 13, 1993.

[168] Houtz, "Everett General Plans Gift," *supra* note 165. Most years, only 5 to 10 abortions per year were performed at General. Ibid. In the year prior to the merger, however, 483 tubal ligations had been performed at General, and it was estimated that three quarters of those would not have been performed under the new policy. Ibid.

[169] Matt Sabo, "Judge Won't Rule on Failed Hospital Plan," *Portland Oregonian*, Mar. 22, 2001.

[170] Matt Sabo, "Church Affiliation Would Not Harm," *Portland Oregonian*, Dec. 29, 2000.

[171] Vince Galloro, "Secular–Church Deal in Oregon Spurs Conflict," *Modern Healthcare* (Dec. 11, 2000).

[172] Matt Sabo, "Court Weighs Health District's Pact With Catholic-Run Hospital," *Portland Oregonian*, Nov. 29, 2000.

[173] Ibid.

[174] Sabo, *supra* note 170.

[175] 280 N.W.2d 73 (Wis. 1979).

[176] Sabo, *supra* note 169.

Chapter Nine: *Ascension Health*

[1] "About Ascension Health: Sponsorship and History." http://www.ascensionhealth.org/about/sponsorship_history.asp (last visited Jan. 11, 2008).

[2] Ibid.

[3] "About Ascension Health." http://www.ascensionhealth.org/about/main.asp (last visited Jan. 11, 2008).

[4] Ibid. The integration of the cultures of the Daughters of Charity and Sisters of St. Joseph was part of the planning process. Ira M. Levin, Deborah Proctor, Thomas Thibault, "The Making of Ascension Health." *Health Progress* (May–June 2001): 48.

[5] Hoover's Company Records — In-Depth Records, Feb. 6, 2008.

[6] Ibid.

[7] Ibid.

[8] 8 Judith VandeWater, "Daughters of Charity, Michigan Firm Will Merge — Deal Will Create One of Nation's Largest Catholic Nonprofit Care Groups." *St. Louis Post-Dispatch*, Sept. 28, 1999, at C6.

[9] Ibid.

[10] Ibid.

[11] Andrew Ward, "The Rise of Ascension." *The Bond Buyer,* Sept. 29, 1999, at 1.

[12] Mary Chris Jaklevic, "IRS Auditing Ascension Deal: Experts Suggest IRS Wants to Learn More About New Ways of Financing Acquisitions." *Modern Healthcare* (May 22, 2000).

[13] Ibid.

[14] Deanna Bellandi, "Catholic Merger Proves Lucrative." *Modern Healthcare* (Nov. 6, 2000), at 2000 WL 8169631.

[15] Ibid.

[16] Ibid.

[17] Ibid.

[18] Vince Galloro, "A Matter of Financial Faith." *Modern Healthcare* (June 24, 2002)

[19] Ibid.

[20] Ibid.

[21] "Ascension Health Finalizes Acquisition of Carondelet Health System Hospitals, Facilities." *Health Care Strategic Management* (Jan. 1, 2003).

[22] Vince Galloro and Patrick Reilly, "Trickling Down: Strong Operational Improvements at Health care Systems Once Again Fail to Show Up on the Bottom Line, According to *Modern Healthcare's* Annual Survey." *Modern Healthcare* (June 2, 2003).

[23] Melanie Evans, "Ascending in Health Care: Roman Catholic Ascension Health Has Made a Fortune 500 Name for Itself with Business Acumen, Risk-taking and Efficiency." *Modern Healthcare*, 37, no. 20 (May 14, 2007).

[24] Laura S. Kaiser, Anthony R. Tersigni, John Serle and James Dover, "A Successful Reconfiguration." *Health Progress* 88, no. 4 (July–Aug. 2007); http://www.chausa.org/Pub/MainNav/News/HP/Archive/2007/07July-Aug/Articles/Features/hp0707g.htm.

[25] Evans, *supra* note 23.

[26] Ibid.

[27] Ibid.

[28] Mike Colias, "Hospital Fighting for Its Life: Board of St. Anthony Scrambles to Stem Losses." *Crain's Chicago Busines* 31, no. 17 (Apr. 28, 2008).

[29] Shane Farley, "Via Christi to Become Ascension Affiliate." *Wichita Business Journal*, Nov. 15, 2006.

[30] Ibid.

[31] Melanie Evans, "Ascension Expands in Joint Deal: Deal to Help Religious Orders Consolidate Their Assets." *Modern Healthcare* (Nov. 20, 2006); Andi Atwater, "New Owners for Via Christi." *Wichita Eagle*, Nov. 16, 2006, C1.

[32] M. William Salganik, "St. Joseph, St. Agnes Form New Health Partnership: Catholic Hospitals Hope Collaboration Expands Services." *Baltimore Sun*, Jan. 19, 2007, 1E.

[33] Anna Velasco, "St. Vincent's, Eastern Health Merging July 1." *Birmingham News*, Apr. 12, 2007.

[34] Chris Parker, "Schuykill Hospitals Agree on Merger: Good Samaritan, Pottsville Could Be Joined by Year End." *The Morning Call*, Apr. 3, 2008, B3.

[35] Melanie Evans and Jessica Zigmond, "The Joint Appeal; Froedtert, Columbia St. Mary's in Milwaukee Choose Joint Operating Agreement." *Modern Healthcare* 38 (Jan. 21, 2008): 14; Guy Boulton, "Can Catholic Ethics Withstand Two Hospitals?" *Milwaukee Journal & Sentinel*, Dec. 11, 2007, D1.

[36] Steve Bailey, "Which Way Is Caritas Headed?" *Boston Globe*, Nov. 14, 2007, C1. Previously, Ascension Health had gone so far as to sign a letter of intent with the Archdiocese of Boston with a planned acquisition date of July 2007. Christopher Rowland, "In Caritas Deal, Fears for Two City Hospitals: Archdiocese Says Ascension Will Strengthen Local System, but Menino Thinks Cuts Could Loom." *Boston Globe*, Feb. 7, 2007, 1D.

[37] Richard A. Webster, "Daughters of Charity and Ascension Health to Open a New Clinic in N.O.." *New Orleans City Business*, Nov. 5, 2007.

[38] Ibid.

[39] Ibid.

[40] Ibid.

[41] Ibid.

[42] Evans, *supra* note 23.

[43] Ibid.

[44] Ibid.

[45] Ibid.

[46] Hoover's Company Records, *supra* note 5.

[47] George C. Stewart, Jr., *Marvels of Charity: History of American Sisters and Nuns* (Huntington, IN: Our Sunday Visitor, 1994), 39.

[48] Christopher J. Kauffman, *Ministry and Meaning: A Religious History of Catholic Health Care in the United States* (Chestnut Ridge, NY: The Crossroads Publishing Company, 1995), 19.

[49] Stewart, *supra* note 47, at 39.

[50] Kauffman, *supra* note 48, at 20.

[51] Ibid., 22.

[52] Ibid., 20–21.

[53] Daughters of Charity History; http://www.doc.org/about/index.htm (last visited Dec. 12, 2008).

[54] Monica Langley, "No Margin, No Mission." *Wall Street Journal*, Jan. 7, 1998, A1.

[55] Kauffman, *supra* note 48, at 23.

[56] Daughters of Charity History, *supra* note 53.

[57] Kauffman, *supra* note 48, at 26.

[58] Kauffman, *supra* note 48, at 34. For a brief description of the founding of the Sisters of Charity by St. Elizabeth Ann Seton, *see* Stewart, *Marvels of Charity*, *supra* note 47, at 55–60.

[59] Ibid. Stewart notes:

> Sisters of Charity from Emmitsburg began their first work in medical institutions at the Baltimore Infirmary in 1823. Father Dubois, their superior, always the careful contractor for the sister's services, insured proper conditions before allowing them to work in the infirmary where Dr. Robert Patterson needed them. The infirmary had three physicians and four surgeons, a special ward for diseases of the eye and one for sailors which later

expanded into a separate Marine hospital. The doctors were affiliated with the medical faculty at the University of Maryland. Working under their supervision, the sisters learned about medicine and treating illnesses and wounds — medical skills they later put to use in their own hospitals (footnotes omitted).

Stewart, *Marvels of Charity, supra* note 47, at 75–76. *See also* Kauffman, *Ministry and Meaning, supra* note 48, at 33–36 for a description of the situation at the Baltimore infirmary.

[60] Stewart, *supra* note 47, at 76.
[61] Kauffman, *supra* note 48, at 51.
[62] Ibid., 43.
[63] Ibid., 50–63.
[64] Ibid., 23. " On July 18,1849, the Council of the Daughters of Charity in Paris voted to admit the American Community." Stewart, *Marvels of Charity, supra* note 47, at 109.
[65] Ibid., 23.
[66] Daughters of Charity History, *supra* note 53.
[67] Langley, *supra* note 54.
[68] Ibid.
[69] Ward, *supra* note 11.
[70] Langley, *supra* note 54.
[71] Ibid.
[72] Ibid.
[73] Ibid.
[74] Ibid.
[75] Deanna Bellandi, "The Old Guard Stands Down: Generation of CEOs That Fostered Systems Is Retiring." *Modern Healthcare* (May 8, 2000).
[76] Ibid.
[77] Ibid.
[78] Ibid.
[79] Ibid.
[80] Langley, *supra* note 54.
[81] Ibid.
[82] Deanna Bellandi, "Ascension Taps No. 2 as New CEO." *Modern Healthcare* (Nov. 6, 2000, at 56).
[83] Ibid.
[84] Ibid.
[85] Cinda Becker and Deanna Bellandi, "Two Systems Restructure: UPHS to Get Spun Off; Ascension Creates Teams." *Modern Healthcare* (Feb. 19, 2001).
[86] Ibid.
[87] Ibid.
[88] Ibid.
[89] Ibid.
[90] About Ascension Health; http://www.ascensionhealth.org/about/national_leadership/anthony_tersigni.asp.
[91] Lucette Lugnado, "Religious Practice: Their Role Growing, Catholic Hospitals Juggle Doctrine and Medicine." *Wall Street Journal*, Feb. 4, 1999.
[92] Ibid.
[93] Ibid.
[94] Ibid.

[95] Nancy A. Fischer, "State Forces Pair of Hospitals to Resuscitate Dead Issue: Hospital Merger Talks Resurface in Niagara Falls and Lewiston." *The Buffalo News*, Dec. 24, 2006, 1.

[96] Nancy A. Fischer, "Hospitals Agree to Share Some Services." *The Buffalo News*, Nov. 3, 2007, D3.

[97] Henry L. Davis, "Hospital Merger Fails over Conflict: Catholic Principles Prevent Agreement." *The Buffalo News*, Sept. 28, 2007, D1.

[98] Cinda Becker, "Full Speed Ahead on Merger: Many Recommendations Ahead of Schedule." *Modern Healthcare* 37, no. 51 (Dec. 24, 2007).

[99] Davis, *supra* note 97.

[100] Lugnado, *supra* note 91.

[101] Ibid.

[102] Ibid.

[103] Ibid.

[104] Ibid.

[105] Directive 68, *Ethical and Religious Directives for Catholic Health Care Services*, 4th ed. (2001), 36-37, provides:

> Any partnership that will affect the mission or religious and ethical identity of Catholic health care institutional services must respect church teaching and discipline. Diocesan bishops and other church authorities should be involved as such partnerships are developed, and the diocesan bishop should give the appropriate authorization before they are completed. The diocesan bishop's approval is required for partnerships sponsored by institutions subject to his governing authority; for partnerships sponsored by religious institutes of pontifical right, his nihil obstat should be obtained.

In addition, Directive 69 provides:

> If a Catholic health care institution is considering entering into an arrangement with another organization that may be involved in activities judged morally wrong by the Church, participation in such activities, must be limited to what is in accord with the moral principles governing cooperation.

Directive 69, *Ethical and Religious Directives for Catholic Health Care Services*, 4th ed. (2001), 37.

[106] *Cf.* Directive 71, *Ethical and Religious Directives for Catholic Health Care Services* 4th ed. (2001), 37, providing:

> The possibility of scandal must be considered when applying the principles governing cooperation. Cooperation, which in all other respects is morally licit, may need to be refused because of the scandal that might be caused. Scandal can sometimes be avoided by an appropriate explanation of what is in fact being done at the health care facility under Catholic auspices. The diocesan bishop has final responsibility for assessing and addressing issues of scandal, considering not only the circumstances in his local diocese but also the regional and national implications of his decision [endnotes omitted].

[107] Ibid. In 1986, Middle Tennessee Medical Center (MTMC) joined with Baptist and St. Thomas Hospital (owned by the Daughters of Charity). "In Jan. 2002, MTMC became a member of Saint Thomas Health Services and Ascension Health and embraced the faith-

based mission, vision, and values of the organization." Middle Tennessee Medical Center, About Us; http://www.mtmc.org/index_home.php?bd=1&title=About%20Us&pth=YWJvdXR1cy9pbmRleC5waHA=&nav=YWJvdXR1cy9fYm9keW5hdl9hYm91dHVzLnBocA (last visited Dec. 12, 2008).

[108] Lugnado, *supra* note 91.
[109] Ibid.
[110] Ibid.
[111] Ibid.
[112] Ibid.
[113] Cinda Becker, "Calling Off the Wedding: Long-Planned Merger Falls Through in New York." *Modern Healthcare* (Nov. 25, 2002).
[114] Ibid.
[115] Ibid.
[116] Jeremy Boyer, "Albany, N.Y., Hospital Sees Affiliation Collapse Due to Merger Issues." *Times Union*, Nov. 12, 2002.
[117] Marco Leavitt, "Amsterdam Hospital Merger to Affect Family Planning Services." *The Business Review* (Albany), Aug. 28, 2007.
[118] Ibid.
[119] Ibid.
[120] Ibid.
[121] Bill Lewis, "St. Thomas Seeks to Block DeKalb Surgery Center." *The Tennessean*, Mar. 24, 2003.
[122] Ibid.
[123] Ibid.
[124] Ibid.
[125] Ibid.
[126] Velasco, *supra* note 33.
[127] Ibid.
[128] Ibid.
[129] Anna Velasco, "Sterilization Issues Surround Medical Center East Changes: Catholic Directives Won't Govern Outpatient Center." *Birmingham News*, Apr. 29, 2007, 17.
[130] Ibid.
[131] Ibid.
[132] Ibid.
[133] Statement, *Birmingham News*, May 7, 2007. It states:

> Saint Vincent's Hospital is a vital part of the healing ministry of the Catholic Church in the Greater Birmingham area. The hospital serves all persons, especially the poor, the unborn, and the elderly. The Daughters of Charity with me continue to ensure the centrality of Jesus Christ in fulfilling our ethical covenants.
>
> I am delighted with the new opportunities taking place bringing other hospitals into the St. Vincent's family. However, this venture has been made possible by the sale of professional buildings adjacent to Medical Center East and an outpatient surgery unit. Saint Vincent's does not and cannot control what goes on in these buildings.
>
> I wish to be clear: direct sterilization of any kind or other unethical medical procedures are not and will not be permitted in any Catholic health care facility or by institutions representing themselves as Catholic in the Diocese of Birmingham in Alabama.
>
> Although it is not possible to police the contraceptive conversations or practices in a physician's office, the Catholic people need to know explicitly that I ask physicians leas-

ing offices in these buildings adjacent to our hospitals to follow the Ethical and Religious Directives.

Saint Vincent's Hospital in Birmingham being a Catholic Hospital from its foundation over a hundred years ago, always has expected these ethical practices with their physicians. They should remain in place as part of the cultural and spiritual undergirding that ensures the highest ideals of health care.

As a Bishop of the Catholic Church and Administrator of the Diocese of Birmingham, I congratulate all who have worked so hard to continue the extension of Saint Vincent's mission to all in need.

Most Reverend David E. Foley, D.D.
Diocesan Administrator
Diocese of Birmingham in Alabama

[134] Gregg Blesch, "Haven't We Met Before?: Don't Call It a Merger — A Spate of New Joint Operating Agreements May Spark '90s *Déjà vu*, but It's Different Now, Executives Say." *Modern Healthcare* 37 (July 16, 2007): 6.

[135] Ibid.

[136] Boulton, *supra* note 35.

[137] Columbia St. Mary's Mission Statement; http://www.columbia-stmarys.org/OPage.asp?PageID=OTH000020 (last visited Dec. 12, 2008).

[138] Ibid.

[139] Ibid.

[140] "Columbia St. Mary's, Froedtert to Merge." *The Business Journal* (Milwaukee), Jan. 16, 2008.

[141] Ibid.

[142] Melanie Evans and Jessica Zigmond, "The Joint Appeal; Froedtert, Columbia St. Mary's in Milwaukee Choose Joint Operating Agreement." *Modern Healthcare* 38, no. 14 (Jan. 21, 2008).

[143] Guy Boulton, "Health Merger Is on Track: System's Boards Back Combining Operations." *Milwaukee Journal & Sentinel*, Jan. 17, 2008.

[144] Evans and Zigmond, *supra* note 142.

[145] Ibid.

[146] Ibid.

[147] "Columbia St. Mary's, Froedtert Put Partnership on Hold." *Milwaukee Journal & Sentinel*, Dec. 20, 2008; http://next-generation-communications.tmcnet.com/news/2008/12/20/3870163.htm.

[148] Boulton, supra note 35. In this regard, Directive 69 provides: "If a Catholic health care institution is participating in a partnership that may be involved in activities judged morally wrong by the Church, the Catholic institution should limit its involvement in accord with the moral principles." *Ethical and Religious Directives for Catholic Health Care Services*, 4th ed. (2001), 27.

[149] Mary Ann Roser, "City-Seton Arrangement Likely to Survive Dispute; No One Else Seems Willing to Run Financially Risky Hospital." *Austin American-Statesman*, Nov. 3, 2001.

[150] Kim Sue Lia Perkes, "Bishops to Weigh Hospital Services: Proposal to Enforce Limits on Reproductive Services Could Affect Brackenridge." *Austin American-Statesman*, Oct. 26, 2000.

[151] Ibid.

[152] Ibid.

[153] Kim Sue Lia Perkes, "Hospital Issues Won't Be on Bishop's Agenda." *Austin American-Statesman*, Nov. 10, 2000.

[154] "Texas Hospital Hit By Church Move." *Modern Healthcare* (June 18, 2001).
[155] Ibid.
[156] Ibid.
[157] Mary Ann Roser and Kim Sue Lia Perkes, "City May Run Birth Control at Brack Austin; Plan Creates a 'Hospital Within a Hospital' for Services Seton Can't Offer." *Austin American-Statesman*, Aug. 22, 2001.
[158] Ibid.
[159] Ibid.
[160] Ibid.
[161] Ibid.
[162] Ibid.
[163] Ibid.
[164] Ibid.
[165] "Brackenridge Plan Is Good for All of Austin." *Austin American-Statesman*, Aug. 23, 2001.
[166] Roser, *supra* note 149.
[167] Ibid.
[168] Ibid.
[169] Ibid.
[170] Jeff Tieman, "Uneasy Truce: Catholic-Run Public Hospital to Walk Fine Line." *Modern Healthcare* (Feb. 18, 2002).
[171] Ibid.
[172] Ibid.
[173] Ibid.
[174] Ibid.
[175] Ibid.
[176] Ibid.
[177] Joe Manning, "Milwaukee Hospital to Perform Sterilizations Despite Catholic Restrictions." *Milwaukee Journal & Sentinel*, Oct. 30, 2001.
[178] Joe Manning, "Columbia Doctors Fear Service Cuts: They Protest Moving Women's Health Care to St. Mary's." *Milwaukee Journal & Sentinel*, Aug. 26, 2000, 1.
[179] Ibid.
[180] Ibid.
[181] Ibid.
[182] Ibid.
[183] Ibid.
[184] Joe Manning, "Merger of Milwaukee Women's Health Services on Hold." *Milwaukee Journal & Sentinel*, Sept. 28, 2000.
[185] Ibid.
[186] Manning, *supra* note 177.
[187] Ibid.
[188] Ibid.
[189] Ibid.
[190] Ibid.
[191] "Merger of Columbia St. Mary's Milwaukee Campus and Columbia St. Mary's Columbia Campus." *Modern Healthcare* (July 11, 2005): 20.
[192] Elizabeth Sanders, "Columbia Birthing Center to Find New Home in Mequon." *The Business Journal* (Milwaukee), June 22, 2007; http://milwaukee.bizjournals.com/milwaukee/stories/2007/06/25/story8.html.

PART FOUR: *Catholic Health Care and the Right of Conscientious Objection*

[1] Jody Feder, "The History and Effect of Abortion Conscience Clause Laws." CRS Report for Congress (Jan. 14, 2005), 2; http://www.law.umaryland.edu/marshall/crsreports/crsdocuments/RS2142801142005.pdf.

[2] Kevin D. O'Rourke, Thomas Kopfensteiner, and Ron Hamel, "A Brief History." *Health Progress* 84 (Nov.–Dec. 2001); http://www.chausa.org/Pub/MainNav/News/HP/Archive/2001/11NovDec/Articles/Features/hp0111G.htm.

[3] Feder, *supra* note 1, at 2.

[4] Maureen Kramlich, "The Assault on Catholic Health Care." United States Conference of Catholic Bishops; http://www.nccbuscc.org/prolife/programs/rlp//kramlich.shtml.

[5] John Witte, *Religion and the American Constitutional Experiment: Essential Rights and Liberties* (Boulder, CO: Westview Press, 2005), 123, discussing *Sherbert v. Verner*, 374 U.S. 398 (1963).

[6] *Employment Division, Department of Human Resources of Oregon v. Smith*, 494 U.S. 872 (1990).

[7] Witte, *supra* note 5, at 123.

[8] *Church of Lukumi v. Hialeah*, 508 U.S. 520 (1992).

[9] 42 U.S.C.A. § 2000b-1 (West, 2008).

[10] *City of Boerne v. Flores*, 521 U.S. 507 (1997).

[11] Christopher C. Lund, "A Matter of Constitutional Luck: The General Applicability Requirement in Free Exercise Jurisprudence." *Harvard Journal of Law & Public Policy* (Spring 2003): 627, 631.

[12] *Gonzales v. O Centro Espirita Beneficente Unia do Vegetal*, 546 U.S. 418 (2006); *see also* Thomas C. Berg, "Religious Liberty in America at the End of the Century." *Journal of Law & Religion* 16 (2001): 187, 193.

[13] *Church of Lukumi v. Hialeah*, 508 U.S. 520 (1993) (striking down law prohibiting sacrificial killing of animals for religious purposes where it was directed only at the Santeria religion).

[14] *Rust v. Sullivan*, 500 U.S. 173 (1991).

[15] In 1953, McFadden noted:

> Only two states in the nation, Massachusetts and Connecticut, have had the courage to hold their ground against the powerful influences demanding the lifting of barriers [to the advertising, sale and distribution of contraceptives]. In these two states, an adequate law exists and diligent effort is made to enforce it. In the November 1948 election, the people of Massachusetts again voted to retain the law.

Charles J. McFadden, *Medical Ethics*, 3rd ed., 81.

[16] *Griswold v. Connecticut*, 381 U.S. 479 (1965).

[17] *Eisenstadt v. Baird*, 405 U.S. 438 (1972).

[18] *Roe v. Wade*, 410 U.S. 113 (1972).

[19] *See, e.g., Lawrence v. Texas*, 539 U.S. 558 (2003).

[20] *See, e.g., Romer v. Evans*, 517 U.S. 620, 634 (1996) (Colorado Constitution amendment prohibiting the enactment of laws protecting homosexuals from discrimination declared unconstitutional). The opinion for the court by Justice Kennedy characterized the motive behind the amendment as a "bare desire to harm" homosexuals, 517 U.S. at 634, while the dissenting opinion by Justice Scalia stated:

> The Court has mistaken a *Kulturkampf* for a fit of spite. The constitutional amendment before us here is not the manifestation of a "bare . . . desire to harm" homosexuals, but is rather a modest attempt by seemingly tolerant Coloradans to preserve traditional sexual mores against the efforts of a politically powerful minority to revise those mores through use of the laws. That objective, and the means chosen to achieve it, are not only unimpeachable under any constitutional doctrine hitherto pronounced (hence the opinion's heavy reliance upon principles of righteousness rather than judicial holdings); they have been specifically approved by the Congress of the United States and by this Court. (citations omitted)

517 U.S. at 636.

[21] 505 U. S. 833 (1992).

[22] Ibid.

[23] 539 U.S. 558, 574 (2003).

[24] Maureen Kramlich, "The Abortion Debate Thirty Years Later: From Choice to Coercion." *Fordham Urban Law Journal* 31 (2004): 783.

[25] Edmund D. Pellegrino, "The Physician's Conscience, Conscience Clauses, and Religious Belief: A Catholic Perspective." *Fordham Urban Law Journal* 30 (2002): 221, 231.

[26] Ibid., 223.

[27] Ibid., 223–24.

[28] Ibid., 224.

[29] James F. Childress, "Appeals to Conscience." *Ethics* 89 (1979): 315, 318.

[30] Pope John Paul II, *Veritatis Splendor,* Par. 59 (1993); http://www.vatican.va/holy_father/john_pa…/hf_jp-ii_enc_06081993_veritatis-splendor_en.htm. Par. 59 states:

> The judgment of conscience is a *practical judgment*, a judgment which makes known what man must do or not do, or which assesses an act already performed by him. It is a judgment which applies to a concrete situation the rational conviction that one must love and do good and avoid evil. This first principle of practical reason is part of the natural law; indeed, it constitutes the very foundation of the natural law, inasmuch as it expresses that primordial insight about good and evil, that reflection of God's creative wisdom which, like an imperishable spark (*scintilla animae*), shines in the heart of every man. But whereas the natural law discloses the objective and universal demands of the moral good, conscience is the application of the law to a particular case; this application of the law thus becomes an inner dictate for the individual, a summons to do what is good in this particular situation. Conscience thus formulates *moral obligation* in the light of the natural law: it is the obligation to do what the individual, through the workings of his conscience, *knows* to be a good he is called to do *here and now*. The universality of the law and its obligation are acknowledged, not suppressed, once reason has established the law's application in concrete present circumstances. The judgment of conscience states "in an ultimate way" whether a certain particular kind of behaviour is in conformity with the law; it formulates the proximate norm of the morality of a voluntary act, "applying the objective law to a particular case." (Footnotes omitted; italics in original.)

[31] Robert John Araujo, S.J., "Conscience, Totalitarianism, and the Positivist Mind." *Mississippi Law Journal* 77 (2007): 571.

[32] Pope John Paul II, *Evangelium Vitae* (The Gospel of Life) (1995), Par.70 http://www.vatican.va/holy_father/john_paul_ii/encyclicals/documents/hf_jp-ii_enc_25031995_evangelium-vitae_en.html.

[33] James Q. Wilson, *The Moral Sense* (New York: Free Press, 1993), 104.

[34] *Veritatis Splendor, supra* note 30, at Par. 101.

[35] Araujo, *supra* note 31, at 611–12.

[36] *Evangelium Vitae, supra* note 32, at Par. 74.

[37] Ibid. For a discussion of a model act developed by Americans United for Life to provide broad conscience protection to individuals and institutions, see Nikolas T. Nikas, "Law and Public Policy to Protect Health Care Rights of Conscience." *National Catholic Bioethics Quarterly* 4 (Spring 2004): 41.

[38] *Evangelium Vitae, supra* note 32, at Par. 74.

[39] Pellegrino, *supra* note 25, at 243–44.

Chapter Ten: *Protection of Conscientious Objection*

[1] 175 U.S. 291 (1899).

[2] William W. Bassett, "Private Religious Hospitals: Limitations Upon Autonomous Moral Choices in Reproductive Medicine." *Journal of Contemporary Health Law & Policy* 17 (2001): 455, 548.

[3] Ibid.

[4] The initial amendment was enacted as part of the Health Programs Extension Act of 1973, Pub. L. No. 93-45. Jody Feder, "The History and Effect of Abortion Conscience Clause Laws." *CRS Report for Congress* 2, n. 3 (Jan. 14, 2005), 2; http://www.law.umaryland.edu/marshall/crsreports/crsdocuments/ RS 2142801142005.pdf. It was codified as 42 U.S.C. A. § 300a-7 (West, 2008).

[5] 42 U.S.C.A. § 300a-7(b) (West, 2008). It states:

> (b) Prohibition of public officials and public authorities from imposition of certain requirements contrary to religious beliefs or moral convictions
>
> The receipt of any grant, contract, loan, or loan guarantee under the Public Health Service Act [42 U.S.C.A. § 201 et seq.], the Community Mental Health Centers Act [42 U.S.C.A. § 2689 et seq.], or the Developmental Disabilities Services and Facilities Construction Act [42 U.S.C.A. § 6000 et seq.] by any individual or entity does not authorize any court or any public official or other public authority to require:
>
> **(1)** such individual to perform or assist in the performance of any sterilization procedure or abortion if his performance or assistance in the performance of such procedure or abortion would be contrary to his religious beliefs or moral convictions; or
>
> **(2)** such entity to:
>
> **(A)** make its facilities available for the performance of any sterilization procedure or abortion if the performance of such procedure or abortion in such facilities is prohibited by the entity on the basis of religious beliefs or moral convictions, or
>
> **(B)** provide any personnel for the performance or assistance in the performance of any sterilization procedure or abortion if the performance or assistance in the performance of such procedures or abortion by such personnel would be contrary to the religious beliefs or moral convictions of such personnel.

[6] Ibid., at § 300a-7(c) (1).

[7] 42 U.S.C.A. § 300a-7(c) (2) (West, 2008).

[8] 42 U.S.C.A. § 300a-7(d) (West, 2008).

[9] 42 U.S.C.A. § 300a-7(e) (West, 2008).

[10] *Chrisman v. Sisters of St. Joseph of Peace*, 506 F.2d 308 (9th Cir. 1974) (relying on Church Amendment; dismissing civil rights lawsuit against Catholic hospital that received Hill-Burton funds brought by woman who was refused sterilization; rejecting establishment clause claim) discussed in Bassett, *Private Religious Hospitals, supra* note 2, at 554.

[11] Feder, *supra* note 4, at 2.

[12] Feder, *supra* note 4, at 2.

[13] Ibid., 2, discussing 20 U.S.C.A. § 1688 (West, 2008).

[14] 42 U.S.C.A. § 238n (West, 2008). This legislation was passed in response to *St. Agnes Hospital v. Riddick* (D-Md., 1990) (upholding withdrawal by Accreditation Council for Graduate Medical Education of accreditation of Catholic hospital's residency program in obstetrics and gynecology because of failure to provide training in elective abortions, sterilizations, and contraception; finding ACGME is state actor but rejecting free exercise claim after determining there is a compelling state interest in providing this type of training).

[15] 42 U.S.C.A. § 1396u-2(3) (B) (West, 2008).

[16] Edmund D. Pellegrino, "The Physician's Conscience, Conscience Clauses, and Religious Belief: A Catholic Perspective." *Fordham Urban Law Journal* 30 (2002): 221, 231; *See also* discussion of mandated contraceptive coverage, *infra*.

[17] Maureen Kramlich, "Coercing Conscience: The Effort to Mandate Abortion as a Standard of Care." *National Catholic Bioethics Quarterly* 4 (Spring 2004): 29.

[18] *Protecting the Rights of Conscience of Health Care Providers and a Parent's Right to Know*, Hearing Before the House Subcommittee on Health of the Committee on Energy and Commerce, 107th Cong. 22, 22–23 (2002) (Statement of Lynn Wardle, J. Reuben Clark Law School, Brigham Young University); http://74.125.113.132/search?q=cache:XYY-7CQWWbwJ:bulk.resource.org/gpo.gov/hearings/107h/80684.pdf+%22Protecting+the+Rights+of+Conscience+of+Health+Care+Providers%22&cd=5&hl=en&ct=clnk&gl=us.

[19] *Valley Hosp. Ass'n, Inc. v. Mat-Su Coalition for Choice*, 948 P.2d 963 (Alaska 1997).

[20] Maureen Kramlich, "The Abortion Debate Thirty Years Later: From Choice to Coercion." *Fordham Urban Law Journal* 31 (2004): 783.

[21] H.R. 4691, 107th Cong. (2002), 2001 CONG US HR 4691 (passed the House Sept. 25, 2002). The legislation never became law. http://www.govtrack.us/congress/bill.xpd?bill=h107-4691.

[22] Letter from Gail Quinn, Executive Director, Secretariat for Pro-Life Activities, United States Conference of Catholic Bishops, July 1, 2002; http://www.usccb.org/prolife/issues/abortion/andah.shtml.

[23] S. 1397, 108th Cong. (2003), 2003 US. S. 1397; H.R. 3664, 108th Cong. (2003), 2003 H.R. 3664. Both bills were declared dead at the end of the 108th Congress; http://www.govtrack.us/congress/bill.xpd?bill=s108-1397.

[24] *Protecting the Rights of Conscience of Health Care Providers and a Parent's Right to Know*, Hearing Before the House Subcommittee on Health of the Committee on Energy and Commerce, 107th Cong. 15, 20 (2002) (Statement of Catherine Weiss, Director, American Civil Liberties Union, Reproductive Freedom Project), http://74.125.113.132/search?q=cache:XYY-7CQWWbwJ:bulk.resource.org/gpo.gov/hearings/107h/80684.pdf+%22Protecting+the+Rights+of+Conscience+of+Health+Care+Providers%22&cd=5&hl=en&ct=clnk&gl=us.

[25] Ibid.

[26] Fact Sheet: ACLU's Misrepresentations About the Abortion Non-Discrimination Act, United States Conference of Catholic Bishops, Secretariat of Pro-Life Activities, July 25, 2002; http://www.consciencelaws.org/Examining-Conscience-Legal/Legal08.htm.

[27] Ibid.

[28] Statement of Catherine Weiss, *supra* note 24, at 20.

[29] Fact Sheet, *supra* note 26, citing to 62 *Federal Register* 8610-01(Feb. 25, 1997).

[30] Letter from Gail Quinn, *supra* note 22.

[31] "Congress Approves Broad Shield to Protect Pro-Life Providers, National Right to Life." http://www.nrlc.org/news/2004/NRL12/congress_approves_broad_shield_t.htm.

[32] *The Campaign to Force Hospitals to Provide Abortions*, Secretariat for Pro-Life Activities, United States Conference of Catholic Bishops; http://www.usccb.org/prolife/issues/abortion/THREAT.PDF.

[33] Consolidated Appropriations Act, 2005, Pub. L. No. 108-447, § 508(d) (1)-(2), 118 Stat. 2809, 3163 (2004). For an excellent discussion of the background of this legislation and its constitutionality, see Judith C. Gallagher, "Protecting the Other Right to Choose: The Hyde-Weldon Amendment." *Ave Maria Law Review* 5 (2007): 527.

[34] Consolidated Appropriations Act, § 508(d)(1)-(2).

[35] Feder, *supra* note 4, at 5.

[36] Ibid.

[37] Ibid.

[38] *See, e.g.*, "Senator Spector's Substitute for the Hyde/Weldon Conscience Protection Amendment." Secretariat for Pro-Life Activities, United States Conference of Catholic Bishops; http://www.usccb.org/prolife/issues/abortion/spectercon.pdf.

[39] Departments of Labor, Health and Human Services, and Education, and Related Agencies Appropriations Act, 2006, Pub.L. No. 109-149, § 508(d), 119 Stat. 2833, 2879–80.

[40] Revised Continuing Appropriations Resolution of 2007, P.L 110-5, §2, 121 Stat. 8, 9; Consolidated Appropriations Act, 2008, Pub. L. No. 110-161, Div. G, § 508(d), 121 Stat. 1844, 2209.

[41] *California v. U.S.*, 2008 WL 744840 (N.D.Cal.) (decided Mar. 18, 2008).

[42] Ibid.

[43] *National Family Planning and Reproductive Health Ass'n, Inc. v. Gonzales*, 468 F.3rd 826 (D.C. Cir. 2006).

[44] Ibid., 830.

[45] Erica L. Norey, "Duty to Fill?: Threats to Pharmacists' Professional and Business Discretion." *New York Law School Law Review* 52 (2007/08): 95, 105–06.

[46] *Pharmacist Conscience Clause: Laws and Legislation*, National Conference of State Legislatures; http://www.ncsl.org/programs/health/conscienceclauses.htm.

[47] Robert F. Card, "Conscientious Objection and Emergency Contraception." *American Journal of Bioethics* 7 (2007): 8; http://www.bioethics.net/journal/j_articles.php?aid=1259.

[48] Ibid. See also Norey, *supra* note 45, at 105–06, noting:

> Some states, including Georgia, Arkansas, South Dakota, and Mississippi, recognize pharmacists' rights to refuse to fill a prescription and place no affirmative duty on them to accommodate the consumer. By contrast, the State of Illinois has chosen to require the timely filling of any valid prescription—no matter what the circumstance. States such as North Carolina, Wisconsin, Texas, and Nevada have chosen a middle-of-the-road approach, allowing pharmacists to refuse to fill a prescription, but placing on them (or on their employer) a duty to have procedures in place to ensure that the patient can still get his medication filled at another pharmacy or by another pharmacist in the same pharmacy. And finally, some states, such as New York, remain silent on the issue (footnotes omitted).

[49] *See, e.g.*, Access to Birth Control Act, H.R. 2596, introduced in the 110th Congress by Congresswoman Carolyn Maloney (D-NY); http://thomas.loc.gov/cgi-bin/query/z?c110:H.R.2596. Congresswoman Maloney had previously introduced the Access to Legal Pharmaceuticals Act, H.R. 1652 in the 109th Congress. http://thomas.loc.gov/cgi-bin/bdquery/D?d109:1:./temp/~bdWtGY:@@@L&summ2=m&|/bss/109search.html. This legislation required a pharmacy to fill a prescription without delay when one of its pharmacists has refused to fill the prescription due to a personal belief. Ibid.

Notes

[50] Joy Wingfield, Paul Bissell, and Claire Anderson, "The Scope of Pharmacy Ethics—an Evaluation of the International Research Literature, 1990–2002." *Social Science & Medicine* 58 (2004): 2383, 2388.

[51] "Moralists at the Pharmacy." Editorial, *New York Times*, Apr. 3, 2005; *see also* Card, *supra* note 86 (arguing against allowing pharmacists to refuse to fill based on a moral objection and refer the patient).

[52] Pellegrino, *supra* note 16, at 238.

[53] *Religious Refusals and Reproductive Rights*, ACLU Reproductive Freedom Project (2002); http://www.aclu.org/FilesPDFs/ACF911.pdf.

[54] Monica Davey, "Illinois Pharmacies to Provide Birth Control." *New York Times*, Apr. 2, 2005. The final rule provides:

> Duty of Division I Pharmacy to Dispense Contraceptives
>
> 1) Upon receipt of a valid, lawful prescription for a contraceptive, a pharmacy must dispense the contraceptive, or a suitable alternative permitted by the prescriber, to the patient or the patient's agent without delay, consistent with the normal timeframe for filling any other prescription. If the contraceptive, or a suitable alternative, is not in stock, the pharmacy must obtain the contraceptive under the pharmacy's standard procedures for ordering contraceptive drugs not in stock, including the procedures of any entity that is affiliated with, owns, or franchises the pharmacy. However, if the patient prefers, the prescription must be transferred to a local pharmacy of the patient's choice under the pharmacy's standard procedures for transferring prescriptions for contraceptive drugs, including the procedures of any entity that is affiliated with, owns, or franchises the pharmacy. Under any circumstances an unfilled prescription for contraceptive drugs must be returned to the patient if the patient so directs.
>
> 2) For the purposes of this subsection (j), the term "contraceptive" shall refer to all FDA-approved drugs or devices that prevent pregnancy.

68 Ill. Adm. Code § 1330.91(j), as amended by 29 Ill. Reg. 13639, 13663 (eff. Aug. 25, 2005) quoted in *Morr-Fitz, Inc. v. Blagojevich*, 867 N.E.2d 1164, 1176–1177 (Ill. App. 2007).

[55] Davey, *supra* note 54.

[56] *Morr-Fitz Inc. v. Blagojevich*, 867 N.E.2d 1164, 1165 (Ill. App. 2007).

[57] Ibid., 1170–1171.

[58] Ibid.

[59] Justice Turner stated:

> I would find plaintiffs have stated a compelling case under the Right of Conscience Act, one that is worthy of and ripe for consideration. In the case *sub judice*, plaintiff pharmacists are alleged to have moral and religious objections to dispensing emergency contraception pursuant to the Rule. The Right of Conscience Act purports to protect their beliefs and prevent "all forms" of coercion on the part of the government to alter those beliefs. Governor Blagojevich, however, has stated pharmacists "are not free to let [religious] beliefs stand in the way" of delivering emergency contraception to customers and "must fill prescriptions without making moral judgments." Further, the Governor has warned pharmacists that the State will "vigorously protect" the right of access to birth control and will take "any and all necessary steps to ensure a woman's access to her health care." The intent of the Governor's statements is clear and undeniable — either comply with the Rule or else. Plaintiffs allege, therefore, they must choose either to violate the Rule or their consciences, a form of coercion expressly prohibited by the Right of Conscience Act. The risk of the

revocation of their professional licenses unless they comply with the Rule is the ultimate in government coercion, threatening their very livelihood in the workforce within the State of Illinois. Accordingly, plaintiffs' claim that the Right of Conscience Act offers them an avenue of relief is ripe for consideration.

Morr-Fitz, Inc., 867 N.E.2d at 1172.

[60] 451 F.Supp.2d 992 (C.D. Ill. 2006).

[61] *Menges*, 451 F.Supp.2d 1000.

[62] 524 F.Supp.2d 1245 (W.D. Wash. 2007).

[63] Ibid., 1248.

[64] Ibid., 1249–50. Health Care Access Act, codified at Wash. Rev. Code § 70.47.160(2). An identical right of conscience is included within the Insurance Reform Act codified at Wash. Rev. Code § RCW 48.43.065.

[65] *Stormans Inc.*, 524 F.Supp.2d at 1250–1251.

[66] Ibid., 1251.

[67] The regulations were adopted by the Board and became effective on July 26, 2007. Wash. Adm. Code § 246-863-095 (4)(d) provides:

Pharmacist's professional responsibilities.

(1) A pharmacist's primary responsibility is to ensure patients receive safe and appropriate medication therapy.

(2) A pharmacist shall not delegate the following professional responsibilities:

(j) Decision to not dispense lawfully prescribed drugs or devices or to not distribute drugs and devices approved by the U.S. Food and Drug Administration for restricted distribution by pharmacies.

. . .

(4) It is considered unprofessional conduct for any person authorized to practice or assist in the practice of pharmacy to engage in any of the following:

(a) Destroy unfilled lawful prescription;

(b) Refuse to return unfilled lawful prescriptions;

(c) Violate a patient's privacy;

(d) Discriminate against patients or their agent in a manner prohibited by state or federal laws; and

(e) Intimidate or harass a patient.

In addition, Wash. Adm. Code § 246-869-010(4)(d) provides:

Pharmacies' responsibilities.

(1) Pharmacies have a duty to deliver lawfully prescribed drugs or devices to patients and to distribute drugs and devices approved by the U.S. Food and Drug Administration for restricted distribution by pharmacies, or provide a therapeutically equivalent drug or device in a timely manner consistent with reasonable expectations for filling the prescription, except for the following or substantially similar circumstances:

(a) Prescriptions containing an obvious or known error, inadequacies in the instructions, known contraindications, or incompatible prescriptions, or prescriptions requiring action in accordance with WAC 246-875-040.

(b) National or state emergencies or guidelines affecting availability, usage or supplies of drugs or devices;

(c) Lack of specialized equipment or expertise needed to safely produce, store, or dispense drugs or devices, such as certain drug compounding or storage for nuclear medicine;

(d) Potentially fraudulent prescriptions; or

(e) Unavailability of drug or device despite good faith compliance with WAC 246-869-150.

(2) Nothing in this section requires pharmacies to deliver a drug or device without payment of their usual and customary or contracted charge.

(3) If despite good faith compliance with WAC 246-869-150, the lawfully prescribed drug or device is not in stock, or the prescription cannot be filled pursuant to subsection (1)(a) of this section, the pharmacy shall provide the patient or agent a timely alternative for appropriate therapy which, consistent with customary pharmacy practice, may include obtaining the drug or device.

These alternatives include but are not limited to:

(a) Contact the prescriber to address concerns such as those identified in subsection (1)(a) of this section or to obtain authorization to provide a therapeutically equivalent product;

(b) If requested by the patient or their agent, return unfilled lawful prescriptions to the patient or agent; or

(c) If requested by the patient or their agent, communicate or transmit, as permitted by law, the original prescription information to a pharmacy of the patient's choice that will fill the prescription in a timely manner.

(4) Engaging in or permitting any of the following shall constitute grounds for discipline or other enforcement actions:

(a) Destroy unfilled lawful prescriptions.

(b) Refuse to return unfilled lawful prescriptions.

(c) Violate a patient's privacy.

(d) Discriminate against patients or their agent in a manner prohibited by state or federal laws.

(e) Intimidate or harass a patient.

[68] *Stormans, Inc.*, 524 F.Supp. 2d. at 1253.

[69] Ibid., 1255.

[70] Ibid., 1256–57.

[71] Ibid., 1259–60. The Court noted:

In actual operation, however, the regulations appear designed to impose a Hobson's choice for the majority of pharmacists who object to Plan B: dispense a drug that ends a life as defined by their religious teachings, or leave their present position in the State of Washington. The evolution of these regulations, as currently described to the Court, convinces the Court that these regulations targeted the religious practices of some citizens and are therefore not neutral. Ibid.

[72] Ibid., 1264.

[73] Ibid.

[74] *Stormans, Inc. v. Selecky*, 526 F.3rd 406 (9th Cir. 2008).

[75] Ibid., 409, stating:

In their application for a stay pending appeal, the Defendant–Intervenors do not controvert these findings. Instead, they cite other evidence — which was before the district court and discussed in its order — of two women who sought Plan B and were refused by a pharmacist, a woman who had heard that Plan B is not available at pharmacies and obtained Plan B from Planned Parenthood, and a woman who has not used Plan B but participated in a Planned Parenthood testing program and made inquiries at five pharmacies. The most serious cases are that of the two women who were refused Plan B by pharmacists; neither woman was unable to obtain Plan B. In the one case, the pharmacist directed the woman to another pharmacy in the area; in the second case, another pharmacist on duty at the store filled the prescription. There is no evidence that any woman who sought Plan B was unable to obtain it. This anecdotal evidence falls short of even the "possibility of irreparable harm" in the absence of a stay pending appeal.

[76] *Noesen v. State Dept. of Regulation and Licensing, Pharmacy Examining Bd.*, 751 N.W.2d 385, 2008 (Wis. App. 2008). The Court stated:

> There is no doubt about, or challenge to, the sincerity of Noesen's religions convictions.... However, the circuit court noted, the discipline imposed here only requires Noesen "to make the extent of his religious belief and objections known to his employer before the commencement of his practice at the pharmacy. This will facilitate, rather than burden, [Noesen's] ability to exercise his conscientious objection in the future." (Ibid. at 393.)

[77] William L. Saunders, Jr., "Washington Insider." *National Catholic Bioethics Quarterly* 8 (Winter 2008): 625, 627.

[78] ACOG Committee Opinion, "The Limits of Conscientious Refusal in Reproductive Medicine." Opinion no. 385, Nov. 2007; http://www.acog.org/from_home/publications/ethics/co385.pdf.

[79] American Board of Obstetrics and Gynecology, *Bulletin* for 2008, "Maintenance of Certification." Nov. 2007; http://www.abog.org/bulletins/MOC2008.pdf. The *Bulletin* states:

> 5. Revoked Certificate
> a. An individual has had their Diplomate status revoked by the American Board of Obstetrics and Gynecology for cause.
> b. Cause in this case may be due to, but is not limited to, licensure revocation by any State Board of Medical Examiners, violation of ABOG or ACOG rules, and/or ethics principles or felony convictions.

Ibid.

[80] AAPLOG Response to the ACOG Ethics Committee Opinion no. 385, Titled "The Limits of Conscientious Refusal in Reproductive Medicine." Feb. 6, 2008; http://www.aaplog.org/downloads/rightofconscience/aaplog%20to%20EthicsComm-Response%20feb%206-pdf.pdf; Letter from Donna Harrison, president, AAPLOG, to Members of the President's Council of Bioethics, Sept 12, 2008; http://www.bioethics.gov/transcripts/sept08/AAPLOG%20letter%20to%20President's%20Council.pdf.

[81] Letter of Michael Leavitt, Secretary Department of Health and Human Services to Norman O. Gant, Executive Director, ABOG, Mar. 14, 2008; http://www.aaplog.org/downloads/rightofconscience/LeavittLettoABOGDrGant3.14.08.pdf.

[82] Letter of Norman O. Gant to Secretary Michael Leavitt, Mar. 19, 2008; http://www.aaplog.org/downloads/rightofconscience/ABOGDrGant%20to%20Leavitt%20Response3.19.08.pdf.

[83] Saunders, *supra* note 77, at 628–29 .On his blog, Secretary Leavitt stated:

> Physician certification is a powerful instrument. Without it, a doctor cannot practice the specialty. Putting doctors (or anyone who assists them) in a position where they are forced to violate their consciences in order to meet a standard of competence violates more than federal law. It violates decency and the core value of personal liberty. Freedom of expression and action are unfit barter for admission to medical employment or training.

Notes

As Secretary of Health and Human Services, I called on the organization that oversees Ob-Gyn board certification to alter its guidelines to assert that refusal to violate conscience will not be used to block board certification. Their answer was dodgy and unsatisfying.

Michael Leavitt, Provider Conscience Blog III, Aug. 21, 2008; http://secretarysblog.hhs.gov/my_weblog/2008/08/physician-con-2.html, discussed in Saunders, "Washington Insider." *Supra* note 116, at 627.

[84] Ensuring That Department of Health and Human Services Funds Do Not Support Coercive or Discriminatory Practices in Violation of Federal Law, Proposed Rules, 73 *Fed. Reg.* 50274-01 (Aug. 26, 2008) (to be codified at 45 CFR pt. 88).

[85] Ibid., 50276.

[86] Ibid.

[87] Ibid.

[88] Ibid., 50277–78.

[89] Ibid., 50278–79.

[90] Letter from Sr. Carol Keehan, D.C., president and CEO, Catholic Health Association, to Michael Leavitt, Sept. 24, 2008; http://www.chausa.org/NR/rdonlyres/6955911E-E1CF-4D9D-960D-7D61EA5E308D/0/080929conscienceClause_nprm.pdf.

[91] Letter from Jon O'Brien, president, Catholics for Choice, to Michael Leavitt; http://www.catholicsforchoice.org/topics/politics/documents/ProviderConscienceRegulation.pdf (last accessed Dec. 17, 2008). The letter stated:

> For any individual provider or institution to lay claim to be the arbiters of any person's good conscience is clearly disingenuous. If conscience truly is one's "most secret core and his sanctuary [where] he is alone with God, whose voice echoes in his depths," as the Catholic *Catechism* states, how can anyone, or any institution for that matter, justify coercing someone into acting contrary to her or his conscience?
>
> Health-care providers must not dismiss the conscience of the person seeking care. In fact, Catholic teaching requires due deference to the conscience of others in making decisions — meaning that, for examples, the pharmacist must not dismiss the conscience of the person seeking emergency contraception or the doctor dismiss the conscience of the woman seeking an abortion. One does not need to deny a patient emergency contraception or abortion in order to remain a good Catholic. When a pharmacist refuses to fill prescriptions for contraception, they are negating the right to conscience of the woman, or man, standing in front of them. This does not fall under anybody's definition of what a good conscience is.

Ibid.

[92] Protecting Patients and Health Care Act; http://thomas.loc.gov/cgi-bin/query/z?c110:S.20.

[93] Ensuring That Department of Health and Human Services Funds Do Not Support Coercive or Discriminatory Practices in Violation of Federal Law, Final Rule; http://federalregister.gov/OFRUpload/OFRData/2008-30134_PI.pdf.

[94] "Bush Threatens Unconscionable Health Regs." *Philadelphia Daily News*, Dec.18, 2008; http://www.philly.com/dailynews/opinion/20081218_Bush_threatens_unconscionable_health_regs.html.

[95] H.R. 1964, 110th Cong. (2007); http://thomas.loc.gov/cgi-bin/query/D?c110:5:./temp/-mdbsdvPTJF:::; S. 1173, 110th Cong. (2007); http://thomas.loc.gov/cgi-bin/query/D?c110:4:./temp/-mdbsdvPTJF::. The operative portion of the legislation states:

Sec. 4 Interference With Reproductive Health Prohibited.

a) Statement of Policy: It is the policy of the United States that every woman has the fundamental right to choose to bear a child, to terminate a pregnancy prior to fetal viability, or to terminate a pregnancy after fetal viability when necessary to protect the life or health of the woman.

(b) Prohibition of Interference: A government may not:

(1) deny or interfere with a woman's right to choose:

(A) to bear a child;

(B) to terminate a pregnancy prior to viability; or

(C) to terminate a pregnancy after viability where termination is necessary to protect the life or health of the woman; or

(2) discriminate against the exercise of the rights set forth in paragraph (1) in the regulation or provision of benefits, facilities, services, or information.

(c) Civil Action: An individual aggrieved by a violation of this section may obtain appropriate relief (including relief against a government) in a civil action.

Ibid.

[96] Ibid., at §§4(a) & 4(b) (1) (B) & (C).

[97] Ibid., at §4(b) (2).

[98] Ibid., at §4(c).

[99] Ibid., at §6.

[100] NARAL Pro-Choice America, Freedom of Choice Act; http://www.prochoiceamerica.org/assets/files/Abortion-Access-to-Abortion-FOCA.pdf.

[101] *The "Freedom of Choice Act": Most Radical Abortion Legislation in U.S. History*, Secretariat for Pro-Life Activities, United States Conference of Catholic Bishops, Sept. 30, 2008; http://www.usccb.org/prolife/issues/FOCA/FOCA_FactSheet08.pdf.

[102] Ibid.

[103] Ibid.

[104] 505 U.S. 833 (1992).

[105] Memorandum by Michael F. Moses, assistant general counsel, United States Conference of Catholic Bishops, Aug. 15, 2008; http://www.usccb.org/prolife/issues/FOCA/analysis.pdf.

[106] Ibid.

[107] Ibid.

[108] Ibid.

[109] Letter from Cardinal Justin Rigali to Members of Congress, Sept. 30, 2008; http://www.usccb.org/prolife/FOCArigaliltr.pdf.

[110] Ibid.

[111] "Advancing Reproductive Rights in a New Administration." Nov. 2008; http://otrans.3cdn.net/3b21d35e246c18a427_d7m6bw2o1.pdf.

[112] Ibid., 2–3.

[113] Ibid., 14–15.

[114] Valerie Schmalz, "Pro-Life Democrats Could Help Hold Line in Congress." *Our Sunday Visitor*, Dec. 14, 2008; http://www.osv.com/OSVNav/OSVNewsweeklyDecember142008/ProlifeDemocratscouldhelpholdline/tabid/7210/Default.aspx.

[115] Laura Meckler, "Bush-Era Abortion Rules Face Possible Reversal." *Wall Street Journal*, Dec. 17, 2008, A5.

[116] Nancy Frazier O'Brien, "Rumors Aside, FOCA No Threat to Catholic Health Care." *National Catholic Reporter*, Jan. 28, 2009; http://ncronline3.org/drupal/?q=comment/reply/3187.

[117] Ibid.
[118] Ibid.
[119] Ibid.
[120] Ibid.
[121] Ibid.
[122] Ron Rychlak, "The Catholic News Service and FOCA." http://www.moralaccountability.com/foca/the-catholic-news-service-and-foca/.
[123] Ibid.
[124] Cathleen Kaveny, "What FOCA Is — and Isn't." *Commonweal*, Jan. 30, 2009; http://www.commonwealmagazine.org/article.php3?id_article=2423.
[125] Ibid.
[126] Michael Stokes Paulsen, "The Legal Consequences of the Freedom of Choice Act." Feb. 3, 2009; http://www.moralaccountability.com/mission/the-legal-consequences-of-the-freedom-of-choice-act/.
[127] *Cf. Doe v. Charleston Area Medical Center,* 529 F.2d 638 (4th Cir. 1975) (holding that a private hospital is a state actor under 42 U.S.C. § 1983 based on receipt of Hill-Burton funds and Medicare and Medicaid; hospital acted "under color of law" when it refused to allow its facilities to be used to perform an abortion).
[128] Denise Burke, "The Freedom of Choice Act." *Ethics & Medics* 34, Feb. 2009.
[129] Prevention First Act, S. 21, 111th Cong. (2009); http://thomas.loc.gov/cgi-bin/query/z?c111:S.21:; Prevention First Act of 2009, H.R. 463, 111th Cong. (2009); http://thomas.loc.gov/cgi-bin/query/z?c111:H.R.463:.
[130] Prevention First Act, § 202, S. 21, 111th Cong. (2009); http://thomas.loc.gov/cgi-bin/query/z?c111:S.21:; Prevention First Act of 2009,§ 202,H.R. 463, 111th Cong. (2009); http://thomas.loc.gov/cgi-bin/query/z?c111:H.R.463:.
[131] Ibid., at § 204.
[132] Prevention First Act, § 402,S. 21, 111th Cong. (2009); http://thomas.loc.gov/cgi-bin/query/z?c111:S.21:; Prevention First Act of 2009, § 402,H.R. 463, 111th Cong. (2009); http://thomas.loc.gov/cgi-bin/query/z?c111:H.R.463:.
[133] Ibid.
[134] "'Prevention First Act' Greater Threat Than FOCA." *Catholic News Agency*, Feb. 4, 2009; http://www.catholicnewsagency.com/new.php?n=14977.

Chapter Eleven: *Mandated Contraceptive Coverage*

[1] Prevention First Act, § 202,S. 21, 111th Cong. (2009); http://thomas.loc.gov/cgi-bin/query/D?c111:1:./temp/~c111qjRvG4; Prevention First Act of 2009,§ 202,H.R. 463, 111th Cong. (2009); http://thomas.loc.gov/cgi-bin/query/D?c111:2:./temp/~c111qjRvG4::. *See also* "Contraceptive Plans Threaten Right to Choose What's Right." *National Catholic Register*, Sept. 8–14, 2002, 1, 12.
[2] "Contraceptive Plans Threaten Right to Choose." *Supra* note 1, at 12.
[3] The NCSL lists laws from 24 states mandating contraceptive coverage, and notes that 21 states have some sort of religious exemption. "State Laws Requiring Insurance Coverage of Contraceptives," National Conference of State Legislatures; http://www.ncsl.org/programs/health/contraceplaws.htm (updated Apr. 2008). *See also* Inimai M. Chettiar, "Contraceptive Coverage Laws: Eliminating Gender Discrimination or Infringing on Religious Liberties." 69 *University of Chicago Law Review* 69 (2002): 1867, 1877, n. 68 (listing statutes from 19 states); "State Policies in Brief: Insurance Coverage of Contraceptives." Guttmacher Institute (June 1, 2008); http://www.guttmacher.org/statecenter/spibs/spib_ICC.pdf.

[4] Chettiar lists four states as having no religious exemption: Georgia, Iowa, New Hampshire, and Vermont. Chettiar, *supra* note 3, at 1878.

[5] Chettiar lists the following states as having laws as containing "broad exemptions": Delaware, Maryland, Missouri, Nevada, New Mexico, and Texas. Chettiar, *supra* note 3, at 1879.

[6] Chettiar lists nine states that provide exemptions based on religiously based objections but further provide a "detailed definition of which employers qualify for the exemption." Chettiar, *supra* note 3, at 1880. She further breaks these "selective exemption" into three categories: (1) Four states (Rhode Island, Connecticut, Massachusetts, and Maine) limiting the exemption to "churches as defined in Section 3121 (w) of the Internal Revenue Code"; (2) Four states (North Carolina, Hawaii, California, and Arizona) focusing on "the purpose of the organization and the people involved in it . . ."; and (3) Washington state's "unique" exemption. Chettiar, *supra* note 3, at 1881.

[7] *See, e.g.*, West's Cal. Health & Safety Code § 1367.25 (2008); N.Y. Ins. Law § 3221 (l) (16) (2008). For example, the New York law provides that "every group or blanket policy which provides coverage for prescription drugs shall include coverage for the cost of contraceptive drugs or devices." Although the law provides an exemption for religious employers, this exemption is narrowly drawn. It provides:

> For purposes of this subsection, a "religious employer" is an entity for which each of the following is true: (a) the inculcation of religious values is the purpose of the entity. (b) The entity primarily employs persons who share the religious tenets of the entity. (c) The entity serves primarily persons who share the religious tenets of the entity. (IV) The entity is a nonprofit organization as described in Section 6033(a) (2) (A) I or iii, of the Internal Revenue Code.

The exemption in the California law is identical to the New York law.

[8] Susan J. Stabile, "State Attempts to Define Religion: The Ramifications of Applying Mandatory Prescription Coverage Statutes to Religious Employers." *Harvard Journal of Law & Public Policy* 28 (2005): 741, 773–74.

[9] Ibid., 775.

[10] Ibid.

[11] Ibid.

[12] Ibid.

[13] Peter J. Cataldo, "Compliance with Contraceptive Insurance Mandates: Licit or Illicit Cooperation in Evil." *National Catholic Bioethics Quarterly* 4 (Spring 2004): 103, 108–09.

[14] Ibid., 111–13.

[15] Ibid., 128–29. Directive 45 provides:

> Catholic health care institutions are not to provide abortion services, even based upon the principle of material cooperation. In this context, Catholic health care institutions need to be concerned about the danger of scandal.

Directive 45, *Ethical and Religious Directives for Catholic Health Care Services*, 4th ed. (2001), 26.

[16] Ibid., 129.

[17] Ibid., 113.

[18] E.E.O.C. Decision on Coverage of Contraception, Dec. 14, 2000; http://www.eeoc.gov/policy/docs/decision-contraception.html.

[19] 141 F.Supp.2d 1266 (W.D. Wash. 2001); Contra: In re Union Pacific Railroad Employment Practices Litigation, 479 F.3rd 936 (8th Cir. 2007) (holding exclusion of all

contraceptive coverage for men and women does not violate PDA or Title VII). *See also Glaubach v. Regence BlueShield*, 74 P.3d 115 (Wash. 2003) (answering certified question; holding failure of health insurer to provide coverage for all methods of contraception did not violate Washington insurance reform act).

[20] The Erickson case was subsequently appealed to the 9th Circuit, but the appeal was dropped when the Bartell Drug Company settled with a class of its female employees. Under the terms of the settlement, Bartell agreed to provide contraceptive coverage to its employees. Sally Roberts, "Plan Agrees to Cover Contraceptive Drugs." *Business Insurance*, Mar. 17, 2003.

[21] Wash. State Atty. Gen. Op. 2002, No. 5, Aug. 8, 2002.

[22] Ibid., referring to 2002 Basic Health Member Handbook, Appendix A, p. 26, 32.

[23] Ibid., referring to Wash. Admin. Code § 284-43-822 (West, 2008).

[24] Wash. Rev. Code Ann. § 48.43.065 (West, 2008).

[25] Wash. State Atty. Gen. Op. 2002, No. 5, Aug. 8, 2002.

[26] Ibid.

[27] Ibid.

[28] 85 P.3d 67 (Cal.). *See also* Carol Hogan, "Catholic Charities Declared a Non-Religious Institution: A Stunning Decision in California." *National Catholic Bioethics Quarterly* 4 (Winter 2004): 711.

[29] Cal. Health & Safety Code § 1367.25 (West, 2008) (governs group health service plan contracts); Cal. Ins. Code § 10123.196 (West, 2008) (governs individual and group disability insurance policies). These two statutes are virtually identical.

[30] Cal. Health & Safety Code § 1367.25 (b)(1) (West, 2008) provides:

> (b) Notwithstanding any other provision of this section, a religious employer may request a health service plan contract without coverage for federal Food and Drug Administration approved contraceptive methods that are contrary to the religious employer's religious tenets. If so requested, a health care service plan contract shall be provided without coverage for contraceptive methods.
>
> (1) For purposes of this section a "religious employer" is an entity for which each of the following is true:
>
> (A) The inculcation of religious values is the purpose of the entity.
>
> (B) The entity primarily employs persons who share the religious tenets of the entity.
>
> (C) The entity serves primarily persons who share the religious tenets of the entity.
>
> (D) The entity is a nonprofit organization as described in Section 6033(a) (2) (A) i or iii, of the Internal Revenue Code of 1986, as amended.

See also Cal. Ins. Code § 10123.196 (d) (West, 2008).

[31] Ibid.

[32] *Catholic Charities*, 85 P.3d 76.

[33] Ibid., 75.

[34] Ibid., 76. The court summarizes the arguments as follows:

> Catholic Charities . . . asserts eight constitutional challenges to the WCEA. All refer to the religion clauses of the federal and state Constitutions . . . Catholic Charities begins with a set of three arguments to the effect that the WCEA impermissibly interferes with the autonomy of religious organizations . . . Next, Catholic Charities claims the WCEA impermissibly burdens its right of free exercise. As part of this claim, Catholic Charities offers four arguments for subjecting the WCEA to strict scrutiny, despite the United States

Supreme Court's holding that the right of free exercise does not excuse compliance with neutral, generally applicable laws. . . . Finally, Catholic Charities contends the WCEA fails even the rational basis test.

Ibid. (citations omitted).
[35] Ibid.
[36] *Catholic Charities of Sacramento, Inc. v. Superior Court,* 109 Cal. Rptr.2d 176 (Cal. App. 2001), *pet for rev granted* 112 Cal. Rptr.2d 258 (Cal. 2001).
[37] Ibid.
[38] *Catholic Charities,* 109 Cal. Rptr.2d 181.
[39] *Catholic Charities of Sacramento, Inc. v. Superior Court,* 112 Cal. Rptr.2d 258 (Cal. 2001).
[40] The following issues are set forth in the Petition for Review:

1. Whether the religious freedom guarantees enshrined in Article 1, Section 4 of the California Constitution continue to trigger "strict scrutiny," as a matter of independent state grounds, where the Legislature has imposed a substantial burden upon religious exercise by deliberately targeting certain religious institutions for coercion of conduct contrary to their religious beliefs.
2. Whether a statutory exemption provision, designed by its authors and sponsors to draw explicit and deliberate distinctions between different religious organizations for the stated purpose of denying the exemption to certain targeted religious organizations, violates the federal and State Establishment Clauses.
3. Whether a statutory exemption provision, which explicitly classifies eligible employers based upon religious criteria, such as the "inculcation of religious values" and the "sharing [of] religious tenets," and was designed by its authors and sponsors to target certain religious organizations that they viewed as holding "particularly objectionable" religious views on the perceived problem at issue, violates the federal Free Exercise Clause.
4. Whether a religious organization, bringing a Free Exercise Clause claim in California state court, may invoke the "hybrid rights" exception to the general rule enunciated in *Employment Division v. Smith,* 494 U.S. 872, 110 S.Ct. 1595 (1990), and, if so, what standard should California courts apply in reviewing such "hybrid rights" claims.

Catholic Charities of Sacramento, Inc., v. Superior Court, 2001 WL 34369289 (Petition for Review), at 1.
[41] Ibid., 2. The Petition states that "what has occurred here is unworthy of a noble democratic institution like the California Legislature." Ibid.
[42] Ibid., 4–12.
[43] Ibid., discussing *Church of Lukumi Babalu Aye, Inc. v. City of Hialeah,* 508 U.S. 520 (1993) (striking down city ordinances prohibiting sacrificial killing of animals for religious purposes where they were directed only at the Santeria religion).
[44] Catholic Charities Petition for Review, *supra* note 40, at 4.
[45] Ibid., 2.
[46] Ibid., 5.
[47] Ibid., 6.
[48] Ibid., 7–8.
[49] Ibid., 6–7 (footnotes omitted).
[50] Ibid., 10.
[51] Ibid., 10.

[52] Ibid., 10, n. 11.
[53] Ibid., 11.
[54] Ibid., 11.
[55] Ibid., 9.
[56] *Catholic Charities*, 85 P.3d 82–83.
[57] Ibid., 84–85.
[58] Ibid., 85–87.
[59] Ibid., 87.
[60] Ibid., 86.
[61] Ibid.
[62] Ibid.
[63] Ibid.
[64] 2001 WL 34369289 (Petition for Review), at 6 (referring to testimony of Kathy Kneer, the CEO of Planned Parenthood of California, before the Senate Insurance Committee).
[65] Ibid., at n. 11. In its brief, Catholic Charities characterizes these assertions as incorrect, but does not provide any specific data on the numbers of Catholic organization providing such coverage for their employees. *Catholic Charities of Sacramento, Inc., v. Superior Court*, 2001 WL 17006644 (Cal.) (Petitioner's Brief on the Merits), at 39.
[66] *Catholic Charities*, 85 P.3d 76–77.
[67] Ibid., 77.
[68] Ibid., 78.
[69] *Catholic Charities*, 2001 WL 34369289 (Petition for Review), at 5.
[70] *Catholic Charities*, 85 P.3d 79–80, citing to *Presiding Bishop v. Amos*, 483 U.S. 3287 (1978).
[71] Ibid., 80. *Cf.* 85 P.3d 96–98 (concurring opinion by Kennard, J.) (expressing doubt as to whether it is permissible under the Establishment Clause for California to limit religious employer exemption to religious organizations engaged in inculcation of religious values).
[72] *Catholic Charities*, 2001 WL 170064 (Brief of Petitioner's on the Merits), at 30.
[73] *Catholic Charities*, 85 P.3d 83.
[74] Ibid.
[75] Ibid., 89–94, citing to West's Ann. Cal. Const., art. 1, § 4 (2008) providing: "Free exercise and enjoyment of religion without discrimination or preference are guaranteed. This liberty of conscience does not excuse acts that are licentious or inconsistent with the peace or safety of the State. The Legislature shall make no law respecting an establishment of religion."
[76] *Catholic Charities*, 85 P.3d 93.
[77] Ibid., 94.
[78] Ibid., 94–95.
[79] Ibid., 95.
[80] *Catholic Charities*, 85 P3d 98 (dissenting opinion by Justice Brown).
[81] Ibid.
[82] Ibid., 99.
[83] Ibid.
[84] Ibid.
[85] Ibid.
[86] Ibid., 100.
[87] Ibid., 99, citing to *Gellington v. Christian Methodist Episcopal Church*, 203 F.3d 1299, 1303 (11th Cir. 2000) (holding that ministerial exception under Title VII survives Smith).
[88] *Catholic Charities*, 85 P.3d 29 (dissenting opinion by Justice Brown).

[89] Ibid., 102.
[90] Ibid., 103.
[91] Ibid.
[92] Ibid., 103, n. 3.
[93] Ibid., 104–105.
[94] Ibid., 105.
[95] Ibid., 106 (footnote omitted).
[96] Ibid.
[97] Ibid., 108.
[98] See, e.g., *North Coast Woman's Care Medical Group v. Superior Court*, 189 P.3d 959 (2008) (holding that neither the United States nor California Constitution required a religious exemption from the Unruh Act's prohibition on sexual orientation discrimination for physicians who refused to provide fertility treatment for a lesbian couple based on a religious objection).
[99] *See Catholic Charities*, 2001 WL 34369289 (Petition for Review), at n. 13, stating:

> Catholic Charities timely filed a Motion for Reconsideration in the trial court, arguing that the approval of RU-486 and Kaiser's intention to add it to the formulary placed the Catholic Church in jeopardy of being complicit in pharmaceutical abortions, masquerading in "post-coital" contraception. . . . In Catholic Charities' view, this expands the issue to include what Catholic Charities regards as abortion. On October 31, 2000, the trial court granted Catholic Charities Motion for Reconsideration, finding that the approval of RU-486 should have been considered by the trial court, and again denied the Motion for Preliminary Injunction.

[100] *Catholic Charities*, 2001 WL 1700664 (Petition for Review), at 39.
[101] *Catholic Charities*, 85 P.3d 89. Commentators have also been critical of the hybrid rights doctrine. *See, e.g.,* Frederick Mark Gedicks, "Three Questions About Hybrid Rights and Religious Groups." *Yale Law Journal*, Pocket Part 117 (2008): 192; http://thepocketpart.org/2008/03/24/gedicks.html.
[102] Directive 70, 2001 *ERD*s, *supra* note 15, at 37. The directive goes on to give specific examples of such intrinsically immoral acts including abortion and direct sterilization, but not contraception.
[103] Janet Smith, Humanae Vitae: *A Generation Later* (Washington, DC: Catholic University of America Press, 1992), 85, stating: "Contraception is intrinsically immoral not because it violates the purpose of the reproductive organs but because it violates the procreative meaning of sexual acts; because it violates the nature of the sexual act."
[104] *Cf.* Directive 71, 2001 *ERD*s, *supra* note 15, at 37, stating:

> "The possibility of scandal must be considered when applying the principles governing cooperation." The Directive cites to the Catechism as follows: "See *Catechism of the Catholic Church*: 'Scandal is an attitude or behavior which leads another to do evil' (no. 2284); 'Anyone who uses the power at his disposal in such a way that it leads others to do wrong becomes guilty of scandal and responsible for the evil that he has directly or indirectly encouraged.'" (Ibid. at n. 45.)

[105] 859 N.E.2d 459 (N.Y. 2006).
[106] See discussion *supra* note 7.
[107] 859 N.E.2d at 462.
[108] Ibid., 463.
[109] Ibid., 463–465.

[110] *McKinney's N.Y. Const.* Art. 1, §3 (McKinney, 2008) provides:

> The free exercise and enjoyment of religious profession and worship, without discrimination or preference, shall forever be allowed in this state to all humankind; and no person shall be rendered incompetent to be a witness on account of his or her opinions on matters of religious belief; but the liberty of conscience hereby secured shall not be so construed as to excuse acts of licentiousness, or justify practices inconsistent with the peace or safety of this state.

[111] Ibid., 467.
[112] Ibid.
[113] Ibid., 468.
[114] Ibid.
[115] Susan J. Stabile, "When Conscience Clashes with State Law and Policy: Catholic Institutions." *Journal of Catholic Legal Studies* 46 (2007): 137, 143.
[116] Ibid.
[117] Ibid., 105.

Chapter Twelve: *Emergency Contraception Laws*

[1] Reza Keshavarz, Roland C. Merchant, and John McGreal, "Emergency Contraception Provision: A Survey of Emergency Department Practitioners." *Academic Emergency Medicine Journal* 9 (2002): 69; *see also Brownfield v. Daniel Freeman Marina Hospital*, 208 Cal. App. 3d 405, 256 Cal. Rptr. 240 (1989) (action for declaratory relief brought by rape victim against Catholic hospital for failing to provide emergency contraception medication to her or refer her; action dismissed but court suggests she might have a malpractice action).

[2] David A. Grimes and Elizabeth G. Raymond, "Emergency Contraception." *Annals of Internal Medicine* 137 (Aug. 6, 2002): E-180, E-181.

[3] Ibid., E-181.

[4] "Emergency Contraceptive Pills ('Morning After' Pills)," http://ec.princeton.edu/info/ecp.html.

[5] Ibid.

[6] Ibid.

[7] Frank Davidoff and James Trussell, "Plan B and the Politics of Doubt." *Journal of the American Medical Association* 296 (Oct. 11, 2006): 1775.

[8] *Statement on the So-Called "Morning After Pill."* Pontifical Academy of Life (Oct. 31, 2000); http://www.vatican.va/roman_curia/pontifical_academies/acdlife/documents/rc_pa_acdlife_doc_20001031_pillola-giorno-dopo_en.html.

[9] Directive 36, *Ethical and Religious Directives for Catholic Health Care Services*, 4th ed. (2001), 21.

[10] Kevin D. O'Rourke, O.P., "Applying the Directives." *Health Progress* 79 (July–Aug. 1998); http://www.chausa.org/Pub/MainNav/News/HP/Archive/1998/07JulyAug/Articles/Features/hp9807e.htm.

[11] Ibid.

[12] Ibid. In December 2008, the Congregation for the Doctrine of the Faith published an instruction on bioethical questions. With respect to pharmaceuticals that could prevent implantation of an embryo, it states:

> Alongside methods of preventing pregnancy which are, properly speaking, contraceptive, that is, which prevent conception following from a sexual act, there are other technical means which act after fertilization, when the embryo is already constituted, either

before or after implantation in the uterine wall. Such methods are *interceptive* if they interfere with the embryo before implantation and *contragestative* if they cause the elimination of the embryo once implanted.

In order to promote wider use of interceptive methods, it is sometimes stated that the way in which they function is not sufficiently understood. It is true that there is not always complete knowledge of the way that different pharmaceuticals operate, but scientific studies indicate that *the effect of inhibiting implantation is certainly present*, even if this does not mean that such interceptives cause an abortion every time they are used, also because conception does not occur after every act of sexual intercourse. It must be noted, however, that anyone who seeks to prevent the implantation of an embryo which may possibly have been conceived and who therefore either requests or prescribes such a pharmaceutical, generally intends abortion. (citations omitted)

Congregation for the Doctrine of the Faith, *Instruction* Dignitas Personae *on Certain Bioethical Questions*, 13–14, Sept. 8, 2008; http://www.usccb.org/comm/Dignitaspersonae/Dignitas_Personae.pdf

[13] Prevention First Act, § 402,S. 21, 111th Cong. (2009); http://thomas.loc.gov/cgi-bin/query/D?c111:1:./temp/~c111qjRvG4:;; Prevention First Act of 2009, § 402, H.R. 463, 111th Cong. (2009); http://thomas.loc.gov/cgi-bin/query/D?c111:2:./temp/~c111qjRvG4::. *See also* Compassionate Care for Female Sexual Assault Victims, H.R. 4113, 107th Cong. (2002); Compassionate Care for Rape Emergencies Act, H.R. 2527, 108th Cong. (2003); Compassionate Care for Rape Emergencies Act, H.R. 2928, 109th Cong. (2004). None of these earlier bills became laws. *See* http://www.govtrack.us/congress/bill.xpd?bill=h107-4113. Similar bills were introduced in the 110th Congress but have not been passed. Compassionate Assistance for Rape Emergencies Act of 2007, H.R. 464, 110th Cong. (2007); Compassionate Assistance for Rape Emergencies Act of 2007, 110th Cong. (2007); http://www.govtrack.us/congress/bill.xpd?bill=s110-1240.

[14] *50 States Summary of Emergency Contraception Legislation,* National Conference of State Legislatures; http://www.ncsl.org/programs/health/ECleg.htm.

[15] Ann. Cal. Penal Code § 13823.11 (e) (2008) (A.B. 1860) (requires health care providers to dispense emergency contraceptive to victims of sexual assault). West's Ann. Cal. Health & Safety Code § 1281 (2008) requires hospitals to comply with this requirement.

[16] Wash. Rev. Code Ann. § 70.41.350 (1) (West, 2008).

[17] Wash. Rev. Code Ann. § 70.41.350 (2) (West, 2008).

[18] Wash. Rev. Code Ann. § 70.41.360 (West, 2004).

[19] N.Y. Pub. Health Law § 2805-p (McKinney, 2008).

[20] Ibid., 2 (c).

[21] Conn. Gen. Stat. Ann. § 19a-112e (3) (West, 2008).

[22] Ibid.

[23] *Statement by Catholic Bishops Regarding Plan B*; http://www.catholicculture.org/library/view.cfm?recnum=7836. It states:

> The Catholic Bishops of Connecticut, joined by the leaders of the Catholic hospitals in the State, issue the following statement regarding the administration of Plan B in Catholic hospitals to victims of rape:
>
> The four Catholic hospitals in the State of Connecticut remain committed to providing competent and compassionate care to victims of rape. In accordance with Catholic moral teaching, these hospitals provide emergency contraception after appropriate testing. Under the existing hospital protocols, this includes a pregnancy test and an

ovulation test. Catholic moral teaching is adamantly opposed to abortion, but not to emergency contraception for victims of rape.

This past spring the Governor signed into a law "An Act Concerning Compassionate Care for Victims of Sexual Assault," passed by the State Legislature. It does not allow medical professionals to take into account the results of the ovulation test. The Bishops and other Catholic health care leaders believe that this law is seriously flawed, but not sufficiently to bar compliance with it at the present time. We continue to believe this law should be changed.

Nonetheless, to administer Plan B pills in Catholic hospitals to victims of rape a pregnancy test to determine that the woman has not conceived is sufficient. An ovulation test will not be required. The administration of Plan B pills in this instance cannot be judged to be the commission of an abortion because of such doubt about how Plan B pills and similar drugs work and because of the current impossibility of knowing from the ovulation test whether a new life is present. To administer Plan B pills without an ovulation test is not an intrinsically evil act.

Since the teaching authority of the Church has not definitively resolved this matter and since there is serious doubt about how Plan B pills work, the Catholic Bishops of Connecticut have stated that Catholic hospitals in the State may follow protocols that do not require an ovulation test in the treatment of victims of rape. A pregnancy test approved by the United States Food and Drug Administration suffices. If it becomes clear that Plan B pills would lead to an early chemical abortion in some instances, this matter would have to be reopened.

[24] Ibid.
[25] Ibid.
[26] NCBC *Statement on Connecticut Legislation Regarding Treatment for Victims of Sexual Assault* (Oct. 3, 2007); http://www.ncbcenter.org/07-10-03-Connecticut.asp.
[27] Steven S. Smugar, Bernadette J. Spina, and Jon F. Merz, "Informed Consent for Emergency Contraception: Variability in Hospital Care of Rape Victims." *American Journal of Public Health* 90 (2000), 1372.
[28] Ibid., 1372.
[29] Ibid., 1373.
[30] Ibid.
[31] Ibid.
[32] Ibid.
[33] Ibid.
[34] Ibid., 1374
[35] Ibid.
[36] Ibid.
[37] Ibid.
[38] Ibid.
[39] Ibid.
[40] *Second Chance Denied: Emergency Contraception in Catholic Hospital Emergency Rooms*, 5; http://www.ibisreproductivehealth.org/downloads/ECcffcStudy.pdf (last accessed June 22, 2008). *See also* Chelsea Polis, Kate Schaffer, and Teresa Harrison, "Accessibility of Emergency Contraception in California's Catholic Hospitals." *Women's Health Issues* 174 (2005): 15 (Sept. 2003 survey of Catholic hospital emergency rooms in California finding access to EC was minimal even for victims of sexual assault).
[41] Ibid., 5.
[42] Ibid., 5.

[43] Ibid.

[44] Telephone Interview with Jan Heller, Ph.D., staff ethicist for Providence Health System, and Sr. Karin Dufault, S.P., Ph.D., R.N, chair of the board, Providence Health System, Sept. 23, 2003.

[45] Telephone interview with Joseph J. Piccione, J.D., Mission Integration and Corporate Ethicist and Attorney, OSF Healthcare, Peoria, Illinois, May 5, 2003.

[46] Directive 36, *Ethical and Religious Directives for Catholic Health Care Services* 20 (4th ed., 2001) provides:

> Compassionate and understanding care should be given to a person who is the victim of sexual assault. . . . A female who has been raped should be able to defend herself against a potential conception from the sexual assault. If, after appropriate testing, there is no evidence that conception has occurred already, she may be treated with medications that would prevent ovulation, sperm capacitation, or fertilization. It is not permissible, however, to initiate or recommend treatments that have as their purpose or direct effect the removal, destruction, or interference with a fertilized ovum.

[47] Ronald P. Hamel and Michael R. Panicola, "Emergency Contraception and Sexual Assault: Assessing the Moral Approaches in Catholic Teaching." *Health Progress* 83 (Sept.–Oct. 2002); http://www.chausa.org/Pub/MainNav/News/HP/Archive/2002/09SeptOct/articles/Features/hp0209i.htm.

[48] Ibid.

[49] *Second Chance Denied*, supra note 40, at 9.

[50] Ibid.

[51] Hamel and Panicola, *supra* note 47.

[52] Daniel P. Sulmasy, "A Reasonable, Realistic, and Ethical Protocol." *Health Progress* 83 (Sept.–Oct. 2002); http://www.chausa.org/Pub/MainNav/News/HP/Archive/2002/09SeptOct/articles/Features/hp0209k.htm. Nonetheless, Sulmasy, a physician and a Catholic priest, endorses the pregnancy approach in light of the delays in treatment that may result from use of the tests called for under the ovulatory approach.

[53] Grimes and Raymond, *supra* note 2; Chris Kahlenborn, Joseph B. Stanford, and Walter L. Larimore, "Postfertilization Effect of Hormonal Emergency Contraception." *Annals of Pharmacology* 36 (2002): 465 (finding that Plan B may act at times by reducing the possibility of implantation).

[54] Horacio B. Croxatto, Luigie Devoto, Marta Durand, Enrique Ezcurra, Fernando Larrea, Carlos Nagle, Maria Elena Ortiz, David Vantman, Margarita Vega, Helena von Hertzen, "Mechanism of Action of Hormonal Preparations Used for Emergency Contraception: A Review of the Literature." *Contraception* 63 (2001): 111. More specifically, they state:

> The most difficult parameter to assess with certainty is endometrial receptivity. Endometrial markers of receptivity have been established so far with certainty only in rodents. Even if endometrial receptivity is shown to be altered by EC, other steps that precede implantation may also be altered enough to interrupt the process at an earlier stage.

Ibid., 119.

[55] "Protect Yourself and Your Future: Important Information for Women About Plan B, Birth Control and Sexually Transmitted Diseases" (from the makers of Plan B, Duramed, a division of Barr Pharmaceuticals); http://www.go2planb.com/PDF/PatientPamphlet.pdf.

[56] Rev. Nicanor Pier Giorgio Austriaco, O.P., "Is Plan B an Abortifacient?" 7 *National Catholic Bioethics Quarterly* 703 (Winter 2007). The author further states:

Studies published in the past few months provide mounting evidence that levonorgestrel has little or no effect on post-fertilization events. In other words, given the limitations of scientific certitude, they suggest that Plan B, when administered once, is not an abortifacient. These human studies correlate well with earlier findings in rodents and monkeys that convincingly showed that the postcoital administration of levonorgestrel in amounts several times higher than typical doses given to women does not interfere with the post-fertilization processes required for mammalian embryo implantation. The evidence also addresses what until now has been a nagging, unanswerable question for pharmacologists: Why would levonorgestrel, a progesterone agonist that mimics the effect of progesterone, prevent implantation, when progesterone produced from the corpus luteum immediately after ovulation actually promotes implantation by converting the endometrium to decidua? Answer: It does not (footnotes omitted).

Ibid. *But see* Rev. Mark Yavarone, O.M.V., "Do Anovulants and IUDs Kill Early Human Embryo?: A Question of Conscience." *National Catholic Bioethics Quarterly* 4 (Spring 2004): 63 (discussing evidence that oral contraceptive may act to prevent implantation).

[57] Correspondence, Letter from Douglas P. Miller, M.D., Catawba Memorial Medical Center, Hickory, N.C., 138 *Annals of Internal Medicine* 237 (2003); http://www.annals.org/cgi/reprint/138/3/237-b.pdf. The letter states in part:

Hormonally mediated contraception, whether pre- or postcoital, is well recognized as having a dual mechanism of action. Sometimes conception itself is prevented and sometimes implantation of an already conceived embryo is prevented, thus precipitating an early abortion. The use of the term *abortion* is appropriate for this type of procedure because a human embryo is genetically a distinct individual from the moment of conception. Ibid.

The Miller letter is a response to an article by Grimes & Raymond, *Emergency Contraception*, supra note 2.

The response by Grimes and Raymond to the Miller letter is interesting in that it disagrees on the point of when a pregnancy begins, but does not take issue with the statement that the effect of emergency contraception may be to prevent implantation. It states in part:

Dr. Miller apparently disagrees with the internationally accepted definition of the beginning of pregnancy that we used in our review. Major medical organizations as well as the federal government concur that implantation defines the beginning of pregnancy. Fertilization is a necessary but insufficient step toward establishing pregnancy (footnotes omitted).

Correspondence, Letter from David A. Grimes, M.D. & Elizabeth G. Raymond, M.D., M.P.H., Family Health International, Research Triangle Park, N.C., 138 *Ann. of Int. Med.* 237-238; http://www.annals.org/cgi/reprint/138/3/237-b.pdf.
[58] O'Rourke, *supra* note 10.
[59] Eugene F. Diamond, M.D., "The Ovulation or Pregnancy Approach in Cases of Rape." *National Catholic Bioethics Quarterly* 3 (Winter 2003): 689, 693.
[60] Hamel and Panicola, *supra* note 47.
[61] Ibid.
[62] Directive 36, 2001 *ERDs*, *supra* note 9, at 20; *see also* O'Rourke, "Applying the Directives." *Supra* note 10.
[63] O'Rourke, *supra* note 10.
[64] Ibid. Ovral is an oral contraceptive that contains progestin and estrogen. Although it is not marketed specifically as an emergency contraceptive, it can be used for that purpose.

"Types of Emergency Contraception: Which Birth Control Pills Can Be Used for Emergency Contraception in the United States." http://ec.princeton.edu/questions/dose.html.

[65] O'Rourke, *supra* note 10.

[66] Interim Protocol Sexual Assault: Contraceptive Treatment Component, OSF Health Care System, Peoria, Illinois, Oct. 1995 (The Peoria Protocol) (on file with author).

[67] O'Rourke, *supra* note 10.

[68] The Peoria Protocol, *supra* note 66.

[69] Ibid.

[70] Hamel and Panicola, *supra* note 47.

[71] Telephone interview with Joseph J. Piccione, J.D., Mission Integration and Corporate Ethicist, OSF Health Care System, Peoria, Illinois, May 5, 2003.

[72] 410 Ill. Comp. Stat Ann. § 70/2.2 (b) (West, 2008).

[73] Ibid.

[74] Ibid.

[75] Ill. Admin. Code tit 77, §545.APPENDIX C, "Emergency Contraception Protocols" (West, 2008).

[76] Ibid.

[77] Ibid.

[78] *Guidelines for Catholic Hospitals Treating Victims of Sexual Assault*, Board of Governors of the Pennsylvania Catholic Conference, Sept. 23, 1998; http://www.ewtn.com/library/BISHOPS/HOSPSEX.HTM.

[79] Ibid.

[80] Ibid.

[81] Ibid.

[82] Ibid.

[83] Ibid.

[84] Hamel and Panicola, *supra* note 47.

[85] Directive 36, 2001 *ERDs*, *supra* note 9, at 20.

[86] Directive 45, 2001 *ERDs*, *supra* note 9, at 26.

[87] Hamel and Panicola, *supra* note 47.

[88] Ibid.

[89] Ibid.

[90] Ibid.

[91] Ibid.

[92] Ibid.

[93] Ibid.

[94] O'Rourke, *supra* note 10.

[95] Hamel and Panicola, *supra* note 47.

[96] Ibid.

[97] Ibid.

[98] Instruction *Dignitas Personae*, *supra* note 12.

[99] Marie Hillard, "*Dignitas Personae* and Emergency Contraception.*Ethics & Medics* 34 (Feb. 2009): 3.

[100] Ibid., 3.

[101] Ibid., 4.

[102] Ibid.

[103] Ibid.

PART V: *End-of-Life Care*

[1] The Catholic bishops of Pennsylvania have stated:

> Bioethics based on philosophy and legal principles provide some guidance through the maze of problems in health care. Yet it is also clear that philosophy and law alone do not adequately address all of the real concerns and pertinent issues. Religious bioethics makes an invaluable contribution to contemporary moral debates by offering insights into human nature, the purpose of life, the meaning of suffering and education to true virtue. These considerations assist doctors and patients alike to make wise choices both in everyday practice and in the most difficult of cases. Religiously grounded bioethics leads people to place their attention on the right thing to do and frees the autonomy of choice from a vision which can easily become narrow and even dreadfully wrong. We can humanize the face of technology by giving it a moral evaluation in reference to the dignity of the human person, who is called to realize the God-given vocation to life and love (footnotes omitted).

Nutrition and Hydration: Moral Considerations — A Statement of the Catholic Bishops of Pennsylvania (rev. ed. 1999; first issued Dec. 12, 1991); http://www.pacatholic.org/statements/nutritionhydration.html.

[2] National Conference of Catholic Bishops, Committee for Pro-Life Activities, *Nutrition and Hydration: Moral and Pastoral Reflections* 1992); http://www.usccb.org/prolife/issues/euthanas/nutindex.shtml.

[3] Ibid., 2.

[4] Directive 59, *Ethical and Religious Directives for Catholic Health Care Services*, 4th ed. (2001), 31–32, states:

> The free and informed judgment made by a competent adult patient concerning the use or withdrawal of life-sustaining procedures should always be respected and complied with, unless it is contrary to Catholic moral teaching.

[5] *See, e.g., Bouvia v. Superior Court*, 225 Cal. Rptr. 297 (Cal. App. 1986) (holding disabled patient in public hospital who expressed desire to starve herself was entitled to court order to remove nasogastric tube). Subsequently, in *Cruzan by Cruzan v. Director, Missouri Dep't. of Health*, 497 U.S. 261, 278 (1990), the United States Supreme Court stated: "The principle that a competent person has a constitutionally protected liberty interest in refusing unwanted medical treatment may be inferred from our prior decisions."

[6] *But see* Kevin D. O'Rourke, O.P., "The Catholic Tradition on Forgoing Life Support." *National Catholic Bioethics Quarterly* 5 (Autumn 2005): 537, 546, stating: "Catholic tradition has always insisted that the patient or the proxy has the right to make the final decision concerning the refusal of health care." O'Rourke does not, however, mention Directive 59, *supra* note 4.

[7] Ibid., 7. See also Directive 59, *supra* note 4.

[8] *Nutrition and Hydration*, *supra* note 2, at 7.

[9] Ibid., 7.

[10] Ibid., 3.

[11] Ibid., 6.

[12] Address of John Paul II to the Participants in the International Congress on "Life-Sustaining Treatments and Vegetative State: Scientific Advances and Ethical Dilemmas" (Mar. 20, 2004); http://www.vatican.va/holy_father/john_paul_ii/speeches/2004/march/documents/hf_jp-ii_spe_20040320_congress-fiamc_en.html.

[13] Ibid., Par. 3.

[14] Ibid., Par. 2.

[15] In *Washington v. Glucksberg*, 521 U.S. 702,734 (2006), Justice Rehnquist commented on euthanasia in the Netherlands as follows:

> This concern [about the slippery slope that would result if physician-assisted suicide is made legal] is further supported by evidence about the practice of euthanasia in the Netherlands. The Dutch government's own study revealed that in 1990, there were 2,300 cases of voluntary euthanasia (defined as "the deliberate termination of another's life at his request"), 400 cases of assisted suicide, and more than 1,000 cases of euthanasia without an explicit request. In addition to these latter 1,000 cases, the study found an additional 4,941 cases where physicians administered lethal morphine overdoses without the patients' explicit consent.... This study suggests that, despite the existence of various reporting procedures, euthanasia in the Netherlands has not been limited to competent, terminally ill adults who are enduring physical suffering, and that regulation of the practice may not have prevented abuses in cases involving vulnerable persons, including severely disabled neonates and elderly persons suffering from dementia.... The New York Task Force, citing the Dutch experience, observed that "assisted suicide and euthanasia are closely linked," ... and concluded that the "risk of ... abuse is neither speculative nor distant." ... Washington, like most other States, reasonably ensures against this risk by banning, rather than regulating, assisting suicide. (citations omitted)

[16] Cf. Paul E. Marik, Joseph Varon, Alan Lisbon, and Harvey S. Reich, "Physician's Own Preferences to the Limitation and Withdrawal of Life-Sustaining Therapy." *Resuscitation* 42 (Nov. 1999): 197–201 (survey of attending physicians at four hospitals inquiring whether they would want active euthanasia if they were suffering from Lou Gehrig's diseases indicated a significant number would favor active euthanasia).

[17] Oregon Death with Dignity Act, Or. Rev. Stat. §§ 127.800 to 127.995 (2008); http://www.oregon.gov/DHS/ph/pas/ors.shtml.

[18] Washington Death with Dignity, Initiative Measure 1000; http://wei.secstate.wa.gov/osos/en/Documents/I1000-Text%20for%20web.pdf. The initiative was passed by the vote of the people. Office of the Washington State Secretary of State, Nov. 4, 2008, General Election; http://vote.wa.gov/elections/wei/Results.aspx?RaceTypeCode=M&JurisdictionTypeID=-2&ElectionID=26&ViewMode=Results.

[19] Or. Rev. Stat. § 127.885(4) (2008) provides:

> No health care provider shall be under any duty, whether by contract, by statute, or by any other legal requirement to participate in the provision to a qualified patient of medication to end his or her life in a humane and dignified manner. If a health care provider is unable or unwilling to carry out a patient's request under ORS 127.800 to 127.897, and the patient transfers his or her care to a new health care provider, the prior health care provider shall transfer, upon request, a copy of the patient's relevant medical records to the new health care provider.

The Washington state measure provides that only willing health care providers can be required to participate in physician-assisted suicide. Initiative Measure 1000, The Washington State Death with Dignity Act, § 19 91(d). There is also a special section dealing with rights of institutional providers:

> (2)(a) A health care provider may prohibit another health care provider from participating under this act on the premises of the prohibiting provider if the prohibiting provider has given notice to all health care providers with privileges to practice on the premises and to

the general public of the prohibiting provider's policy regarding participating under this act. This subsection does not prevent a health care provider from providing health care services to a patient that do not constitute participation under this act.

(b) A health care provider may subject another health care provider to the sanctions stated in this subsection if the sanctioning health care provider has notified the sanctioned provider before participation in this act that it prohibits participation in this act:

(i) Loss of privileges, loss of membership, or other sanctions provided under the medical staff bylaws, policies, and procedures of the sanctioning health care provider if the sanctioned provider is a member of the sanctioning provider's medical staff and participates in this act while on the health care facility premises of the sanctioning health care provider, but not including the private medical office of a physician or other provider;

(ii) Termination of a lease or other property contract or other nonmonetary remedies provided by a lease contract, not including loss or restriction of medical staff privileges or exclusion from a provider panel, if the sanctioned provider participates in this act while on the premises of the sanctioning health care provider or on property that is owned by or under the direct control of the sanctioning health care provider; or

(iii) Termination of a contract or other nonmonetary remedies provided by contract if the sanctioned provider participates in this act while acting in the course and scope of the sanctioned provider's capacity as an employee or independent contractor of the sanctioning health care provider. Nothing in this subsection (2)(b)(iii) prevents:

(A) A health care provider from participating in this act while acting outside the course and scope of the provider's capacity as an employee or independent contractor; or

(B) A patient from contracting with his or her attending physician and consulting physician to act outside the course and scope of the provider's capacity as an employee or independent contractor of the sanctioning health care provider.

(C) A health care provider that imposes sanctions under (b) of this subsection shall follow all due process and other procedures the sanctioning health care provider may have that are related to the imposition of sanctions on another health care provider.

[20] *Baxter v. Montana*, Decision and Order, Cause No. ADV 2007-787, Montana First Judicial District Court, Lewis and Clark County, Dec. 5, 2008; http://www.compassionandchoices.org/documents/McCarter_Opinion_Montana.pdf.

Chapter Thirteen: *Catholic Teaching on End-of-Life Care*

[1] William E. May, *An Introduction to Moral Theology*, 2d ed. (Huntington, IN: Our Sunday Visitor, 2003), 106.

[2] Ibid., 251–52

[3] Ibid., 252–53.

[4] Richard M. Doerflinger and Carlos Gomez, M.D., Ph.D., *Killing the Pain, Not the Patient: Palliative Care vs. Assisted Suicide*, United States Conference of Catholic Bishops Office of Pro-Life Activities; http://www.usccb.org/prolife/programs/rlp/98rlpdoe.shtml. Doerflinger and Gomez restate the traditional Catholic teaching, but also note: "[W]hen dosages of painkilling drugs are adjusted to relieve patients' pain, there is little if any risk that they will hasten death. This fact alone should put to rest the myth that pain control is

euthanasia by another name." Gerald Kelly notes that under the principle of double effect, an action is deemed morally licit if the following requirements are met:

> 1) *The action, considered by itself and independently of its effect, must not be morally evil.* . . . 2) *The evil effect must not be the means of producing the good effect.* The principle underlying this condition is that a good end cannot justify the use of an evil means. . . . 3) *The evil effect is sincerely not intended, but merely tolerated.* . . . In the cases we are considering, therefore, neither the patient nor the physician may intend the loss of fetal life or the sterilization. The attitude toward these effects must be one of mere tolerance. 4) *There must be a proportionate reason for performing the action, in spite of its evil consequences.* In practice, this means that there must be a sort of balance between the total good and the total evil produced by an action. Or, to put it another way, it means that, according to a sound prudential estimate, the good to be obtained is of sufficient value to compensate for the evil that must be tolerated.

Gerald Kelly, S.J., *Medico-Moral Problems* (St. Louis: The Catholic Hospital Association, 1958), 13–14; *see also* Charles J. McFadden, *Medical Ethics*, 3rd ed., 33.

[5] Ronald Hamel and Michael Panicola, "Must We Preserve Life?" *America* 190 (Apr. 19–26, 2004): 6, 7.

[6] Ibid., 7.

[7] Ibid., 7.

[8] William E. May, *Catholic Bioethics and the Gift of Human Life* (Huntington, IN: Our Sunday Visitor, 2000), 258.

[9] Ibid., discussing two essays by Richard McCormick.

[10] Pope Pius XII, address to those taking part in Ninth Congress of the Italian Anaesthesiological Society (Feb. 24, 1957); http://www.lifeissues.net/writers/doc/doc_31resuscitation.html.

[11] Ibid.

[12] *Declaration on Euthanasia* (1980).

[13] Ibid., 1.

[14] Ibid., 3.

[15] Ibid., 4.

[16] Ibid., 3.

[17] Ibid.

[18] Ibid., 4.

[19] Ibid., 8.

[20] Ibid.

[21] Ibid., 9. The problem with this terminology is that it risks confusion with the proportionalist methodology. Benedict M. Guevin, O.S.B., "Ordinary, Extraordinary, and Artificial Means of Care." *National Catholic Bioethics Quarterly* 5 (Winter 2005): 471, 475. Guevin also notes that Ashley and O'Rourke have noted similar concerns with this possibility of confusion. Ibid., *citing to* Benedict M. Ashley, O.P. and Kevin D. O'Rourke, O.P., *Health Care Ethics: A Theological Analysis*, 4th ed. (Washington, DC: Georgetown University Press, 1997), 420–21.

[22] Kevin D. O'Rourke, O.P., "The Catholic Tradition on Forgoing Life Support." *National Catholic Bioethics Quarterly* 5 (Autumn 2005): 537,– 543.

[23] Ibid., 9.

[24] Ibid.

[25] *Catechism of the Catholic Church* (1995), Pars. 2276–79.

[26] Ibid., 608.

[27] Ibid.
[28] Ibid.
[29] Ibid.
[30] Ibid.
[31] Pope John Paul II, *Evangelium Vitae* (The Gospel of Life) (1995), Par. 65; http://www.vatican.va/holy_father/john_paul_ii/encyclicals/documents/hf_jp-ii_enc_25031995_evangelium-vitae_en.html.
[32] Ibid.
[33] Ibid., Par. 15.
[34] Ibid.
[35] Ibid., Par. 65.
[36] Ibid.
[37] Ibid.
[38] Ibid. *See also* Hamel and Panicola, "Must We Preserve Life?" *supra* note 25, at 7 (discussing this passage and arguing that even for traditional moralists the benefits and burdens of treatment must be assessed "relative to the persons overall situation").
[39] *Charter for Health Care Workers* (1994) (*issued by the* Pontifical Council for Pastoral Assistance to Health Care Workers).
[40] Ibid., 11.
[41] Ibid., 65.
[42] Ibid.
[43] Ibid., 105.
[44] *Ethical and Religious Directives for Catholic Health Care Services,* 4th ed. (2001), at 29-33.
[45] Ibid., 31, at Directive 56.
[46] Ibid., 31, at Directive 57.
[47] Ibid., 31, at Directives 56 and 57.

Chapter Fourteen: *The Controversy over Withdrawing Artificial Nutrition and Hydration from Patients in a Persistent Vegetative State*

[1] *See, e.g.,* William E. May, *Catholic Bioethics and the Gift of Human Life* (Huntington, IN: Our Sunday Visitor, 2000), 268–70.
[2] Ibid.
[3] Ibid., 258–59, discussing "Richard McCormick's 'Quality of Life' Position." May refers to two seminal articles by McCormick: Richard McCormick, S.J., "To Save or Let Die: The Dilemma of Modern Medicine." *Journal of the American Medical Association* 229 (1974): 171, abridged version in Nancy S. Jecker, Albert R. Jonsen, and Robert A. Pearlman, *Bioethics: An Introduction to the History, Methods and Practice* (Sudbury, MA: Jones and Bartlett, 2007), 57; and Richard McCormick, S.J., "The Quality of Life, The Sanctity of Life." *Hastings Center Report* 8 (1978), 30. McCormick states: "But often enough it is the kind of, the quality of life thus saved... that establishes the means as extraordinary. *That* type of life would be an excessive hardship for the individual. It would distort and jeopardize his grasp on the overall meaning of life." McCormick, "To Save or Let Die." *Supra*, at 60.
[4] *See, e.g.,* "Open Letter to Bishop McHugh, Father Kevin D. O'Rourke on Hydration and Nutrition." *Origins* 19 (1989): 351, stating: "In sum, I would consider the use of artificial hydration to prolong the life of persons with permanent and irreversible cessation of function of the cerebral cortex as an ineffective means of care or therapy." Ibid., 352.

[5] William E. May, Robert Barry, O.P., Msgr. Orville Griese, Germain Grisez, Brian Johnstone, C.Ss.R., Thomas J. Marzen, Bishop James T. McHugh, S.J.D., Gilbert Meilander, Mark Siegler, and Msgr. William Smith, "Feeding and Hydrating the Permanently Unconscious and Other Vulnerable Persons." *Issues in Law & Medicine* 3 (1987): 203, reprinted in James J. Walter and Thomas A. Shannon, eds., *Quality of Life: The New Medical Dilemma* (Mahwah, NJ: Paulist Press, 1990), 195.

[6] May, et al., in *Quality of Life*, *supra* note 5, at 196.

[7] Ibid., 197.

[8] Ibid., 199.

[9] Ibid., 198.

[10] Ibid., 198.

[11] Ibid., 199.

[12] Ibid., 199.

[13] Ibid., 200.

[14] Ibid., 200.

[15] Ibid., 201.

[16] Benedict Ashley, O.P., and Kevin D. O'Rourke, O.P., *Health Care Ethics: A Theological Analysis* (Washington, DC: Georgetown University Press, 1997), 419–26.

[17] Kevin O'Rourke, O.P., "The A.M.A. Statement on Tube Feeding: An Ethical Analysis." *America* 155 (Nov. 22, 1986), 321.

[18] Ibid., 322.

[19] Ibid., 322.

[20] Ibid., 322.

[21] Ibid., 322.

[22] Kevin D. O'Rourke, O.P., *Development of Church Teaching on Prolonging Life* (St. Louis, MO: Catholic Health Association, 1988), 12–14.

[23] Ibid., 13.

[24] Ibid., 12.

[25] Ibid., 14.

[26] Ibid., 12 *quoting from* Pope Pius XII, address to those taking part in Ninth Congress of Italian Anaesthesiological Society, Nov. 24, 1957; http://www.lifeissues.net/writers/doc/doc_31resuscitation.html.

[27] O'Rourke, *supra* note 22, at 12–13.

[28] Kevin D. O'Rourke, O.P., "When to Withdraw Life Support." *National Catholic Bioethics Quarterly* (Winter 2008): 663, 671.

[29] Ibid., 664–65.

[30] Ibid., 671.

[31] May, *supra* note 1, at 255–56.

[32] Ibid., 256.

[33] Ibid.

[34] Ibid.

[35] The Most Reverend James McHugh, Bishop of Camden, N.J., "Artificially Assisted Nutrition and ANH." *Origins* 19 (Sept. 21, 1989), 314–16.

[36] Ibid., 315.

[37] Ibid.

[38] Ibid.

[39] Ibid.

[40] Ibid.

[41] Ibid.

[42] Ibid., 316.
[43] O'Rourke, "Open Letter" *supra* note 4, at 352.
[44] Ibid.
[45] Ibid.
[46] Ibid.
[47] Ibid.
[48] Ibid.
[49] Ibid.
[50] Ibid.
[51] Thomas A. Shannon and James J. Walter, "The PVS Patient and the Forgoing/Withdrawing of Medical Nutrition and ANH." *Theological Studies* 49 (Dec. 1998): 623, reprinted in James J. Walter and Thomas A. Shannon, eds., *Quality of Life: The New Medical Dilemma* (Mahwah, NJ: Paulist Press, 1990), 203.
[52] "Quality of Life: The New Medical Dilemma." *supra* note 51, at 212.
[53] Ibid., 212.
[54] Ibid., 214.
[55] Ibid., 214.
[56] David F. Kelly, *Contemporary Catholic Health Care Ethics* (Washington, DC: Georgetown University Press, 2004), 187.
[57] Ibid., *citing to* Gerald Kelly, S.J., "The Duty of Using Artificial Means of Preserving Life." *Theological Studies* 11 (1950): 203.
[58] Ibid., 218–19.
[59] Ibid., 219.
[60] Ibid.
[61] Ibid.
[62] Ibid., 219–20.
[63] Ibid., 189.
[64] Most Reverend Louis Gelineau, Bishop of Providence, R.I., "Statement on Removing Nutrition and Hydration from Comatose Woman." *Origins* 17 (Jan. 21, 1988), 546.
[65] Texas Conference of Catholic Bishops, "On the Care of Vegetative Patients." *Origins* 20 (May 7, 1990): 53. Two Texas bishops dissented from the statement. Ibid., 53. *See also* Bishop Rene H. Gracida, "Interim Pastoral Statement on Artificial Nutrition and Hydration: A Dissent Issued By the Texas Conference of Catholic Health Facilities and Some of the Bishops of Texas"; http://www.ewtn.com/library/BISHOPS/GRACIDA.HTM.
[66] *Nutrition and Hydration: Moral Considerations — A Statement of the Catholic Bishops of Pennsylvania* (rev. ed. 1999; first issued Dec. 12, 1991); http://www.pacatholic.org/statements/nutritionhydration.html.
[67] National Conference of Catholic Bishops Committee for Pro-Life Activities, *Nutrition and Hydration: Moral and Pastoral Reflections* (1992); http://www.usccb.org/prolife/issues/euthanas/nutindex.shtml
[68] *Nutrition and Hydration*, *supra* note 67, at 1.
[69] Ibid.
[70] Ibid.
[71] Ibid.
[72] Ibid. [footnote omitted]
[73] Ibid. [footnote omitted]
[74] Ibid.
[75] Ibid.
[76] Ibid.

[77] Ibid.
[78] Ibid.
[79] Ibid.
[80] Ibid.
[81] Ibid.
[82] Ibid.
[83] Ibid.
[84] Ibid.
[85] Ibid.
[86] Ibid.
[87] Ibid.
[88] Ibid.
[89] Ibid.
[90] Ibid.
[91] Ibid.
[92] Ibid.
[93] Ibid.
[94] Ibid.
[95] Ibid.
[96] *Ethical and Religious Directives for Catholic Health Care Services* (1994), 22.
[97] Ibid.
[98] Directive 58, ibid., 23.
[99] Directive 58, *Ethical and Religious Directives for Catholic Health Care Services*, 4th ed. (2001), 31.
[100] Ibid. at 30 and 1994 *ERD*s, *supra* note 96, at 22 citing to *Nutrition and Hydration*, *supra* note 67.
[101] Address of John Paul II to the Participants in the International Congress on "Life-Sustaining Treatments and Vegetative State: Scientific Advances and Ethical Dilemmas." Par. 4 (Mar. 20, 2004); http://www.vatican.va/holy_father/john_paul_ii/speeches/2004/march/documents/hf_jp-ii_spe_20040320_congress-fiamc_en.html.
[102] Ibid., Par. 4.
[103] Ibid., Par. 2.
[104] Ibid., Par. 2.
[105] Ibid., Par. 4.
[106] Ibid., Par. 4.
[107] Ibid., Par. 5.
[108] Cathy Lynn Grossman, "Pope Declares Feeding Tube a 'Moral Obligation.'" *USA Today*, Apr. 4, 2004; http://www.usatoday.com/news/religion/2004-04-01-pope-usat_x.htm.
[109] Ibid.
[110] Rev. Germain Kopaczynski, O.F.M. Conv., "Initial Reactions to the Pope's March 20, 2004 Allocution." *National Catholic Bioethics Quarterly* 4 (Autumn 2004): 473, 479.
[111] Richard M. Doerflinger, "John Paul II on the 'Vegetative State,'" *Ethics & Medics* 29 (June 2004): 2. *See also* Peter J. Cataldo, "Pope John Paul II on Nutrition and Hydration: A Change of Catholic Teaching?" *National Catholic Bioethics Quarterly* 4 (Autumn 2004): 513 (arguing papal allocution does not represent a change in Catholic teaching).
[112] Doerflinger, *supra* note 111.
[113] John F. Tuohey, "The Pope on PVS: Does JPII's Statement Make the Grade?" *Commonweal*, June 18, 2004.
[114] Ibid., 10.

[115] Ibid.
[116] Ibid.
[117] Ibid.
[118] Ibid.
[119] Ibid.
[120] Ibid.
[121] Thomas A. Shannon, James J. Walter, "Artificial Nutrition, Hydration: Assessing Papal Statement." *National Catholic Reporter*, Apr. 16, 2004; http://findarticles.com/p/articles/mi_m1141/is_24_40/ai_n6049668?tag=artBody;col1.
[122] Ibid.
[123] Ibid.
[124] Ibid.
[125] Ibid.
[126] Ibid.
[127] Ibid.
[128] Ibid.
[129] David Kelly, *supra* note 56, at 194.
[130] Ibid.
[131] Kevin D. O'Rourke, O.P., "The Catholic Tradition on Forgoing Life Support." *National Catholic Bioethics Quarterly* 5 (Autumn 2005): 537, 542, quoting from Bishops Committee on Doctrine and Morals (Australian Catholic Bishops' Conference), Bishops Committee for Health Care (Australia), and Catholic Health Australia, "Briefing Note on the Obligation to Provide Nutrition and Hydration" (Sept. 3, 2004), n. 3; http://www.acbc.catholic.org.au/documents/2004090316.pdf.
[132] O'Rourke, *supra* note 131, at 543.
[133] Ibid., 547.
[134] Kevin D. O'Rourke, "Artificial Nutrition and Hydration and the Catholic Tradition." *Health Progress* 88 (May–June 2007); http://www.chausa.org/Pub/MainNav/News/HP/Archive/2007/05MayJune/Articles/Features/hp0705i.htm.
[135] Ibid.
[136] Ronald Hamel and Michael Panicola, "Must We Preserve Life?" *America* 190 (Apr. 19–26, 2004): 6, 10.
[137] Ibid., 10
[138] Ibid., 12
[139] Congregation for the Doctrine of the Faith, *Responses to Certain Questions of the United States Conference of Catholic Bishops Concerning Artificial Nutrition and Hydration* (August 1, 2007); http://www.usccb.org/prolife/tdocs/anhresponses.shtml.
[140] Ibid. The complete questions and response state:

First question: Is the administration of food and water (whether by natural or artificial means) to a patient in a "vegetative state" morally obligatory except when they cannot be assimilated by the patient's body or cannot be administered to the patient without causing significant physical discomfort?

Response: Yes. The administration of food and water even by artificial means is, in principle, an ordinary and proportionate means of preserving life. It is therefore obligatory to the extent to which, and for as long as, it is shown to accomplish its proper finality, which is the hydration and nourishment of the patient. In this way suffering and death by starvation and dehydration are prevented.

Second question: When nutrition and hydration are being supplied by artificial means to a patient in a "permanent vegetative state," may they be discontinued when competent physicians judge with moral certainty that the patient will never recover consciousness?

Response: No. A patient in a "permanent vegetative state" is a person with fundamental human dignity and must, therefore, receive ordinary and proportionate care, which includes, in principle, the administration of water and food even by artificial means.

Ibid.

[141] Ibid.

[142] Commentary from the Congregation of the Doctrine of the Faith; http://www.usccb.org/prolife/tdocs/anhcommentary.shtml

[143] Q&A from the USCCB Committee on Doctrine and Committee on Pro-Life Activities regarding the Holy See's *Responses on Nutrition and Hydration for Patients in a "Vegetative State."* http://www.usccb.org/comm/archives/2007/07-143.shtml.

[144] Ibid.

[145] Ibid.

[146] Ibid.

[147] Melanie Evans, "Moral Obligations: Catholic Officials Differ Over Vatican Feeding-Tube Rules." *Modern Health Care* 37 (Oct. 1, 2007).

[148] Ibid.

[149] John L. Allen, Jr., "A Matter of Life and Death: Ethicists Ponder Practicality, Rightness of Vatican Rules on Artificial Feeding." *National Catholic Reporter*, Oct. 5, 2007, 5.

[150] Ibid.

[151] Nancy Frazier O'Brien, "Catholic Leaders Welcome Vatican Documents on Artificial Nutrition." *Catholic News Service,* Sept. 18, 2007; http://www.catholicnews.com/data/stories/cns/0705284.htm.

[152] Ibid.

[153] Ibid.

[154] John J. Hardt, Ph.D., and Kevin D. O'Rourke, O.P., J.C.D., S.T.M., "Nutrition and Hydration: The CDF Response, in Perspective." *Health Progress* 88 (Nov.–Dec. 2007); http://www.chausa.org/Pub/MainNav/News/HP/Archive/2007/11Nov-Dec/Articles/Features/hp0711g.htm.

[155] Ibid.

[156] Ibid. Their argument is based on Canon 18, which states: "Laws which establish a penalty or restrict free exercise of rights . . . are subject to strict interpretation." Ibid. They then argue that that CDF response amounts to a limitation on a right and thus should be limited only to PVS cases and not to all patients "who are unable to assimilate food and water without artificial assistance." Ibid.

Chapter Fifteen: *A Case Study in End-of-Life Care: Terri Schiavo*

[1] *Cf.* Daniel P. Sulmasy, "Terri Schiavo and the Roman Catholic Tradition of Forgoing Extraordinary Care." *Journal of Law, Medicine & Ethics* 33 (2005): 359.

[2] Abby Goodnough, "The Schiavo Case: The Overview." *New York Times*, Apr. 1, 2005, A1.

[3] Ibid.

[4] Ibid.

[5] Manuel Roig-Franzia, "Long Legal Battle Over as Schiavo Dies." *Washington Post*, Apr. 1, 2005, A1.

[6] Goodnough, *supra* note 2.

[7] Order, *In Re: The Guardianship of Theresa Marie Schiavo,* In the Circuit Court for Pinella County, Florida, Probate Division, File No. 90-2908GD-003; http://www6.miami.edu/ethics/schiavo/pdf_files/021100-Trial_Ct_Order_0200.pdf (order authorizing removal of tube).

[8] Ibid.

[9] *Guardianship of Schiavo*, 792 So.2d 551 (Fla. App. 2001).

[10] Excerpt of Trial Testimony of Fr. Murphy, Jan. 24, 2000, Before Judge W. Greer; http://www6.miami.edu/ethics/schiavo/timeline.htm.

[11] Ibid., 3.

[12] Ibid., 12.

[13] Ibid., 16.

[14] Ibid., 16.

[15] Ibid., 16.

[16] Ibid., 16.

[17] Ibid., 38.

[18] Ibid., 39.

[19] *Guardianship of Schiavo*, 789 So.2d 176, 180 (Fla. App. 2001).

[20] Ronald Hamel and Michael Panicola, "Must We Preserve Life?" *America* 190 (Apr. 19–26, 2004): 6, 10.

[21] Official Statement of the Catholic Diocese of St. Petersburg Regarding Terri Schiavo (Oct. 15, 2002); http://www6.miami.edu/ethics/schiavo/pdf_files/Offical_Statement_of_Petersburg_Diocese.pdf.

[22] Ibid.

[23] Order authorizing removal of feeding tube, *supra* note 7.

[24] Official Statement, *supra* note 21.

[25] Statement of Bishop Robert N. Lynch Concerning the Terri Schiavo Case (Aug. 12, 2003); http://www6.miami.edu/ethics/schiavo/STATEMENT_OF_BISHOP_ROBERT_N.html.

[26] Ibid.

[27] Ibid.

[28] Order authorizing removal of feeding tube, *supra* note 7.

[29] Ibid. But cf. Rev. Donald E. Henke, "Consciousness, Terri Schiavo, and the Persistent Vegetative State." *National Catholic Bioethics Quarterly* 8 (Spring 2008): 69 (discussing conflicting medical testimony over Terri Schiavo's medical condition).

[30] 30 Florida Catholic Conference, *Florida Bishops Urge Safer Course for Terri Schiavo* (Aug. 27, 2003); http://www.flacathconf.org/Publications/Statements/2003/schiavo.pdf.

[31] Ibid.

[32] Ibid.

[33] Florida Bishops, *Statement on the Life, Death and the Treatment of Dying Patients* (Apr. 27, 1989); http://www.flacathconf.org/Publications/Statements/1989/dyingtreatment.pdf.

[34] Address of John Paul II to the Participants in the International Congress on "Life-Sustaining Treatments and Vegetative State: Scientific Advances and Ethical Dilemmas." Par. 4 (Mar. 20, 2004); http://www.vatican.va/holy_father/john_paul_ii/speeches/2004/march/documents/hf_jp-ii_spe_20040320_congress-fiamc_en.html.

[35] Rita L. Marker, "Terri Schiavo and the Catholic Connection." *National Catholic Bioethics Quarterly* 4 (Autumn 2004): 555, 566.

[36] Order, *In Re: the Guardianship of Theresa Marie Schiavo, Schiavo v. Schindler,* in the Circuit Court for Pinellas County, Florida, Probate Division, No. 90-2908-GD-003 (order denying motion to reopen case based on papal allocution); http://www6.miami.edu/eth-

ics/schiavo/pdf_files/102204-denymotion.pdf. The District Court of Appeals subsequently denied an application for writ of certiorari to review the Circuit's order. *Schindler v. Schiavo*, 2004 WL 2726107 (Fla. App. 2004).

[37] *In Re: Guardianship of Theresa Marie Schiavo, Michael Schiavo, Petitioner v. Robert Schindler and Marie Schindler, Respondents,* in the Circuit Court for Pinellas County, Florida, Probate Division (File No. 90-2908GD-003), Motion for Relief from Judgment and Motion to Reconsider; http://www6.miami.edu/ethics/schiavo/pdf_files/Filed_07-19-2004_ReliefFromJudgment.pdf.

[38] *In Re: Guardianship of Theresa Marie Schiavo, Michael Schiavo, Petitioner v. Robert Schindler and Marie Schindler, Respondents,* in the Circuit Court for Pinellas County, Florida, Probate Division (File No. 90-2908GD-003), Appendix to Schindler's Motion for Relief from Judgment and Motion to Reconsider, Affidavits of Robert Schindler, Sr., Mary Schindler, and Frances L. Casler; http://www6.miami.edu/ethics/schiavo/pdf_files/Filed_07-19-2004_ReliefFromJudgmentAppendix.pdf.

[39] *Guardianship of Schiavo*, 789 So.2d 176, 180 (Fla. App. 2001).

[40] Order denying motion to reopen, *supra* note 36. The District Court of Appeals subsequently denied an application for writ of certiorari to review the Circuit's order. *Schindler v. Schiavo*, 2004 WL 2726107 (Fla. App. 2004).

[41] Letter to Jon R. Thogmartin, M.D., District 6 Medical Examiner, from Stephen J. Nelson, M.A., M.D., F.C.A.P., Chief Medical Examiner, 10th Judicial Circuit of Florida, In Re: Theresa Marie ("Terri") Schiavo, deceased, Your Medical Examiner Case No. 5050439, at 5; http://www.sptimes.com/2005/06/15/schiavoreport.pdf.

[42] Ibid., 9.

Notes

PART SIX: *Social Justice and Health Care Reform*

[1] Robert Steinbrook, "Election 2008 — Campaign Contributions, Lobbying, and the U.S. Health Care Sector." *N. Eng. J. Med.* 357(8): 736-739 (Aug. 23, 2007).

[2] According to the results of a CBS News/*New York Times* poll taken February 23–27, 2007, and released March 1, 2007:

> Two-thirds [of Americans] say it is the responsibility of the federal government to guarantee that all Americans have health insurance. This sentiment is little changed from 2000 and even higher than it was ten years ago. Most say they still believe this even if it meant the cost of their own care would go up.

SHOULD GOVERNMENT GUARANTEE HEALTH INSURANCE FOR ALL?

	Now	7/2000	8/1996
Yes	64%	62%	56%
No	27%	29%	38%

CBS News/*New York Times* Poll, U.S. Politics (Mar. 1, 2007); http://www.cbsnews.com/htdocs/CBSNews_polls/health_care.pdf.

[3] "The Obama Health Care Express." *Wall Street Journal,* Dec. 9, 2008; http://online.wsj.com/article/SB122878091745389615.html.

[4] Rev. Rul. 56-185, 1956-1 C.B. 202, modified by Rev. Rul. 69-545, 1969-2 C.B. 117.

[5] "Present Law and Background Relating to the Tax-Exempt Status of Charitable Hospitals." Prepared by the Staff of the Joint Committee on Taxation 5 (Sept. 12, 2006).

[6] Ibid., 6.

[7] Rev. Ruling 69-545, 1969-2 C.B. 117.

[8] Ibid.

[9] John Carreyou and Barbara Martinez, "Nonprofit Hospitals, Once for the Poor, Strike It Rich." *Wall Street Journal*, Apr. 4, 2008.

[10] Ibid.

[11] Ibid.

[12] Ibid.

[13] Taking the Pulse of Charitable Care and Community Benefit at Nonprofit Hospitals, Hearing before the Senate Finance Committee, Sept. 13, 2006, proceedings; http://finance.senate.gov/sitepages/hearing091306.htm; The Tax Exempt Hospital Sector, Hearing before the House Ways and Means Committee, May 26, 2005; http://waysandmeans.house.gov/hearings.asp?formmode=detail&hearing=415.

[14] John D. Colombo, "The Role of Access in Charitable Tax Exemption." *Washington University Law Quarterly* 82 (2004): 343.

[15] John Carreyou and Barbara Martinez, "Grassley Targets Nonprofit Hospitals on Charity Care." *Wall Street Journal*, Dec.18, 2008, A5.

[16] Ibid.

[17] *Provena Covenant Medical Center v. Department of Revenue of State*, 894 N.E.2d 452 (Ill. App. Ct. 2008). In November 2008, the Illinois Supreme Court agreed to hear the hospital's appeal. Barbara Martinez, "Pursuing Charitable Mission Leaves a Hospital Struggling." *Wall Street Journal*, Dec. 12, 2008; http://online.wsj.com/article/SB122893293185295179.html.

[18] "Overcharging Patients Suit Settles for $423 Million." *National Law Journal* (Jan. 22, 2007): 16.

[19] Colombo, *supra* note 14, at 344. See also, M. Gregg Bloche, "Health Policy Below the Waterline: Medical Care and the Charitable Exemption." *Minnesota Law Review* 80: 299, 318. "Studies of comparable nonprofit and for-profit hospitals, matched on the basis of community demographics and patient characteristics, have not shown a significant difference in rates of uncompensated care" (footnotes omitted). Cited in Colombo, *supra* note 14, at 344, n. 5.

[20] Jill R. White, "Why We Need the Independent Sector: The Behavior, Law, and Ethics of Not-for-Profit Hospitals." *UCLA Law Review* 50 (2003): 1345, cited in Colombo, *supra* note 14, at 344, n. 5.

[21] Kenneth R. White and James W. Begun, "How Does Catholic Hospital Sponsorship Affect Services Provided?" *Inquiry* 35 (Winter 1998/1999): 398.

[22] Ibid.

Chapter Sixteen: *The United States Health Care System*

[1] Four separate National Health Systems exist in England, Scotland, Wales, and Northern Ireland. There have been substantial similarities among these four systems, but with the policy of devolution there may be more divergence among them. Arthur Morris, "BMJ Should Stop Confusing Its Readers Over National Differences." *British Medical Journal* 318 (1999): 1221.

[2] About the NHS, NHS Structure; http://www.nhs.uk/aboutnhs/HowtheNHSworks/Pages/NHSstructure.aspx (last accessed Dec. 19, 2008).

[3] *See, e.g.*, Private Health Care U.K.; http://www.privatehealth.co.uk/ (last accessed Dec. 19, 2008).

[4] Health Care System, Health Canada; http://www.hc-sc.gc.ca/hcs-sss/index-eng.php (last accessed Dec. 19, 2008).

[5] *Chaoulli v. Quebec*, [2005] 1 S.C.R. 791, 2005 SCC 35 (CanLII) (Canadian Supreme Court decision striking down Quebec law banning private health insurance). *See also* "Unsocialized Medicine: a Landmark Ruling Exposes Canada's Health Care Inequity." *Wall Street Journal Online*, June 13, 2005; http://www.opinionjournal.com/editorial/feature.html?id=110006813 (discussing Canadian Supreme Court decision striking down Quebec's ban on private health insurance).

[6] Alexandra Shimo, "The Rise of Private Health Care in Canada: All the Health Care Money Can Buy." Maclean's, Apr. 25, 2006; http://www.macleans.ca/article.jsp?content=20060501_125881_125881.

[7] *See, e.g.*, Lawrence O. Gostin and Peter D. Jacobson, *Law and the Health System* (Foundation Press, 2006), 222. The authors state:

> The United States spends some $1.6 trillion each year on medical care—more per capita than any other nation in the world. Health care spending now accounts for nearly 15% of the nation's gross domestic product (GDP), and is expected to rise to 20% over the next decade. Despite this vast spending, physicians and patients alike, not to mention insurers, lawmakers, and the media, are quick to point to failures of the American health care system. The very nature of their complaints belies a fundamental problem regarding the provision of health care in this country — specifically the fact that there is no American health care "system" as such. Unlike some countries, most notably Canada and the United Kingdom, which are known for their national health systems, the United States lacks either a central organizing apparatus for delivering health care or an organizational plan to determine how health care resources should be distributed. (Ibid.)

[8] A Rube Goldberg machine is "any exceedingly complex apparatus that performs a very simple task in a very indirect and convoluted way. Rube devised and drew several such paraphysical devices. The term also applies as a classification for generally overcomplicated apparatus or software." *Webster's Online Dictionary*; http://www.websters-online-dictionary.org/definition/RUBE+GOLDBERG+MACHINE (last accessed Dec. 19, 2008).

[9] Uwe E. Reinhardt, Peter S. Hussey, and Gerald F. Anderson, "U.S. Health Care Spending in an International Context." *Health Affairs* 23 (2004): 10, 10–12.

[10] *See* Gerald F. Anderson, Uwe E. Reinhardt, Peter S. Hussey, and Varduhl Petroysan, "It's the Prices, Stupid: Why the United States Is So Different from Other Countries." *Health Affairs* 22 (2003): 89, 93–94.

[11] The 13 countries, first listed being best, are: Japan, Canada, Sweden, France, Australia, Spain, Finland, Netherlands, U.K., Denmark, Belgium, U.S., Germany. Barbara Starfield, "Is U.S. Health Really the Best in the World?" *Journal of the American Medical Association* 284 (2000): 483; http://jama.ama-assn.org/cgi/reprint/284/4/483.pdf.

[12] Ibid.

[13] Anderson, et al., *supra* note 10, at 98–99.

[14] John D. Finch, *Health Services Law* (London: Sweet & Maxwell, 1981), 4.

[15] Her Majesty's Government, Department of Health, "Working for Patients" (1989).

[16] The Conservative party platform for the 2006 election stated:

> The Conservative Party is committed to ensuring that all Canadians have access to timely, quality health care services regardless of their ability to pay. We are committed to a universal, publicly funded health care system that respects the five principles of the Canada Health Act and the Canadian Charter of Rights and Freedoms. Twelve years of Liberal government have done nothing to improve health care for Canadians. It is harder to find a family doctor. Canadians wait longer for access to critical surgery and specialist services. Hospitals get dirtier and dirtier. And more Canadians cross the border or seek out private clinics in Canada to get the care they need. The Supreme Court of Canada recently declared, "access to a waiting list is not access to health care"... A Conservative Government will ... in conjunction with the provinces, allow for a mix of public and private health care delivery, as long as health care remains publicly funded and universally accessible.
>
> *Stand Up For Canada: Conservative Party of Canada Federal Election Platform* 2006, 17; http://www.cbc.ca/canadavotes2006/leadersparties/pdf/conservative_platform20060113.pdf.

[17] Volker Amelung, Sherry Glied, and Angelina Topan, "Health Care and the Labor Market: Learning from the German Experience." *Journal of Health Politics, Policy, & Law* 28 (2003): 693, 695.

[18] Christa Altenstetter, "Insights from Health Care in Germany." *American Journal of Public Health* 93 (2003): 38.

[19] *See* Norman Barry, "Conservative Thought and the Welfare State." *Political Studies* XLV (1997): 331.

[20] Congressional Budget Office, "Key Issues in Analyzing Major Health Insurance Reform Proposals" (Dec. 2008), ix; http://www.cbo.gov/ftpdocs/99xx/doc9924/12-18-KeyIssues.pdf.

[21] Ibid., 10.

[22] Ibid.

[23] Ibid., xv.

[24] Ibid., 6.

[25] Ibid.

[26] Melissa A. Thomasson, "From Sickness to Health: The Twentieth Century Development of U.S. Health Insurance." *Explorations in Economic History* 39 (July 2002): 233; http://www.sba.muohio.edu/thomasma/Research%20Papers/from%20sickness%20to%20health.pdf. *See also* Terree P. Wasley, "Health Care in the Twentieth Century: A History of Government Interference and Protection." *Business Economics* (Apr. 1993); http://findarticles.com/p/articles/mi_m1094/is_n2_v28/ai_13834930/pg_1?tag=artBody;col1.

[27] Thomasson, *supra* note 26.

[28] Ibid.

[29] Ibid.

[30] Ibid.

[31] Ibid. *See also* "History of Blue Cross and Blue Shield." http://www.bcbs.com/about/history/ (last accessed Dec. 30, 2008).

[32] Thomasson, *supra* note 26.

[33] Ibid.

[34] Ibid.

[35] Ibid.

[36] Ibid.

[37] Ibid.

[38] For example, coverage is available for those eligible for Aid to Families with Dependent Children under requirements in effect on July 16, 1996; SSI recipients; children in low-income families; caretakers for children; low-income pregnant women and their children; couples and persons living in medical institutions with less than 300% of the SSI income standard. "Medicaid At-a-Glance 2005: A Medicaid Information Source," 2. Department of Health and Human Services, Centers for Medicare and Medicaid Services, Center for Medicaid and State Operation; http://www.cms.hhs.gov/MedicaidGenInfo/Downloads/MedicaidAtAGlance2005.pdf.

[39] This permits states to expand eligibility, and the requirements vary some from state to state. The medically needy include low-income persons who do not meet requirements for the "categorically needy," but meet state requirements for coverage of medically needy. If the state elects to provide this coverage, then certain persons must be covered. Generally, "children under age 19 and pregnant women who are medically needy must be covered, and prenatal and delivery care for pregnant women, as well as ambulatory care for children, must be provided."

"Medicaid Program — General Information, Technical Summary." Centers for Medicare and Medicaid Services, Department of Health and Human Services; http://www.cms.hhs.gov/MedicaidGenInfo/03_TechnicalSummary.asp#TopOfPage (last accessed Dec. 18, 2008).

[40] For example, Medicaid pays Medicare premiums for certain low-income persons. It also may provide coverage for the working disabled, women with breast or cervical cancer, and persons with tuberculosis who are uninsured. "Medicaid At-a-Glance 2005: A Medicaid Information Source," 2–3. Department of Health and Human Services, Centers for Medicare and Medicaid Services, Center for Medicaid and State Operation; http://www.cms.hhs.gov/MedicaidGenInfo/Downloads/MedicaidAtAGlance2005.pdf.

[41] "Medicaid Program — General Information, Technical Summary." Centers for Medicare and Medicaid Services, Department of Health and Human Services; http://www.cms.hhs.gov/MedicaidGenInfo/03_TechnicalSummary.asp#TopOfPage (last accessed Dec. 18, 2008).

[42] Ibid. According to the Centers for Medicare and Medicaid Services (CMS):

Long-term care is an important provision of Medicaid that will be increasingly utilized as our nation's population ages. The Medicaid program paid for over 41 percent of the total cost of care for persons using nursing facility or home health services in 2001. National data for 2001 show that Medicaid payments for nursing facility services (excluding ICFs/MR) totaled $37.2 billion for more than 1.7 million beneficiaries of these services—an average expenditure of $21,890 per nursing home beneficiary. The national data also show that Medicaid payments for home health services totaled $3.5 billion for more than 1 million beneficiaries — an average expenditure of $3,475 per home health care beneficiary. With the percentage of our population who are elderly or disabled increasing faster than that of the younger groups, the need for long-term care is expected to increase.

Ibid.

[43] In 1982, Arizona became the last state to receive federal money for the care of its poor. At that time it established an alternative program that received federal funding. H.E. Freeman and B.L Kirkman-Liff, "Care Under AHCCCS: An Examination of Arizona's Alternative to Medicaid." *Health Services Resources* 20 (1985): 245; http://www.pubmedcentral.nih.gov/picrender.fcgi?artid=1068880&blobtype=pdf.

[44] "Medicaid Program — General Information, Technical Summary." Centers for Medicare and Medicaid Services, Department of Health and Human Services; http://www.cms.hhs.gov/MedicaidGenInfo/03_TechnicalSummary.asp#TopOfPage (last accessed Dec. 19, 2008).

[45] Craig Caplan, "The Medicare Program: A Brief Overview." 1, AARP Public Policy Institute (Feb. 2005); http://assets.aarp.org/rgcenter/health/fs103_medicare.pdf.

[46] Ibid., 1.

[47] Ibid., 1.

[48] Thomas R. Oliver, Philip R. Lee, and Helene Tipton, "A Political History of Medicare and Prescription Drug Coverage." *Milbank Quarterly* 82 (2004): 283, 291.

[49] Ibid.

[50] Ibid., 283–84.

[51] Caplan, *supra* note 45, at 3.

[52] "State Children's Health Insurance Program (SCHIP) at a Glance." Kaiser Family Foundation (Jan. 2007) http://www.kff.org/medicaid/upload/7610.pdf.

[53] Ibid.

[54] Ibid.

[55] Ibid.

[56] "A Decade of SCHIP Experience and Issues for Reauthorization." Kaiser Family Foundation (Jan. 2007); http://www.kff.org/medicaid/upload/7574-2.pdf.

[57] Ibid.

[58] Ibid.

[59] Ibid.

[60] Brigitte C. Madrian, "Employment Health Insurance and Job Mobility: Is There Evidence of Job-Lock?" *Quarterly Journal of Economics* 109 (1999): 27, 28–29.

[61] "Present Law and Analysis Relating to Tax Treatment of Health Savings Accounts and Other Health Expenses," 3. Prepared by Staff of Joint Committee on Taxation (June 27, 2006); http://www.house.gov/jct/x-27-06.pdf.

[62] Ibid., 7.

[63] Ibid., 5.

[64] Ibid., 8.

[65] Congressional Budget Office Report, *supra* note 20, at 36.

[66] Congressional Budget Office Report, *supra* note 20, at 48.

[67] Ibid.

[68] "Eliminating Racial and Ethnic Disparities." Office of Minority Health, Centers for Disease Control; http://www.cdc.gov/omhd/About/disparities.htm (last accessed Dec. 19, 2008).

[69] Ibid.

[70] Ibid.

[71] Ibid.

[72] S.J. Kunitz and I. Pesis-Katz, "Mortality of White Americans, African Americans, and Canadians: The Causes and Consequences for Health of Welfare State Institutions and Policies." *Milbank Quarterly* 83 (2005): 5.

[73] Ibid.

[74] Ibid.

[75] Sara Rosenbaum, "The Proxy War — SCHIP and the Government's Role in Health Care Reform." *New England Journal of Medicine* 358 (Feb. 28, 2008): 869; http://content.nejm.org/cgi/reprint/358/9/869.pdf.

[76] I am indebted to Loretta Kopelman for this concept of "theories of justice." This discussion of the SCHIP controversy is a response to her presentation at the 2008 HEAL conference at Samford University. Her presentation and my response are available at: http://www.samford.edu/heal/proceedings2008.html.

[77] "State Children's Health Insurance Program (SCHIP): Reauthorization History" (Rev. Nov. 2008), The Kaiser Commission on Medicaid and the Uninsured; http://www.kff.org/medicaid/upload/7743.pdf.

[78] SCHIP Veto Message to the House of Representatives, George W. Bush, The White House (Oct. 3, 2007); http://www.msnbc.msn.com/id/21117054/.

[79] Ibid.

[80] Ibid.

[81] "State Children's Health Insurance Program," *supra* note 77.

[82] Statement of Administration Policy (Oct. 25, 2007), Executive Office of the President, Office of Management and Budget; http://www.whitehouse.gov/omb/legislative/sap/110-1/hr3963sap-h.pdf.

[83] Medicare, Medicaid, and SCHIP Expansion Act of 2007, 110th Cong. (2007); http://www.govtrack.us/congress/bill.xpd?bill=s110-2499.

[84] Rosenbaum, *supra* note 75, at 869.

[85] Ibid., 870.

[86] Remarks as delivered by The Honorable Mike Leavitt, Secretary of Health and Human Services, AEI Speech (Apr. 24, 2007); http://www.aei.org/docLib/20070426_LeavittRemarks.pdf.

[87] Robert B. Helms, John E. Calfee, and Joseph Antos, "SCHIP Guidelines: Principles for Health Insurance Coverage for Children and Families" (May 22, 2007); http://www.aei.org/publications/filter.all,pubID.26224/pub_detail.asp.

[88] Michael Cannon, "Sinking SCHIP: A First Step Toward Stopping the Growth of Governmental Health Programs." Cato Institute (Sept. 13, 2007); http://www.cato.org/pubs/bp/bp99.pdf.

[89] Henry J. Aaron, "Template for Health Care Coverage." Brookings (Nov. 25, 2007); http://www.brookings.edu/opinions/2002/1125useconomics_aaron.aspx.

[90] *9 Million Children and Counting: The Administration's Attack on Health Coverage for America's Children.* Issue Brief, Families USA (Feb. 2008); http://familiesusa.org/assets/pdfs/chip-9-million-and-counting.pdf.

[91] Rahm Emanuel, "A New Deal for the New Economy." *Wall Street Journal*, Mar. 19, 2008, A17.

⁹² Jonathan Kaplan, "House Dems See Political Win on SCHIP." *The Hill*, Sept. 7, 2007; http://thehill.com/leading-the-news/house-dems-see-political-win-on-schip-2007-09-07.html.

⁹³ Jeffrey Young, "Baucus Wants SCHIP, Health IT in Stimulus." *The Hill*, Dec. 10, 2008; http://thehill.com/leading-the-news/baucus-wants-schip-health-it-in-stimulus-2008-12-10.html.

Chapter Seventeen: *Health Care Reform Proposals*

¹ Derek Bok, "The Great Health Care Debate of 1993–1994" (1998), Penn National Commission on Society, Culture, and Community; http://www.upenn.edu/pnc/ptbok.html.

² Ibid. *See also* Paul Starr, "What Happened to Health Care Reform?" *The American Prospect* 20 (Winter 1995): 20–31; http://www.princeton.edu/~starr/20starr.html.

³ Steven A. Schroeder, "The Clinton Health Plan: Fundamental or Incremental Reform?" *Annals of Internal Medicine* 119 (Nov. 1993): 945; http://www.annals.org/cgi/content/full/119/9/945.

⁴ Ibid.

⁵ "A Detailed Timeline of the Health care Reform Debate in 'the System': Events Following Clinton's Health care Address to Congress Through March 1994." *Online NewsHour*; http://www.pbs.org/newshour/forum/may96/background/health_debate_page2.html (last accessed Dec. 20, 2008).

⁶ John Goodman and Mark Pauly, "Tax Credits for Health Insurance and Medical Savings Accounts." *Health Affairs* 14 (Spring 1995): 126.

⁷ *Health Savings Accounts*. CRS Report for Congress (Updated Mar. 23, 2005); http://www.law.umaryland.edu/marshall/crsreports/crsdocuments/rl3246701212005.pdf.

⁸ Ibid.

⁹ Stuart Butler, "The Conservative Agenda for Health Care Reform." *Health Affairs* 14 (1995): 150.

¹⁰ Daniel Miller, "An Analysis of Senator Kerry's Health Plan." Joint Economic Committee, (Oct. 2004); http://papers.ssrn.com/sol3/papers.cfm?abstract_id=659121; Ceci Connoly, "Kerry Plan Could Cut Insurance Premiums." *Washington Post*, June 5, 2004, A1; http://www.washingtonpost.com/wp-dyn/articles/A16748-2004Jun4.html.

¹¹ Gerard J. Widig and Ming Tai-Seale, "The Effect of Report Cards on Consumer Choice in the Health Care Market." *Journal of Health Economics* 21 (2002): 1031.

¹² Proposal of the Physician's Working Group for Single-Payer National Health Insurance, *Journal of the American Medical Association* 290 (2003): 798.

¹³ Ibid.

¹⁴ Ibid.

¹⁵ Ibid.

¹⁶ Ibid.

¹⁷ Theodore R. Marmor, *Understanding Health Care Reform* (New Haven, CT: Yale University Press, 1994), 134–35.

¹⁸ Stuart Butler and Henry J. Aaron, "A Bipartisan Attempt to Break the Health-reform Stalemate." *Brookings,* Jan. 1, 2007; http://www.brookings.edu/opinions/2007/0101useconomics_aaron.aspx?rssid=aaronh.

¹⁹ Ibid.

²⁰ Chapter 58, Acts of 2006, Chapter 151F, § 2; http://www.mass.gov/legis/laws/seslaw06/sl060058.htm.

[21] Ibid. See David A.Hyman, "The Massachusetts Plan: The Good, the Bad, and the Ugly." *Policy Analysis,* No. 595; http://www.cato.org/pubs/pas/pa-595.pdf.

[22] "'Pay-or-play' refers to states using their tax authority to assess employers (pay) while giving them the option to avoid the fee by providing health care or coverage to their workers (play)." "2006–2007 Fair Share Health Care Fund or 'Pay or Play' Bills: Can States Mandate Employer Health Insurance Benefits?" National Conference of State Legislatures; http://www.ncsl.org/programs/health/payorplay2006.htm.

[23] "Massachusetts Passes Universal Health Care Package." *supra* note 21. *See also Retail Industry Leaders Association v. Fielder,* 475 F.3d 180 (4th Cir. 2007) (striking down Maryland's fair share law as preempted by ERISA).

[24] *Health Care Access and Affordability,* Massachusetts Legislature, Conference Committee Report, Apr. 4, 2006; http://www.mass.gov/legis/summary.pdf.

[25] Ibid.

[26] Chapter 58, Acts of 2006, Chapter 111m, § 2 (a) & (b); http://www.mass.gov/legis/laws/seslaw06/sl060058.htm.

[27] Chapter 58, Acts of 2006, Chapter 111m, § 1 (a); http://www.mass.gov/legis/laws/seslaw06/sl060058.htm.

[28] Alice Dembner, "State Gives More Time for Bids on Insurance." *Boston Globe,* Feb. 2, 2007; http://www.boston.com/news/local/articles/2007/02/02/state_gives_more_time_for_bids_on_insurance/.

[29] Ibid.

[30] Julie Appleby, "Mass Pioneering Health Plan Turns 1." *USA Today,* June 30, 2008; http://www.usatoday.com/news/health/2008-06-29-massreform_N.htm.

[31] "Access to Health Care and the Uninsured." National Conference of State Legislatures; http://www.ncsl.org/programs/health/h-primary.htm (last accessed Dec. 20, 2008).

[32] Hawaii — Prepaid Health Care Act, National Conference of State Legislatures; http://www.ncsl.org/programs/health/hawaiipp.htm (last accessed Dec.20, 2008). Hawaii is the only state that has an employer mandate. This may be due in part to the impact of the Employee Income Retirement Security Act (ERISA), which is generally understood to preempt such laws. Hawaii is the only state that has been granted an exemption from ERISA because its law was passed the same year as ERISA. Ibid.

[33] Expanding Health Care Coverage in the United States: A Historic Agreement, Health Care Coalition for the Uninsured (HCCU), Families USA; http://www.familiesusa.org/issues/uninsured/hccu/about-hccu.html (last accessed Dec. 20, 2008). HCCU participating organizations include AARP, America's Health Insurance Plans, American Academy of Family Physicians, American Hospital Association, American Medical Association, American Public Health Association, Blue Cross and Blue Shield Association, Catholic Health Association, Families USA, Federation of American Hospitals, Health care Leadership Council, Johnson & Johnson, Kaiser Permanente, Pfizer, United Health Foundation and U.S. Chamber of Commerce. Ibid.

[34] Ibid.

[35] Ibid.

[36] Ibid.

[37] Ibid.

[38] Ibid.

[39] Ibid.

[40] Ibid.

[41] Jonathan Oberlander, "The Partisan Divide — The McCain and Obama Plans for U.S. Health Care Reform." *New England Journal of Medicine* 359 (Aug. 21, 2008): 781,

782. *See also* "Barack Obama and Joe Biden's Plan to Lower Health Care Costs and Ensure Affordable, Accessible Health Coverage for All." http://www.barackobama.com/pdf/issues/HealthCareFullPlan.pdf (last accessed Dec. 20, 2008).

[42] Obama–Biden Plan, *supra* note 41.
[43] Ibid.
[44] Ibid.
[45] Ibid.
[46] Ibid.
[47] Ibid.
[48] Oberlander, *supra* note 41, at 782.
[49] Ibid.
[50] "National Catholic Leaders Call on Congress to Strengthen Child Insurance Program." United States Conference of Catholic Bishops, Mar. 20, 2007; http://www.usccb.org/comm/archives/2007/07-050.shtml.
[51] *Our Vision for U.S. Health Care*, Catholic Health Association (2007); http://www.chausa.org/NR/rdonlyres/F844C0E2-5E66-4D03-9051-96178F20380C/0/HealthCareVision.pdf.
[52] Anthony R. Tersigni, "Covering the Uninsured Is America's Problem." *Health Progress* 88 (May–June 2007); http://www.chausa.org/Pub/MainNav/News/HP/Archive/2007/05MayJune/Articles/SpecialSection/hp0705c.htm.
[53] Ibid.
[54] "Advocacy and Public Policy." Providence Health System, at http://www.providence.org/phs/advocacy/default.htm (last accessed Dec. 20, 2008).
[55] Fr. Kenneth Himes, O.F.M., Ph.D., "Health Care Access for All." *Health Progress* 88 (May–June 2007); http://www.chausa.org/Pub/MainNav/News/HP/Archive/2007/05MayJune/Articles/SpecialSection/hp0705d.htm.
[56] Dennis P. McCann, "Catholic Social Teaching and the Economics of Health Care Management." *Christian Bioethics* 6 (2000): 231, 241.
[57] Gustav Niebuhr, "The Health Care Debate: The Catholic Church." *New York Times*, Aug. 25, 1994.
[58] Ibid.
[59] Ibid.
[60] *Our Vision for U.S. Health Care, supra* note 51.
[61] Ibid.
[62] Ibid.
[63] Ibid.
[64] Ibid.
[65] "Continuing the Commitment: A Pathway to Health Care Reform." Catholic Health Association (2000); http://www.chausa.org/NR/rdonlyres/BC5971B9-13DF-4FA4-858F-E96244A3E865/0/Commitment.pdf.
[66] Ibid., 10–12.
[67] "Health Care in America: A Catholic Proposal for Renewal." *Linacre Quarterly* 72 (2005): 92; http://www.cathmed.org/publications/Health%20Care.pdf.. See also Mary J. McDonough, *Can a Health Care Market Be Moral?: A Catholic Vision* (Washington, DC: Georgetown University Press, 2007), 57–62 (discussing CHA and CMA proposals).
[68] "Health Care in America: A Catholic Proposal for Renewal." *supra* note 67, at 103.
[69] Ibid., 104.
[70] Ibid., 92.
[71] Ibid., 93–96.
[72] Ibid., 106–12.
[73] Ibid., 98.

[74] McDonough, *supra* note 67, at 62.
[75] Ibid.
[76] Ibid., 62–63.
[77] "The State Legislators' Guide to Health Insurance Solutions." American Legislative Exchange Council (2003), 12 http://www.cahi.org/cahi_contents/resources/pdf/statelegislatorsguide.pdf.
[78] *See, e.g.*, H.R. 5262, 109th Congress; http://www.govtrack.us/congress/billtext.xpd?bill=h109-5262. This legislation never became law. http://www.govtrack.us/congress/bill.xpd?bill=h109-5262.
[79] "Catholic Health Association Statement on the Naming of Tom Daschle and Jeanne Lambrew to Health Leadership Positions in Obama's Administration." Catholic Health Association, Dec. 11, 2008; http://www.chausa.org/Pub/MainNav/Newsroom/NewsReleases/2008/r081211a.htm.
[80] Kathleen Gilbert, "Catholic Health Association Applauds Pro-Abortion Cabinet Picks Lamented by Pro-lifers." LifeSiteNews.com, Dec. 18, 2008; http://www.lifesitenews.com/ldn/2008/dec/08121805.html.
[81] Ibid.
[82] Jeff Zeleny, "Daschle Ends Bid for Post; Obama Concedes Mistake." *New York Times,* Feb. 3, 2009; http://www.nytimes.com/2009/02/04/us/politics/04obama.html?hp.
[83] Tim Townsend, "Burke Calls Sebelius HHS Appointment an "Embarassment,'" *St. Louis Post-Dispatch,* Mar. 13, 2009; http://www.stltoday.com/blogzone/civil-religion/general/2009/03/burke-calls-sebelius-hhs-appointment-an-embarrassment/.

Conclusion

[1] *Ex Corde Ecclesiae* (On Catholic Universities); http://www.ewtn.com/library/PAPALDOC/JP2UNIVE.HTM.

[2] Beverly Catherine Dunn, S.P., *Sponsorship of Catholic Institutions, Particularly Health Care Institutions, by the Sisters of Providence in the Western United States* (1995; unpublished dissertation submitted to the faculty of Canon Law, Saint Paul University, Ottawa, Canada, in partial fulfillment of the requirements for the degree of Doctor of Canon Law), 189. Dunn notes: "Neither canon law nor civil law contains the concept of sponsorship. Rather, it has developed as a practical means for adapting to changing conditions." Ibid., 189. Dunn further states:

> In order to find an expression of Catholic identity applicable to health care, though, one must look to the realm of Catholic education, as legislative texts, including the Code, and most other ecclesial documents do not directly address Catholic institutions of social welfare, except in terms of medical ethics. The Apostolic Constitution on Catholic Universities, *Ex Corde Ecclesiae*, presents two aspects of the Catholic identity of institutions: fidelity to the mission of Jesus in the tradition of the Catholic Church; and a communio relationship with the entire Church and the local bishop, either through a formal juridical bond or through the recognition of an institution as Catholic by competent ecclesial authority. (Ibid., 189–90.)

[3] *Cf.* William W. Basset, "The American Civil Corporation, The 'Incorporation Movement' and the Canon Law of the Catholic Church." *Journal of College & University Law* 25 (1999): 721. Professor Basset states:

> The "incorporation movement" was born after the Second Vatican Council, after the Land O'Lakes Declaration on Academic Freedom led by Father Theodore Hesburgh, in the wake of the strike and firing of liberal philosophers and theologians at St. John's University on Long Island, and the trial of the dissenting theologians at the Catholic University. It spanned the aftermath of the Encyclical Letter *Humanae Vitae* of Pope Paul VI and the agreement of the United States Catholic Bishops Conference to approve the Ethical and Religious Directives for Catholic Health Care Services and place Catholic hospitals under the moral governance of local ordinaries. (Ibid. at 725.)

See also Burton Bollag, "Who Is Catholic?" *Chronicle of Higher Education*, Apr. 9, 2004, A26 (discussing the *Land O'Lakes Declaration* and a new generation of Conservative Catholic colleges).

[4] *Ex Corde Ecclesiae*, *supra* note 1, at Art. 4, Par. 3.

[5] Canon 812 reads: "It is necessary that those who teach theological disciplines in any institute of higher studies have a *mandatum* from the competent ecclesiastical authority." James A. Coriden, ed., *The Code of Canon Law: A Text and Commentary* (Mahwah, NJ: Paulist Press, 1985), Canon 812, at 575. The *National Catholic Register* did a series of articles on the refusal of Catholic universities and ecclesiastical authorities to disclose who has received the *mandatum*. *See, e.g.,* Tim Drake, "Who Teaches with the Church?: Georgetown Won't Tell Parents." *National Catholic Register*, June 15–21, 2003.

[6] A Higher Education Research Institute study recently conducted by the University of California-Los Angeles showed that after four years on a Catholic campus, Catholic students' moral views were weaker, rather than stronger. At 38 of the Catholic colleges surveyed, 37.9% of Catholic freshmen said in 1997 that abortion should be legal. Four years later, as seniors, 51.7% supported legalized abortion. Tim Drake, "Mandatum Cover-up?: Parents

Feel Left in the Dark About Professors at Catholic Colleges." *National Catholic Register*, June 1–7, 2003.

[7] Kevin O'Rourke, O.P., "Catholic Hospitals and Catholic Identity." *Christian Bioethics* 7 (2001): 15, 25.

[8] *See, e.g., Lawrence v. Texas*, 123 S. Ct. 2472, 2480 (2003), in which the court refers to an "emerging awareness that liberty gives substantial protection to adult persons in deciding how to conduct their private lives in matters pertaining to sex." In the same opinion, Justice Kennedy also quotes the infamous mystery passage from *Planned Parenthood v. Casey*, 505 U.S. 833, 851 (1992):

> Those matters [referring to "marriage, procreation, contraception, family relationships, child rearing, and education"] involving the most intimate and personal choices a person may make in a lifetime, choices central to personal dignity and autonomy, are central to the liberty protected by the Fourteenth Amendment. At the heart of liberty is the right to define one's own concept of existence, of meaning, of the universe, and of the mystery of human life. Beliefs about these matters could not define the attributes of personhood were they formed under the compulsion of the state.

[9] *Cf.* Stephen L. Carter, "Liberalism's Religion Problem." *First Things* 121 (Mar. 2002). Professor Carter notes:

> The liberal state is uncomfortable with deep religious devotion—and, for the most part, so is its product, liberal law. Religious belief is reduced to precise parity with all other forms of belief, an act of leveling that is already threatening to religion itself. In practice, liberalism often reduces religion to an even smaller role than other belief systems, seeking to limit or shut off its access to the public square and often deriding the efforts of the religious to live the lives they think the Lord requires when those efforts seem to conflict with other liberal goals.

[10] Several provisions of the *Ethical and Religious Directives for Catholic Health Care Services*, 4th ed. (2001), refer to the risk of scandal. Directive 45 instructs Catholic health care institutions to "be concerned about the danger of scandal in any association with abortion providers." Ibid., 26. Directive 67 states that decisions entailing a "high risk of scandal should be made in consultation with the diocesan bishop or his health care liaison." Ibid., 36. And Directive 71 states, "The possibility of scandal must be considered when applying the principles governing cooperation." Ibid., 37 (footnote omitted).

[11] *See, e.g.*, Dennis Brodeur, "Catholic Health Care: Rationale for Ministry." *Christian Bioethics* (1999): 5, 20.

[12] Richard A. McCormick, "The End of Catholic Hospitals." *America* 179 (July 4, 1998): 5, 12.

[13] Daniel P. Sulmasy, O.F.M., *Catholic Health Care: Not Dead Yet*, National Catholic Bioethics Quarterly 1 (Spring 2001): 41.

[14] Ibid., 50.

[15] Martien A.M. Pijnenburg and Henk A.M.J. ten Have, M.D., "Catholic Hospitals and Modern Culture: A Challenging Relationship." *National Catholic Bioethics Quarterly* 4 (Spring 2004): 73, 74.

[16] Rev. Romanus Cessario, O.P., "Catholic Hospitals in the New Evangelization." *National Catholic Bioethics Quarterly* 5. (Winter 2005): 675.

[17] Ibid., 676, quoting from *Charter for Health Care Workers*, Pontifical Council for Pastoral Assistance to Health Care Workers (1995), Par. 1.

[18] Clark E. Cochran, "Institutional Identity: Sacramental Potential: Catholic Health Care at Century's End." *Christian Bioethics* 5 (1999): 26, 37.

[19] *Cf.* Corinna Delkeskamp-Hayes, "Christian Credentials for Roman Catholic Health Care: Medicine versus the Healing Mission of the Church." *Christian Bioethics* 7 (2001): 117, 137–39.

[20] "Divine Mercy Care." Fox News, Dec. 23, 2008; http://www.foxnews.com/video-search/m/21708885/divine_mercy_care.htm#seek=38.909.

[21] Anne Hendershott, "How Support for Abortion Became Kennedy Dogma." *Wall Street Journal,* Jan. 1, 2009; http://online.wsj.com/article/SB123086375678148323.html.

[22] Albert R. Jonsen, *The Birth of Bioethics* (New York: Oxford University Press, 1998), 290–91.

[23] Ibid., 291.

[24] Ibid.

[25] Mario M. Cuomo, "Religious Belief and Public Morality." speech delivered Sept. 13, 1984 at the University of Notre Dame, *American Rhetoric: The Top 100 Speeches*; http://www.americanrhetoric.com/speeches/mariocuomoreligiousbelief.htm.

[26] Ibid.

[27] Charles J. Chaput, *Render Unto Caesar* (New York: Doubleday, 2008), 231.

[28] Robert M. Cover, "Nomos and Narrative." *Harvard Law Review* 97 (1993): 4, 32, 46–53.

[29] Speech by Father Smith, fictional character portrayed in Walker Percy's *The Thanatos Syndrome* (New York: Ivy Books, 1987), 393. The following is a summary of the novel:

> Dr. Tom More, from *Love in the Ruins* . . . , now middle-aged, returns to Feliciana after spending two years in prison for selling prescriptions of Dalmane and Desoxyn at a truckstop. On his return to his psychiatric practice, More observes that two of his former patients are acting strangely. In his own words: "In each there has occurred a sloughing away of the old terrors, worries, rages, a shedding of guilt like last year's snakeskin, and in its place is a mild fond vacancy, a species of unfocused animal good spirits."
>
> More observes that his wife Ellen and his children have also undergone some mysterious personality change. More, the scientist-physician, with the help of his cousin Dr. Lucy Lipscomb, launches a search for the cause of these and other observations. More and Lucy discover that John Van Dorn, head of the computer division of the nearby Grand Mer nuclear power plant and Dr. Bob Comeaux, director of the Quality-of-Life Division of the Federal Complex overseeing euthanasia programs, are involved in social engineering, releasing Heavy Sodium into the water supply to "improve" the social welfare.
>
> Throughout the novel, Dr. Tom More returns several times to evaluate and talk with Father Rinaldo Smith, a parish priest who has exiled himself to a firetower overlooking the vast pine forest of Feliciana. More has been asked by Comeaux, who sits on the probationary board overseeing More's return to practice, to declare Father Smith crazy, so that Comeaux can take over Father Smith's hospice and put it to better use. The conversations between More and Father Smith contain the philosophic and moral themes that support the plot and action of the novel.
>
> Perhaps Percy's most ambitious novel, his sixth and last, *The Thanatos Syndrome* revisits old themes found in his previous works, while giving perhaps his most rambunctious and outrageous commentary upon the post-modern predicament. The novel moves from existential themes found in his earlier novels to those subjects that most concerned him as a Catholic near the end of his life.

The protagonist, a wayfarer, confused and disoriented in a world bordering on catastrophe, begins a search, and comes to the values of commitment, relationships, ordinary life, and faith. Percy satirizes the do-gooders and grand social solutions of our age, and reminds readers that moral good emerges in the space between two people struggling and talking together. Dr. More, like Percy, "renders the unspeakable speakable," . . . and in so doing, offers the reader reflection upon themes of healing, moral good, and hope in the "age of thanatos." [Citations omitted]

Richard Martinez, *Literature Annotations,* Literature, Arts, and Medicine Database, New York University; http://litmed.med.nyu.edu/Annotation?action=view&annid=1366.

Index

A

abortifacient, 72, 152, 163, 165-172
abortion, 9-19, 21-28, 30-34, 36-40, 43, 45-46, 48, 51-54, 57-59, 61, 64-66, 71-73, 77, 80, 82-83, 88, 97, 101, 110-111, 114-117, 124-128, 130-143, 145-150, 152, 160, 165-166, 169, 172, 217-221, 225-229
Abortion Non-Discrimination Amendment (ANDA), 139-141
absolute moral norms, 21, 25, 29, **33-41**, 225
Alzheimer's disease, 195
agenesis, 77, 113
aggressive medical treatment, 34, 39, 180
American Association of Pro-Life Obstetricians and Gynecologists, 146
American Board of Obstetricians and Gynecologists (ABOG), 146
American Civil Liberties Union (ACLU), 10, 12, 135, 140, 142, 148
American College of Obstetricians and Gynecologists (ACOG), 19, 145-146, 148
American Hospital Association, 81
American Life League, 150
American Society for Bioethics and Humanities, 44
anencephalic infant, 44, 114
anencephaly, 77, 113
Araujo, Robert, S.J., 136
artificial contraception 22, 24, 27-29, 31, 33-34, 53, 60, 62-63, 67, 161, 163
Ascension Health Care, 101, **118-130**, 217
Ashley, Benedict, 24, 28, 114
artificial insemination, 30, 56, 60-61, 63, 72

assisted nutrition and hydration (ANH), 19, 74, 176-177, 181, **182-195**
assisted suicide, 23, 39, 46, 48, 52, 75, 77, 80, 117, 142, 176-177
Augustine, Saint, 14
Australian bishops, 193

B

Biden, Joseph, 14, 148
bioethics, 18, 21, 25, **42-52**, 110, 175
bishop, local, 13, 55, 57, 61, 63-65, 70-71, 75, 79-80, 90, 92, 96, 97, 101, 121, 124, 128, 152, 165, 199, 224, 226
Blagojevich, Rod, 143
Blue Cross and Blue Shield, 206
Bourke, Michael, 56
Bradfield v. Roberts, 85, 138
Brackenridge case, 77, 127-130
Brown, Judie, 150
business, Catholic hospital as a, 9, 17, 19, 81-83, **84-89**
Burke, Raymond L., Archbishop, 13-15
Bush, George W., 141, 145, 209-210

C

canon law, 34, 39, 79-80, **90-99**, 104-105, 109, 195, 223-224
casuistry, 48-49, 65
Cataldo, Peter J., 152
Catechism of the Catholic Church, 28, 33-34, 180
Catholic Charities v. Serio, **161-162**
Catholic Charities of Sacramento, Inc. v. Superior Court, **154-160**
Catholic Charities USA, 217

345

Catholic Health Association of the United
    States (CHA), 11, 18, 55, 60, 64, 81, 91,
    97-98, 108, 141, 146, 148, 183, 190-191,
    193, 195, 201, 216-221
Catholic Healthcare West, 202-203
Catholic Hospital Association, 170; see
    Catholic Health Association
Catholic identity, 10, 11, 19, 69-70,
    79-130, 203, 223,-225
Catholic Medical Association, 197, 219
Catholics for Choice, 146, 148
Catholics for a Free Choice, 31, 112, 116,
    166-167
Catholics in Political Life, 14
Catholic Theological Society of America,
    31, 192
Catholic University of America, 16, 31
Center for Health Care Ethics, 69, 124
Chaput, Charles, O.F.M. Cap., Archbishop,
    16, 228
Charter for Health Care Workers, 181, 226-227
Childress, James, 136
Church Amendments, 131, 138, 145
City of Boerne v. Flores, 132
*Church of Lukumi Babalu Aye, Inc. v. City of
    Hialeah*, 133, 155, 158
Clinton, Bill, 115
Clinton Health Plan, 115, 213, 217
Clinton, Hillary, 146, 213
COBRA, 208
Colombo, John, 202
Committee on Pro-Life Activities (NCCB,
    USCCB), 74, 147, 187, 190, 194
Congregation for the Doctrine of the Faith
    (CDF), 54-55, 68-69, 76, 78, 172, 176,
    179, 194-195, 200

Congregation for Institutes of Consecrated
    Life and Societies of Apostolic Life
    (CICLSAL), 92
Connecticut Catholic Conference, 164-165
conscience, 13, 14, 18-19, 26, 35, 40, 63-65,
    70-71, 75, 131-132, 135-136, 143-144
conscience clause/consience-clause (legisla-
    tion, law, protection, statutes), 9, 12, 16,
    19, 64-66, 132, 135, **138-150**, 151, 153,
    155, 160-161, 164-165, 218-219, 223
conscientious objection, right of, **131-137**
consequentialism, 29, 36
conception, moment of, 15, 33, 37, 58, 111
contraceptive coverage, mandated, **151-162**
contraception laws, emergency, **163-173**
contraceptive sterilization, 28, 31, 34, 60,
    65, 67
contraceptives, oral, 26, 152
Coats Amendment, 139-140
Corrada, Alvaro, S.J., Bishop, 54
culture of death, 9, 19, 33, 37-39, 81, 219,
    228-229
culture of life, 9, 17, 38-39, 226, 228
Cuomo, Mario, 228
Curran, Charles, 30-31, 66, 73, 228

D

Danforth Amendment, 139
Daschle, Tom, 221
Daughters of Charity, *see* Ascension Health
    Care
deBlois, Jean, C.S.J., 70, 72-73, 98
Declaration on Euthanasia, 179-180, 194
Death With Dignity, 117, 181
dementia, 47, 195
deontologists, 28
disabled, 38, 46-47, 182-183
Divine Mercy Care, 227
DNR, 44
doctors, 16, 18, 25-26, 46, 51, 125, 143,
    145, 178, 229
Doerflinger, Richard, 191
Dunn, Beverly, S.P., 96, 105, 109

E

ectopic pregnancy, 31, 58, 67
Eisenstadt v. Baird, 134
elderly, 38, 47, 185, 201, 207, 211, 226
election, presidential, 13-18, 201, 212
Employee Retirement Income Security Act
    (ERISA), 151-152, 206

Employment Division, Department of Human Resources of Oregon v. Smith, 132-134, 154, 156-157, 159, 162
end-of-life-care, **175-200**
end-of-life care, Catholic teaching on, **178-181**
end-of-life care, case study in, Terri Schiavo, **196-200**
Engelhardt, Tristram, 52
ERDs, *see Ethical and Religious Directives for Catholic Health Care Services*
Erickson v. Bartell Drug Co., 152-153
Establishment Clause, 85, 138, 155, 158-161
Ethical and Religious Directives for Catholic Health Care Services (*ERD*s), 12, 18, 22, 24, 27, 33, **53-78**, 80, 82-83, 88, 90, 92, 94, 98, 101, 110-111, 114-117, 123-124, 126-127, 130, 131, 132-133, 135, 152, 163, 165, 166, 167, 175, 177, 181, 189, 190, 197, 203, 218, 223-228
ethical relativism, 37-38, 44, 52, 136, 219, 225
ethics, medical, 22, 25, 27, 55, 58, 62, 135
euthanasia, 22, 25, 34, 38-40, 46-47, 52-53, 58-59, 68, 74-75, 77, 80, 110, 135-136, 142, 175-176, 178-181, 185, 187, 189, 190-192, 194-195, 218
Evangelium Vitae, 9, 33, 37-41, 180
Ex Corde Ecclesiae, 223-224
extraordinary care or treatment, 39, 59, 68, 74, 175, 178-181, 183-188, 192-194
extrauterine pregnancy, 66, 72

F
FDA, 142, 163
Federal Employees Health Benefits Program (FEHBP), 214, 217-220
finis operis, finis operantis, 24, 27

Florida bishops, 198-199
FOCA, *see* Freedom of Choice Act
formal cooperation, 15, 34, 76-77
foundationalism, 48
Free Exercise Clause, 134, 144, 161-162, 199

Freedom of Choice Act (FOCA), 9, 16-19, 132, **147-150**, 225-226
Freud, Sigmund, 136

G
Gelineau, Louis, Bishop, 187
geographical morality, 63, 65
George, Francis, O.M.I. Cardinal, 15, 17
Gregoire, Christine, 144
Griswold v. Connecticut, 134
Guidelines for Catholic Hospitals Treating Victims of Sexual Assault, 170

H
handicapped, 34, 38, 180, 227
Hamel, Ronald, 193, 195
Hardt, John, 195
Hatch Amendment, 228
Healey-Sedutto, Mary, 11
Health and Human Services, U.S. Department of, 141, 145, 146, 221
health insurance in U.S., employer provided, 206-207
health care, government programs in U.S., 207-208
health care reform, social justice and, **201-203**
health care reform proposals, **213-221**
health care system in the United States, **204-212**
health care systems in Canada and Great Britain, 204-206
Hehir, Brian, 11
Hill-Burton Act, 51, 82, 85, 107
Hippocratic Oath, 219
Holy Communion, 13, 14, 221
Holy See, *see* Vatican
"hospital within a hospital," 127-129
Humanae Vitae, 21, 29, 31, 43, 61-64

I-J
incest, 32, 228
individual autonomy, 35, 37-38, 44, 52, 175, 225
infallibility, papal, 39-40

infant mortality rates, 204, 209
infanticide, 16, 38
Internal Revenue Code 501(c)(3), 86, 202
Internal Revenue Service (IRS), 86, 118, 202, 206
John Paul II, 9, 22, 28, 33-37, 39-40, 95, 136, 176-177, 179-180, 190, 192-194
Johnson, Lyndon, 207
Jonsen, Albert, 25, 42-43, 49-50, 227-228

K-L

Kaczor, Christopher, 28
Kaufman, Christopher, 94, 121
Kaveny, Kathleen, 17, 149
Keehan, Carol, D.C., 148, 195
Kelly, David, 21-22, 25, 55, 58, 73, 186-187, 193
Kelly, Gerald, S.J., 21, 25, 56-59, 186
Kerry, John, 13, 214
Kennedy Institute of Ethics, 43, 69
Kopfensteiner, Thomas, 195
Kramlich, Maureen, 139
Krol, John, Cardinal, 64
Land O' Lakes Declaration, 223-224
Lawrence v. Texas, 135
Lynch, Robert, Bishop, 148, 198

M

Magisterium 23, 24-25, 30, 34-37, 39-40, 50, 63, 74, 180, 184, 187, 190, 194, 224
mandatum, 224
material cooperation, 18, 61-62, 65, 72, 76-77, 83, 127, 133, 161, 173
Martino, Joseph, Bishop, 15
May, William, 23-24, 27, 29, 39, 182-185
McCarrick, Theodore, Cardinal, 13

McCormick, Richard, 36-37, 61-62, 64, 94, 226, 228
McGrath-Maida controversy, 90, 93-95
McFadden, Charles J., O.S.A., 21, 25-26
McHugh, James, Bishop, 185-186
Medicaid, 13, 51, 82, 86, 107, 139, 149, 202, 207-211, 216, 218, 228
Medical-Moral Board of the Archdiocese of San Francisco, 69

Medicare, 51, 82, 86-87, 107, 122, 133, 149, 202, 207-208, 211, 213-214, 218
Medical Ethics, 25
medical schools in U.S. associated with Catholic university, 97-99
Medico-Moral Problems, 57
Menges v. Blagojevich, 143
moral absolutes, 22-23, 29, 35, 44, 57, 62, 64-65
"morning-after pill,"163
Morrisey, Francis, 80-81, 92
Murray, Patty, 147

N

NARAL, 115
National Catholic Bioethics Center (NCBC), 69, 114, 165
National Catholic Bioethics Quarterly, 168
National Conference of Catholic Bishops (NCCB), 12, 53, 60, 64, 68-69, 74, 76, 187-190
National Organization for Women, 31, 128
natural family planning, 73, 219, 227
natural law, 13, 18, 21, 23-33, 35-36, 39, 48, 50-51, 53, 56-57, 63, 65, 68, 136, 161, 175, 178, 180, 186
natural-law tradition, Catholic, **23-26**
natural-law tradition, Catholic, challenges to, **27-32**
Naumann, Joseph, Archbishop, 226
Nazis, 47
Netherlands, 46-47
Notre Dame, University of, 7, 17, 36, 149, 228
nurses, 18, 25-26, 42, 84, 112, 224

O

Obama, Barack, 9, 16-18, 132, 142, 146, 148-149, 201, 212, 216-217, 221
Obey, David, 13
O'Donnell, Thomas J, S.J.,. 21, 27, 64-68, 73
organ donation, 44, 68-69
O'Rourke, Kevin, O.P., 24, 28, 70, 72-73, 114, 169, 172, 179, 183-185, 193. 195, 225

P

palliative care, 34, 218
Papal Commission for the Study of Population, the Family, and Natality, majority report of, 29-31
Paprocki, Thomas, Bishop, 17
Paulsen, Michael Stokes, 149
Pavone, Frank, 196
Pellegrino, Edmund, 43, 50, 135, 139
Pelosi, Nancy, 14
Pennsylvania, Catholic Bishops of, 50, 187
Pennsylvania Catholic Conference, 72, 171
Peoria Protocol, 169-172
persistent vegetative state (PVS), 19, 43, 46, 74, 176, 181, **182-195**, 196-200, 227
physicalism, 21, 35
Pius XII, 178-179, 184-185
Place, Michael, 191
Plan B, 132, 142, 144-145, 163, 167-168, 219
Planned Parenthood v. Casey, 134, 147
Planned Parenthood, 117, 123, 127, 134, 147-148, 156-157
politicians, Catholic, 12-13, 32, 227-228
politicians, "pro-choice," 12, 14-15, 32, 221, 227
Pontifical Academy of Life, 163
Pontifical Council for Pastoral Assistance to Health Care Workers, 181, 226
Pregnancy Discrimination Act, 152-153
Prevention First Act, 132, 150, 164
principle of double effect, 26, 29-31, 39, 55, 57-59, 63, 66, 68, 73, 75, 166, 172, 178
principle of proportionate good, 27-28
principles of cooperation, 62, 77
principle of totality, 27-28, 63, 67-68
principlism, 48
pro-choice activists, groups, lobby, 10-11, 31, 96, 110, 123, 134-135, 137
proportionalism, 29, 33, 36
proportionalist, 21, 28, 33-37, 77
Provena Covenant Medical Center, 203
Providence Health System, 101, **103-117**, 122, 217
prudential judgment, 14, 65, 228

Q-R

Quaecumque Sterilizatio, 78
quality of life, 45, 50, 178, 181-183, 186-188, 190, 198
Quinlan, Karen Ann, 43-44, 200
Quinn, Gail, 151
rape, 10, 32, 66, 71, 112, 129, 140, 150, 163-172, 228
Ratzinger, Joseph, Cardinal, 40
Reich, Warren T., 62-64, 94
Religious Coalition for Abortion Rights, 148
Religious Freedom Restoration Act, 132
religious orders, 10, 55, 69, 79-80, 82, 84-86, 90-93, 101, 118, 224
respirator, 43, 189
revisionist theologians, 22-23, 27-29, 60
Rigali, Justin, Cardinal, 97-98, 147
Rome, *see* Vatican
Roe v. Wade, 13, 16, 64, 72, 110, 131, 134, 138, 147, 228
Rosenbaum, Sara, 209-210
RU-486, 152, 160,
Rust v. Sullivan, 133

S

salpingostomy, 59, 67, 73
Schiavo, Terri, 19, 176, **196-200**,
Schindler, Robert and Mary, 196, 200
Schwietz, Roger, Archbishop, 114
Sebelius, Kathleen, 221
Secretariat for Pro-Life Activities (NCCB, USCCB), 141, 147, 151, 191
sexual assault, 71-72, 112, 129, 150, 163-165, 167, 170-173
Shannon, Thomas A., 186, 192
Sheen, Fulton J., Archbishop, 25
Singer, Peter, 44-47
Sisters of Providence, *see* Providence Health System
Sisters of St. Joseph of Carondelet, *see* Ascension Health Care
Sisters of Saint Joseph of Nazareth, *see* Ascension Health Care
Smith, Janet, 37
social justice and health care reform, **201-203**
Stabilization Act, 204

State Children's Health Insurance Program (SCHIP), 208-212, 216-218
stem cell research, 135
sterilization, 18, 21, 24-37, 43, 47, 51-57, 59-63, 65-68, 72-73, 77-78, 80, 82-83, 88, 97, 101, 110-111, 115, 117, 124-132, 137-139, 160, 217, 219, 220, 225-227
Stormans, Inc. v. Selecky, 144-145
suicide, 39, 46, 75, 77, 80, 142, 175, 178-180
suicide, physician-assisted, 23, 48, 52, 117, 176
Sullivan, Francis, S.J., 40
Sulmasy, Daniel, 226
surrogate decision maker, 175-176
surrogate motherhood, 72

T

tax-exempt status, 10, 201-203
teleologism 29, 36
teleologists 28
Texas Conference of Catholic Bishops, 187
therapeutic abortion, 26, 57-58, 115
Thomas Aquinas, Saint, 14, 23
Thomasson, Melissa, 204
Tradition, 35, 39, 224
traditionalist, 21-22, 24-25, 28, 33
tubal ligation, 55, 64, 116, 125-126, 130
Tuohey, John F., 73, 191

U-V

United States Catholic Conference (USCC), 27, 53, 72
United States Conference of Catholic Bishops (USCCB), 14, 17, 53, 140-141, 147-148, 187, 189, 191, 217
universal health care, 203, 211

University of Notre Dame 7, 17, 36, 149, 228
Vatican, 13, 32, 58, 68, 77, 92, 95, 97-98, 115, 128-129, 191, 194-196, 223
Vatican Council I, 40
Vatican Council II, 21, 29-30, 35, 39-40, 51, 63, 85-86
Veritatis Splendor, 28-29, 33, 34-37, 13

W-X-Y-Z

Walter, James J., 186
Wardle, Lynn, 10, 139
Weigel, George, 16
Weldon Amendment, 141-142
Wildes, Kevin, S.J., 48-49
Women's Contraception Equity Act (WCEA), 154, 157,
Women's Health and Wellness Act (WHWA), 161-162
Wuerl, Donald, Archbishop, 13
Zavala, Gabino, Bishop, 15